2nd Fully Revised and

Livestock Eco
Marketing, Entreprene
Management and A

NIPA GENX ELECTRONIC RESOURCES & SOLUTIO
New Delhi-110 034

2nd Fully Revised and Enlarged Edition

Livestock Economics Marketing, Entrepreneurship Business Management and Accountancy

K.S. Gangadhar, B.sc., M.V.Sc., Ph.D.
Former Director of Extension, KVAFSU
Professor and Head
Department of Veterinary and Animal Husbandry Extension
Veterinary College, KVAFSU, Hebbal, Bangalore – 560 024 , Karnataka

K. Satyanarayan, M.V.Sc., Ph.D.
Professor and Head
Department of Veterinary and Animal Husbandry Extension
Veterinary College, KVAFSU, Hebbal, Bangalore – 560 024 , Karnataka

K.C. Veeranna, M.V.Sc., Ph.D.
Registrar
Karnataka Veterinary, Animal and Fisheries Sciences University
Bidar - 585401, Karnataka

V. Jagadeeswary, M.V.Sc., Ph.D.
Associate Professor
Department of Veterinary and Animal Husbandry Extension
Veterinary College, KVAFSU, Hassan - 573 202, Karnataka

J. Shilpa Shree, M.V.Sc.
Assistant Professor
Department of Animal Husbandry Economics
Faculty of Basic Sciences, Madras Veterinary College
TANUVAS, Vepery, Chennai – 600 00707, Tamilnadu

NIPA GENX ELECTRONIC RESOURCES & SOLUTIONS P. LTD.
New Delhi-110 034

NIPA GENX ELECTRONIC RESOURCES & SOLUTIONS P. LTD.

101,103, Vikas Surya Plaza, CU Block
L.S.C.Market, Pitam Pura, New Delhi-110 034
Ph : +91 11 27341616, 27341717, 27341718
E-mail:newindiapublishingagency@gmail.com
www: www.nipabooks.com

For customer assistance, please contact
Phone: + 91-11-27 34 17 17 Fax: + 91-11- 27 34 16 16
E-Mail: feedbacks@nipabooks.com

ISBN: 978-93-91383-11-4

Composed and Designed by NIPA.

Preface to the First Edition

The course entitled Livestock Economics, Marketing and Business Management incorporating fundamentals of accountancy is offered to first year B.V.Sc. & A.H. students during the second semester of the concerned academic year. The course curriculum is as per the Veterinary Council of India regulations. It is a well known fact that each of the components of the course namely, economics, marketing, business management and accountancy forms an independent and separate study by itself. Hence the teacher offering the course has to draw information from varied and diversified sources to cater to the task of teaching the subject covering the fundamental and applied aspects of all the four components of the course. Further students also have to refer separate text books for each of the component, if they have to update the knowledge pertaining to the course. The libraries in the agricultural universities and veterinary universities are also not very much equipped with more number of books in these subjects. Hence, in order to make the task of teaching and learning comparatively easier, an attempt has been made to bring out a compilation of various topics connected to livestock economics, marketing, business management and accountancy in the form of a handbook. In doing so, the authors do not claim any originality in the subject matter. The information is drawn from various text books, the list of which is presented at the end. However, the authors believe that the handbook will serve the needs of the teachers and students who are involved in this course work. The narration is done in a very simple way without complicating the information presented with many graphs and mathematical expressions.

K.S. Gangadhar
K. Satyanarayan
K.C. Veeranna

25 Nov. 2008

Preface to the Second Edition

Livestock provides nutritious food, cash income and opens up employment opportunities. Livestock ownership also significantly impacts on agricultural productivity through provision of required draft power and manure as fertilizer in crop production. Livestock holding helps farmers in sustained farming and economic stability. The first chapter of this book focuses on livestock population and production status which has changing facts but still readers should know the livestock wealth of the nation. Currently in India, majority of the livestock production is handled by small farmers with limited resources and the productivity is very low which might be due to poor management practices. The second chapter in this textbook has been designed to study the economic concepts in livestock farming. As we know, no product can be produced with single input and also input availability is very competitive in this world. So this chapter helps us to know various economic concepts, various inputs required for farming and how the inputs and outputs are related with each other.

Along with production, marketing is the other challenge faced by farmers. Both the backward linkage of input acquirement and forward linkage of marketability to reach final users are very important to farmers. The third chapter helps in sharing the information related to market and marketing concepts. The demand for livestock products in India has increased tremendously and has a strong potential to rise at a very fast rate in future. This is a continuing challenge of supplying food to ever-expanding human population especially safe, nutritious, convenient, economical and satisfiable to the consumer. In order to meet this demand, livestock farming must enter as business enterprise which in turn, is a key driver for employment opportunities, wealth creation, economic growth and for final target group i.e. farmers to increase their standard of living whereas at present, this sector also helps to sustain their livelihood. Thus, the industry will have to shift to larger producers of livestock.

Education is essential for farmers to know about steps to shift from farming to business enterprise which should provide opportunities for people to earn and lead a full productive life. With this background, this second edition of the book includes livestock entrepreneurship concepts as fourth chapter in simple and lucid form. The fourth chapter focuses on concept of entrepreneurship, entrepreneur skills, enterprising opportunities in livestock sector, forms of livestock business, bank support to start an enterprise, entrepreneurial training, livestock entrepreneurial project preparation and its feasibility , sales promotion and marketing communication.

Though the factors are made available, managing them is an important task for farmers/entrepreneurs to take business enterprise towards a successful end. The fifth chapter deals about livestock business management concept i.e. management skills, farm management, resource management, personnel management, financial management and product management in livestock business. Recording is also an important management function. It is important to check frequently whether the business is progressing in proper direction for which knowledge on financial recording is very important. Thus, the sixth chapter focuses on accountancy which deals with how to record the data in a journal, ledger, cash book, subsidiary books, different financial statements, assessing liquidity and solvency position of livestock business.

This textbook has been designed based on latest guidelines of Veterinary Council of India and is extremely useful to Veterinary students as the content of the book is prepared based on the course outline of livestock economics, marketing, entrepreneurship, business management and accountancy which is offered for IIIrd Professional year of BVSc & AH degree students. It is a well known fact that each of the components of the course namely, Livestock economics, Marketing, entrepreneurship, business management and accountancy, forms an independent and separate study by itself. Hence the teacher offering the course has to draw information from varied and diversified sources to cater to the task of teaching the subject covering the fundamental and applied aspects of all the four components of the course. Further students also have to refer separate text books for each of the component, if they have to update the knowledge pertaining to the course. The libraries in the agricultural universities and veterinary universities are also not very much equipped with more number of books in these subjects. Hence, in order to make the task of teaching and learning comparatively easier, an attempt has been made to bring out a compilation of various topics connected to livestock economics, marketing, entrepreneurship, business management and accountancy in the form of a handbook. In doing so, the authors do not claim any originality in the subject matter. The information is drawn from various text books, the list of which is presented at the end. However the authors believe that the handbook will serve the needs of the teachers and students who are involved in this course work. The narration is done in a very simple way without complicating the information presented with many graphs and mathematical expressions.

This book would also benefit veterinary professionals and extension officers who are involved in promoting livestock entrepreneurship activities in India as well as in other developing countries. We sincerely acknowledge people from whom we have taken help in writing this book from various articles, reports, books and websites. The authors are also obliged to New India Publishing Agency for bringing out this second edition to benefit teachers, students and graduates in a shorter duration.

Authors

Contents

Preface to the First Edition .... *v*

Preface to the Second Edition .... *vii*

Part A: Introduction to Livestock Sector in India

Introduction to Livestock Sector and Its Contribution to Indian Economy 3

Part B: Livestock Economics

1. Introduction to Livestock Economics 13
2. Basic Economics: Terms and Concepts 23
3. Factors of Production and Their Rewards 35
4. Theory of Demand and Supply 49
5. Theory of Production 59
6. Theory of Cost 81

Part C: Livestock Marketing

7. Basic Terms and Importance of Studying Livestock Marketing 93
8. Classification of Markets 95
9. Concepts of Marketing 103
10. Price Determination Under Perfect Competition 105
11. Marketing Functions 109
12. Market Information 123
13. Marketing of Livestock Products and Defects in Livestock Marketing 133

14. Marketing Agencies, Institutions and Channels for Livestock and Livestock Products 137

15. Government Interventions and Role in Marketing of Livestock and Livestock Products 161

16. Trade Performance of Livestock Sector in India 171

Part D: Livestock Entrepreneurship

17. Entrepreneur and Entrepreneurship 181

18. Entrepreneur 185

19. Theories and Forms of Entrepreneurship 195

20. Basic Requirements for Entrepreneurship Initiatives in Livestock & Allied Sectors 203

21. Avenues of Livestock Entrepreneurship 213

22. Livestock Entrepreneurship Training and Development Programmes 217

23. Essential Criteria for Development of Entrepreneurship in Livestock and Allied Sectors 221

24. Financial Credit & Its Management: General Principles and Practices 237

25. Bank Support and Insurance for Livestock Enterprises 247

26. Approaches to Preparation of Entrepreneurial Projects on Livestock..255

27. Procurement Management, Quality Issues, Standardization, Grading and Packaging 261

28 Retail Marketing, Sales Operations and Management, Advertising, Marketing of Services 269

29 Expectations From A Veterinary Professional 285

30 Eco Jobs and Sustainable Development Through Livestock Production 289

Part E: Livestock Business Management

31. Management 297

Functions of Management 298

Farm Management 309

Financial Management 319

Product Management 323

Personnel Management / Labour Management 326

Risk Management 341

Part F: Accountancy

32. Book Keeping 347

Glossary of Commercial Terms 352

Accountancy 356

References 409

Part A
Introduction to Livestock Sector in India

Introduction to Livestock Sector and Its Contribution to Indian Economy

Animal husbandry is the most important economic activity in rural areas as livestock plays a vital role in the economy. Over 90 per cent of the milk production comes from small farmers, who are located in rural areas. Growing human population, increasing urbanisation, rising domestic incomes and changing lifestyles in the country have led to increasing demand for dairy products (Anita and John, 2001). The dairy sector stretch its hand to 150 million farm households by providing nutritive food, supplementary income and productive employment for family labour, mainly for women (Payal *et al.* 2018 and Rais *et al.* 2007). Dairying is also an important secondary source of income for millions of rural families. Indian Dairying is unique in more than one ways. Contributing about 5.3 per cent to India's agricultural GDP, milk is a leading agricultural produce (Satish and Soumyakant, 2016). During the post independence period, the dairy sector showed increase in growth rate (Ashish, 2017). This impressive growth effort speaks volume about the co-coordinated efforts of large number of milk producing farmers, scientists, planners, NGO's and industry in achieving self-sufficiency in milk production. The country is the world largest milk producer, contributing 18.5% of the world's total milk production (FAO Agricultural Outlook 2016-2025, Economic Survey 2015-16). It is the world's largest consumer of dairy products, consuming almost 100% of its own milk production. Dairy products are considered as cheap and nutritious food to millions of people in India and the only acceptable source of animal protein for large vegetarian segment of Indian population (Amit and Monojit, 2015). In India, Dairy sector helps in alleviating the poverty and unemployment status. Livestock sector provides employment to 18 million people and nearly 70 per cent of them are women (Ramesh et al. 2018). Further, dairy sector is the major source of income for an estimated 27.6 million people. Among these, 65 to 70 per cent are small, marginal farmers and land-less labor (Satish and Soumyakant, 2016). The dairy sector supports around 10 million members / farmers through one lakh cooperative societies existing in the country (Amarja, 2013). Apart from employment generated by rearing of animals, the procurement of milk and its processing also provides substantial employment. Dairy Industry showed its impact on society, increase in economic status of farmers, better infrastructure facilities, improved food aid security and nutrition (Shilpa and Prabu, 2019).

Bovine Population

The bovine population in India has increased continuously since 1950's and the growth was more prominent during the inter census period of 1977-1982 and 1997-2003. In India, the bovine population was 198.7 millions in 1951 which had increased to 235.7 millions in the year 1972, 288.8 millions in 1992 and 302.4 millions in 2019.

Bovine Population in India

Year	India (in millions)			% change
	Cattle	Buffalo	Total Bovine	
1951	155.3	43.4	198.7	
1956	158.7	44.9	203.6	2.5
1961	175.6	51.2	226.8	11.4
1966	176.2	53.0	229.2	1.1
1972	178.3	57.4	235.7	2.8
1977	180.0	62.0	242.0	2.7
1982	192.5	69.8	262.2	8.4
1987	199.7	76.0	275.7	5.2
1992	204.6	84.2	288.8	4.8
1997	198.9	89.9	288.8	0
2003	185.2	97.9	283.1	-2.0
2007	199.1	105.3	304.4	7.5
2012	190.9	108.7	299.6	-1.6
2019	192.5	109.9	302.4	0.9

Milk Production Trend in India

Dairy development is one of the important activities in livestock sector. The total milk production in the country was at 17 million tonnes in the year 1950-51 and since then the production of milk continues to rise over the period. As can be observed in the graph, there is a steady increase in production of milk and it reached 187.7 million tonnes in the year 2018-19. The per capita availability of milk was 130 grams per day during the period 1950-51. There has been steady increase in per capita availability of milk since then till 1980-81 with marginal fluctuations in the intermittent periods. The per capita availability of milk in the year 2000-01 was 217grams per day from against 128grams per day in the year 1980-81. Further there is a substantially increasing trend has been observed in the per capita availability of milk from 2000-01 to 2016-17. As a result, the per capita availability of milk reached 394 grams per day in the year 2018-19. The reasons for the increase in the milk production was mainly due to operation flood which connected rural production centres with urban consumption centres followed by the liberalization policy which paved the way for the entry of private sectors in the dairy industry.

Milk Production Trend in India

Year	Milk Production (in Million Tonnes)	Percapita Availability (grams/day)
1950-51	17.0	130
1980-81	31.6	128
1990-91	53.9	176
2000-01	80.6	217
2010-11	121.8	281
2011-12	127.9	290
2012-13	132.4	299
2013-14	137.7	307
2014-15	146.3	322
2015-16	155.5	337
2016-17	165.4	355
2017-18	176.3	375
2018-19	187.7	394

Contribution of Dairy sector to the National Economy

Milk contributes more than 60 per cent of the total livestock production and accounts for nearly 67.69 per cent of the value of the output of the livestock sector's contribution to the national GDP. Likewise, Beef contributes 2.92 per cent of the value of the output of the livestock sector's contribution to the national GDP. The value of output from dairy sector was more than Rs. 549 billions and accounts for 67.69 per cent of the value of the livestock sector output in the year 2015-16.

Value of Output from Dairy Sector - At Constant Prices

Year	Value of Milk group produced in Crores	Percentage share of Milk group in Livestock Sector	Value of Beef produced in Crores	Percentage share of Beef in Livestock Sector	Value of Output from Livestock Sector in Crores
2011-12	327767	67.20	11754	2.41	487751
2012-13	339240	66.77	12997	2.56	508074
2013-14	352247	66.34	13243	2.49	530953
2014-15	374267	66.59	15255	2.71	562026
2015-16	396662	66.64	16886	2.84	595242
2016-17	421495	65.78	16267	2.54	640811
2017-18	448970	66.22	16288	2.40	677960

Source: Basic Animal Husbandry Statistics, 2019

Poultry farming in India has grown rapidly in the last 20 years from backyard farming activity to highly scientific commercial enterprises (Landes *et al.,* 2004). It has registered maximum growth rate among all the sectors of agriculture and has been recognised by the government as one of the growth engines of the Indian economy. The potential in this sector is due to a combination of factors like growth in per capita income, a growing urban population and falling real poultry prices (Shilpa *et al.*2017). This sector has shown phenomenal growth averaging about 10 per cent in egg production and 15-20 per cent in broiler production annually (FAO, 2007). Over 90 per cent of the poultry production comes from small poultry farmers, who are located in rural areas (Chatterjee and Rajkumar. 2015). Growing human population, increasing urbanisation, rising domestic incomes and changing lifestyles in the country have led to increasing demand for poultry products. Nonetheless, village or backyard production can make a useful contribution to dietary protein intake and incomes of resource poor households (Acamovic et al., 2005, Rajkumar et al., 2010). The development of livestock sector leads to many other socio-economic spin offs like slowdown of rural-urban migration, mitigation of farmers' suicides, empowerment of rural women and protection of environment. Animal production contributes about 40 per cent of the total value to agriculture globally. Poultry farming has tremendous potential for expansion and employment generation (Sharma and Chatterjee, 2009; Rajkumar *et al.,* 2010). Youth in general and educated unemployed youth in particular can take up this profession easily. The inputs required for poultry farming are available locally in rural areas. Simple equipment for feeding, watering and sheltering for small units can be manufactured from materials locally available in the villages with the help of local artisans. Land required for starting poultry units is small. Women are also engaged in decision-making related to poultry production. According to the ICAR Vision- 2025, an increase in per capita availability of one egg will generate 50,000 more jobs. Similar increase in employment generation is anticipated due to acceleration in broiler production, marketing of eggs and meat, processing, etc. Poultry sector can absorb competent manpower at a rate of above 6.5 per cent per annum. Seetharaman (1996) studied the pattern of poultry development in India.

Poultry Population

The poultry population in India has increased continuously since 1950's and the growth was more prominent during the inter census period of 1977-1982 and 1997-2003. In, India the poultry population was 73.5 million in 1951 which had increased to 138.5 million in the year 1972, 307.07 million in 1992 and 851.81 million in 2019.

Poultry Population in India

Year	INDIA	
	Poultry (in millions)	Percentage change
1951	73.5	
1956	94.8	28.98
1961	114.2	20.46
1966	115.4	1.05
1972	138.5	20.02
1977	159.2	14.95
1982	207.74	30.49
1987	275.32	32.53
1992	307.07	11.53
1997	347.61	13.20
2003	489.01	40.68
2007	648.83	32.68
2012	729.21	12.39
2019	851.81	16.81

Poultry Production

Poultry development is one of the important activities in livestock sector. The total egg production in the country was at 1832 million in the year 1950-51 and since then the production of egg continues to rise over the period. There is a steady increase in production of egg upto the year 1999-2000. From the year 1999-2000 onwards the production of egg improved substantially and it reached 103318 million numbers in the year 2018-19. The per capita availability of egg was 5 eggs per annum during the period 1950-56. There has been steady increase in per capita availability of egg since then till 1979-80 with marginal fluctuations in the intermittent periods. There has been sudden jump in the per capita availability of egg in the year 2000-01 which registered 36 eggs per annum from 30 eggs per annum in the year 1999-2000.Thereafter from 2000-01 to 2003-04, there is a marginal increase in the per capita availability of egg and further there is a substantially increasing trend has been observed in the per capita availability of eggs from 2004-05 to 2018-19. As a result, the per capita availability of eggs reached 79 eggs per annum in the year 2018-19.

The increase in the egg production in the country could be attributed to the technological interventions and production management systems introduced in late 80's. New hybrid layer was introduced in the country whose productivity was very high when compared to native birds. Likewise, management changes such as deep litter system (later replaced by cages), automatic feeder, waterer, new vaccines, new feeds such as layer mash, grower, starter, etc. were introduced which were responsible for the increase in the egg production. More importantly, the growth in layer industry was largely catapulted by the private industry with little support/intervention by the government.

Egg Production Trend in India

Year	Egg Production (in Million Numbers)	Percapita Availability
1950-51	1832	5
1980-81	10060	15
1990-91	21101	25
2000-01	36632	36
2010-11	63024	53
2011-12	65480	55
2012-13	69731	58
2013-14	74752	61
2014-15	78484	63
2015-16	82929	66
2016-17	88137	69
2017-18	95217	74
2018-19	103318	79

Poultry sector contribution to the National Economy

Poultry meat contributes 40 per cent of the total meat production and accounts for nearly 8.6 per cent of the value of the output of the livestock sector's contribution to the national GDP (Table 4). Likewise, egg contributes 3.25 per cent of the value of the output of the livestock sector's contribution to the national GDP. The value of output from Poultry sector is more than Rs. 963

billion and accounts for 11.86 per cent of the value of the livestock sector output in the year 2015-16. Similar results were reported by Rajendran *et al.*, 2014 which assessed the value of output from poultry industry.

The table reveals that the share of poultry meat in the livestock sector has been gradually increasing from 6.73 per cent in 2004-05 to 8.60 per cent in 2015-16 which indicates the growth of poultry sector. Likewise, the consumption pattern of people is also slowly changing from red meat to lean meat. Further, per capita consumption of meat in India has been slowly increasing due to rising per capita income.

Value of Output from Poultry Sector - At Constant Prices

Year	Value of Poultry Meat produced in Crores	Percentage share of Poultry Meat in Livestock Sector	Value of Egg produced in Crores	Percentage share of Egg in Livestock Sector	Value of Output from Livestock Sector
2004-05	12118	6.73	5850	3.25	180034
2008-09	23002	7.87	10445	3.58	292146
2009-10	27768	8.02	13373	3.86	346147
2010-11	34839	8.48	15493	3.77	410937
2011-12	39583	8.12	16633	3.41	487751
2012-13	42470	8.36	17364	3.42	508074
2013-14	49681	9.36	18308	3.45	530953
2014-15	53120	9.45	19080	3.39	562026
2015-16	60066	10.09	19829	3.33	595242
2016-17	72873	11.37	20346	3.18	640811
2017-18	76924	11.35	21876	3.23	677960

Source: Basic Animal Husbandry Statistics, 2019

Part B
Livestock Economics

1

Introduction to Livestock Economics

Economics

The term "Economics" is derived from the Greek words 'OIKOS' and 'NOMAS' or 'NEMEIN'. 'Oikos' means house hold and Nomas or Nemein means management. So in its original sense economics means house hold management; i.e. satisfying as many wants of the house hold or family as possible by allocating the limited resources at the disposal of the family wisely among different wants. In the modern and practical sense Economics means management of day to day problems arising from unlimited wants and limited resources by wisely allocating limited resources to satisfy maximum wants. In other words economics is the study of how man manages his limited resources as it satisfies as many wants as possible.

Definition of economics

There are many definitions which may be grouped under four different categories based on their stresses or emphasis given on different aspects of the subject.

The four groups of definitions are:

1. Classical or Wealth definition.
2. Neoclassical or Welfare definition.
3. Scarcity definition.
4. Modern or Growth oriented definition.

1. **Classical or wealth definition**

Adam Smith who is considered as father of economics was the first to give a systematic definition in his book "Wealth of nations" in the year 1776. Later on other economists like J.B. Say, J.S. Mill and F.A. Walker also defined economics on the similar lines as that of Adam Smith. They are as follows:

Adam Smith (1776): (Father of Economics)	Economics is "An enquiry into nature and causes of wealth" or economics is the science of wealth.
J.B. Say: (French Economist)	"Economics is the science which treats wealth"
J.S. Mill:	Economics is the practical science of production and distribution of wealth.
F.A. Walker: (American Economist)	Economics is that body of knowledge which relates to wealth.

According to these definitions the main object of human activity is to acquire wealth and the study of how wealth is produced, distributed and exchanged for human consumption. Probably these economists might have not meant wealth as just meaning richness or money. By wealth they would have meant all economic goods that would satisfy human wants.

Criticism on wealth definition: Many philosophers like Dickens, Ruskin, Carlyle and Mathew Arnold strongly criticised the wealth definition. They said that the science which concentrates only on the study of wealth is a "Selfish Science", " Mundane Science", "Bastard Science", "Bread and butter Science", "The Science of getting riches", "The gospel of mammon"(song of the devil), "a science of illth and not wealth" etc. These philosophers were highly critical of the wealth definition because they at that time were highly influenced by the religious sentiments and spiritual values. They considered that mere acquisition of wealth is not the object of all human activity and they looked at acquiring wealth with great contempt.

Defects of wealth definition: The stress in the wealth definition is only on acquiring wealth. But in reality the human life and activity consists of other considerations like love, affection, charity, social obligation, family obligation etc. Wealth is only a means and not an end to human activity. The end of human activity is his welfare i.e. welfare of man. Wealth definition did not include the services of various professionals like teachers, doctors, veterinarians, lawyers etc.

2. Neoclassical or welfare definition

Prof. Alfred Marshall in his book Principles of economics Published in 1890 defined economics as "the study of mankind in the ordinary business of life. It examines that part of the individual and social action which is mostly connected with the attainment and use of material requisites of well-being. Thus it in on the one side a study of wealth and on the other and more important side a part of the study of man". Other economists of his time also held similar view.

Prof. Edwin Cannan-: Economics is the study of the causes of material welfare.

Prof. Pigou-: Economics is the study of economic welfare.

Prof. Ely-: Economics is the science which treats those social phenomenon that are due to the wealth getting and wealth utilising activities of man.

Main points of Welfare definition

Economics is;

a) a social science,

b) a study that stresses on human welfare rather than wealth, and,

c) about how man earns and spends his income to increase his welfare.

3. Scarcity definition

Prof. Lionel Robbins in 1932 in his book 'The nature and significance of economic science' defined economics as a science which studies human behaviour as a relationship between ends and scarce means, which have alternative uses.

Ends i.e. human wants are Unlimited Means i.e. the resources are limited and can be used for alternative purposes. Hence there are problems. These problems are solved by people by adjusting their limited resources which can be put to alternative uses to their unlimited wants. They choose most urgent ones first and sacrifice the less urgent ones.

Limitations of scarcity definition

1. Resources are limited but scarcity definition has not taken into account the possibility of improving resources due to scientific and technological development.
2. Scarcity definition is silent about the role of resources towards human welfare.
3. Problems can arise not necessarily due to scarcity of resources but also due to abundance. For example more production of eggs and milk than the demand will bring down the price to such an extent that even the production cost may not be met.
4. Scarcity definition does not discuss about employment, economic growth, determination of value or price etc.

4. Modern definition or growth oriented definition

The following are some of the definitions given by various economists, which conform to the modern or growth oriented definitions of economics.

Keynes: "Economics is a study of the administration of scarce resources and of the determinants of employment and national income."

Samuelson: "Economics is the study of how men and society choose with or without the use of money to employ scarce producing resources which will have alternative uses, to produce various commodities over time and distribute them for consumption now and in the future among the various people and groups of society."

Benham: Economics is the study of the factors affecting the size, distribution and stability of a country's national income.

M.L. Jhingham: Economics is a social science concerned with the proper uses and allocation of resources for the achievement and maintenance of growth with stability.

It can be concluded that a practical and correct definition should encompass the theory of wealth acquisition, welfare aspect of wealth, careful allocation of scarce resources for satisfying unlimited wants, theory of national income, employment and economic growth. Thus the definitions given by Prof. Samuelson and Jhingham are very close to the ideal definition of economics.

Livestock economics

In the light of definitions discussed above, the term livestock economics may be defined as the study of how people in a country or peoples of different countries of the world employ the scarcely available resources towards the production of livestock and their products for the best advantage of mankind of the present and of the future. The best advantage of human kind may include various aspects of human life like:

a) Meeting food requirements in the form of milk, meat, fat, eggs, etc.

b) Providing sustainable employment,

c) Providing stable income,

d) Maintenance of ecological balance,

e) Maintenance of sentimental aspects of human-animal companionship,

f) Sustenance of interest in animal sporting activity,

g) Meeting the manure requirements of the soil,

h) Meeting the requirements of hides, skin, wool, etc.

i) Efficient conversion of non edible crop residues into valuable edible products, and

j) Meeting the draught (for ploughing the land etc.) and transport requirements especially in rural areas of certain countries.

Scope of economics

It is the subject matter of economics. It refers to boundaries with in which the subject matter of economics is studied. It means what we study in economics.

The scope of economics is very wide. It includes the following aspects.

a) What is the subject matter of economics?

b) What type of science is it?

c) Is economics, a science or art or both?

d) Is economics a positive science or a normative science or both?

a) Subject matter of economics:

i) It studies the behaviour of man in society.

ii) It does not study all aspects of human behaviour like his birth, growth, death etc.

iii) Wants lead to efforts or economic activities. Efforts lead to income and income enables man to satisfy wants.

i.e. wants – efforts – satisfaction ® constitute the subject matter of economics.

Approaches to study the subject matter of economics

There are two approaches 1) Traditional approach 2) Modern approach

Traditional approach: Economics is studied under the following head lines in traditional approach;

a) Production, b) Distribution, c) Exchange, d) consumption, e) Public finance and f) Economic planning.

Modern approach: In the modern approach, economics is studied under

(a) Micro economics and (b) Macro economics

Traditional approach

Production: This includes the study of production, types of production, factors of production namely Land, Labour, Capital and Organisation,

Laws governing production, division of labour, Theories of population, Role of entrepreneurs.

Distribution: Study of National income, study of how the rewards of four factors of production are distributed among people, The theories of rent, wages, interest, profit etc. are studied in this part.

Exchange: Study of how the produced goods and services are exchanged among people, Market conditions, price determination, trade, money, branding etc.

Consumption: This includes the study of human wants, their characteristics and their satisfaction, the Law of diminishing utility, Law of demand and elasticity of demand, Law of substitution, the Law of family expenditure, concept of consumer surplus.

Public finance: Public finance deals with the sources of public revenue, principles of taxation, items of public expenditure, items of public borrowing or debt, etc.

Economic planning: Here objectives of economic planning and techniques of economic planning are studied. Developing countries plan to promote economy and growth. Developed countries plan to maintain the already existing stable economy.

Modern approach

Micro economics: It is the study of the economic behaviour of any particular decision making unit such as a dairy farm, a poultry farm, a sheep unit etc. Micro economics is also called "Price theory"

Macro economics: It is the study of the behaviour of economic system as a whole or all the decision making units put together. For example, National income, per capita income, per capita consumption etc. It is also called "Income theory".

Nature of the subject of economics

There has been considerable argument both in favour and against recognising the subject of economics as science. However as the subject of economics generates a lot of data which can be collected, analysed and generalised conclusions drawn as in any other science subject. Economics is also accepted as a science more so as social science as it studies the human activities pertaining to utilisation of resources to fulfill human wants of the present and future. It may not be an exact science as that of physics, chemistry of biology, nevertheless its laws are also generalised conclusions drawn from careful analysis of data and hence also have universal application.

Economics is considered as both positive science and a normative science. It is positive science because it positively explores the problems of economy, causes of such problems and their effects more in a fact finding spirit of science. It is also a normative science because the subject of economics also gives suggestions to find remedial measures for various economical problems in the society thus playing a normalising role. Because of this nature of the subject namely the subject of economics suggests solutions for practical problems of society like unemployment, inflation, poverty etc., it is also considered as one which prescribes remedies or practical solutions to a problem. Finally we can conclude that economics is both an art and science and is both a positive and normative science.

Importance of the study of economics in general and livestock economics in particular

Among social sciences the subject of economics is more scientific and exact. Economists world over are most respected lot and outstanding contributors in the field of economics are also recognised and honoured by way of Nobel Prize and other awards. All economic activities are interdependent and these activities are aimed at satisfying human wants for the ultimate welfare of mankind. Economics as a subject tries to find out the basic principles and laws behind these activities, which are a part of human behaviour. When grossly viewed the magnitude of various economic activities not only appears to be of mammoth proportion but also appears to be highly intricate and complicated. Nevertheless, behind these seemingly complicated activities there lies certain tendencies and general patterns which can be started in the form of economic laws whose reliability can be subjected to scrutiny through scientific methods. All this gives an excellent mental discipline to one who persues the study of the subjects of economics. With proper understanding of the various laws of economics one can predict the economic behaviour that is likely to emerge at a future date. Its study helps producers, traders, consumers, labourers, labour leaders, statesmen and common persons in the society as all these are involved in one or the other economic activity. The study of economics helps in solving many national and international problems arising out of improper distribution of resources.

Livestock population status

India with its more than 100 crore population and about more than 70 per cent of them residing in over 6 lakh villages with Agriculture as major vocation has adopted livestock production as one of the major allied agriculture economic activity. Mixed farming involving crop production and livestock production with the latter contributing at least 10 to 15 per cent of the farm income is the most common system of farming adopted in India.

The cattle population of India grows steadily and reaches 192.49 million in the year 2019 with the overall Compound annual growth rate (CAGR) of India's cattle population is 0.32 per cent. The Buffalo population of India grows steadily and reaches 109.85 million in the year 2019 with the overall CAGR of India's Buffalo population is 1.38 per cent. The Sheep population of India grows significantly and reaches 74.20 million in the year 2019 with the overall CAGR of India's Sheep population is 0.95 per cent. The Goatpopulation of India grows significantly and reaches 148.80 million in the year 2019 from 47.20 millions from the year 1951. The overall CAGR of India's Goat population is 1.70 per cent. The Pig population of India grows steadily and reaches 9.06 million in the year 2019. The overall CAGR of India's Pig population is 1.07 per cent. The total Indian livestock population increases by 83 per cent when compared to total livestock population of the year 1951. More specifically after the year 1982, the percentage growth in Indian livestock population is more than 50 per cent. Among the various livestock species, the highest percentage of growth is observed in Goats (223.14 per cent) followed by Buffalo population (153.11 per cent), Sheep (89.92 per cent), Pigs (105.91 per cent) and cattle (23.97 per cent). The population of poultry increases by 1058.93 per cent.

Total Milk production of India is 198.43 million in the year 2019-20. Out of total india's Milk production 48.70 per cent (96.94 Million) contributed by Total Cow milk and 48.35 per cent (95.94 Million) is contributed by Total Buffalo milk and remaining 2.95 per cent (5.85 million kgs) contributed by goat milk. The milk production has increased by 6.5% over the previous year. The per-capita availably of milk is 394 grams per day. The average yield per animal per day for exotic/crossbred is 7.95 Kg per day and for indigenous/non-descript is 3.01 Kg per day. The milk production from exotic/crossbred cattle has increased by 8.7% and indigenous/non• descript cattle has increased by 5.7% as compared to previous year. The milk production from buffaloes also increased by 6.4% as compared to previous year. Top 5 Milk producing States are : Uttar Pradesh (16.3%), Rajasthan (12.6%), Madhya Pradesh (8.5%), Andhra Pradesh (8.0%), Gujarat (7.7%). They together contribute 53.1% of total Milk production in the country.

The total egg production in the country is 103.32 Billion numbers. The egg production has increased by8.5% as compared to previous year. The per-capita availability of egg is 79 eggs per annum. Top 5 egg producing States are Andhra Pradesh (19.1%), Tamil Nadu (18.2%), Telangana (13.2%), West Bengal (8.3%). Haryana (5.9%). They together contributes 65% of total egg production in the country. The total egg production from commercial poultry is 84.91 Billion numbers and backyard poultry is 18.41 Billion numbers contributing 82.2% and 17.8% of total production of egg, respectively.

The total meat production in the country is 8.11 Million tonnes.The meat production has increased by 6.0% as compared to previous year. The meat production from poultry is 4.06 Million tonnes, contributing about 50% of total meat production. The poultry meat production has increased by 7.8% over previous year. The top 5 meat producing States are Uttar Pradesh (15.1%), Maharashtra (12.6%), West Bengal (10.2%), Andhra Pradesh (9.6%} and Telangana (9.3%}. They together contribute56.9% of total meat production in the country.

The total wool production in the country is 40.42 million Kgs. The wool production has declined by 2.5% as compared to previous year. The top 5 wool producing States are Rajasthan (35.9%), Jammu & Kashmir (18.9%), Telangana (10.5%), Karnataka (7.6%) and Gujarat (5.6%). They contribute78.5% of total wool production in the country. Livestock sector contributes 4.9 per cent to total GDP value whereas contributes 28.4 per cent to Agricultural GDP.

2

Basic Economics Terms and Concepts

Human wants

Human wants refer to person's desires for commodities or goods and services.

Importance of the study:

Human wants are the main cause of all economic activities like Agriculture, Livestock production, trading etc. Wants are satisfied through consumption of commodities and services.

It is from the characteristics of wants several economic laws or theories are developed. The following are some of them.

a) Law of demand
b) Law of substitution
c) Law of family expenditure
d) Law of diminishing marginal utility

Origin of human wants

Its origin is as old as human existence. In olden days wants were few. But due to civilisation wants have multiplied. Wants arise due to various desires which include desire for security, affection, recognition, adventure, necessities, comforts, luxuries, and to satisfy certain customs and cultural wants.

Characteristics of wants

a) Wants are unlimited
b) All wants cannot be satisfied
c) Only a few wants can be satisfied
d) Wants are competitive

While human wants are unlimited, the resources to satisfy these wants are limited leading to a situation where human beings have to make choice between the most urgent and needy wants(to be satisfied) and the ones not so important.

Wants are complementary: There are certain commodities or goods which cannot be put to their intended uses unless they are complemented with their closely connected goods. For example the fountain pen cannot be used for writing without ink or a ball point pen without refill.

Wants are alternative: There are always alternative means or ways by which a particular want can be satisfied. For example, breakfast can be made with milk and bread, eggs only, eggs in the form of omelets, dosas, iddlies or some rice preparation. Similarly a drink can be satisfied with a cup of tea, coffee, milk or fruit juice etc.

Most wants are recurring: A person sleeps every day, eats every day, drinks every day, thus these wants are regularly recurring in one's life.

Wants vary in intensity and urgency: Salt is required only to taste, but more salt in the food instead of satisfying the want leaves one dissatisfied. Some wants like taking or drinking water are satisfied more urgently compared to owning a house or a motor car. Thus wants vary in their urgency.

Wants Vary with person, place and time: A vegetarian loves to eat vegetarian food compared to non vegetarian whose love will naturally be for a meat preparation. Clothing requirements of a cold country are different from warm countries. Wants of present day people are different from old times.

Wants may change into habits: Drinking a cup of coffee or tea in the morning or smoking a cigarette after food etc., when such wants are fulfilled regularly they tend to become habits later on.

Classification of human wants

Human wants are classified in two ways.

I. Primary wants & secondary wants

Primary wants refer to necessities of life like food, water, clothing etc.

Secondary wants refer to those wants other than the necessities of life.

II. Necessities, comforts and luxuries.

Necessities include; (a-1) Necessities of life like food, shelter and clothing.

(a-2) Necessities of efficiency like provision of good transport to work place, providing proper lighting while reading, using suitable audiovisual aids while teaching etc. are good examples of necessities of efficient and (a-3) Necessities of convention like offering a cup of tea or coffee to guests.

Comforts: Use of fan in summer, woolen garments in winter are good examples of comforts which enhance the physical wellbeing and efficiency of people.

Luxuries: Very costly cars, palatial bungalows, expensive jewelry etc constitute luxuries without which men can live. They will not add comfort or efficiency.

Luxuries may be further classified into a) harmful luxuries like smoking cigarettes, excessive drinking of alcohol etc., b) defence luxuries like raising a huge military in the name of defence and owning excessive gold or silver in the name of security and c) harmless luxuries like wearing very costly clothes, spending huge sums of money on the decoration of house etc.

Goods

Goods in the ordinary language means material things like cement, building materials, land equipments, food grains etc. But in economics goods refer to commodities which have physical existence and also services like the services of a veterinarian, dentist, teacher, lawyer etc.

Classification of goods

Free goods and economic goods

Free goods: Free goods are gifts of nature which are available in plenty and freely available in nature without paying a price. *Eg:* Air, sunshine, water etc.

Economic goods: Economic goods are the goods which can be obtained only by paying a price. These goods are scarce in relation to demand, they are man made and have value in utility . *Eg:* Milk, meat, food, clothes, car etc.

However, there is no rigid line between free goods and economic goods. Because what is free in one place may be an economic goods else where. *Eg*: Water is free from drinking by the riverside but the same water when supplied through pipes, taps or bottles it becomes economic goods.

Air is free in nature for breathing but the same air when supplied in cylinders for deep sea divers, miners, it becomes economic goods.

b) Consumer goods and producer goods

Consumer goods: They are the goods which are consumed directly by the user and they satisfy the human wants directly. *Eg:* Food, clothes, books etc.

Producer goods: These goods are capitable goods or investment goods which are not directly consumed by the consumers but they are used for production of some other goods. These goods satisfy the human wants not directly but indirectly. *Eg:* Fuels like coal, petrol or diesel, factory building, machines etc.

Even the above classification into consumer goods and producer goods is also not rigid. *Eg*: Rice, wheat etc when used as food they are consumer goods but when used as seeds for producing respective crops they become producer goods.

c) Single use goods and durable use goods

Single use goods: Single use goods are those which get used up in a single act of consumption. Once they are used they disappear altogether or change their form. They may be single use consumer goods or single use producer goods.

Eg: Single use consumer goods: Food, milk, eggs, tea, ink, match stick etc.

Single use producer goods: Raw materials like sowing seeds, fuels etc.

Durable use goods: These are goods which can be used again and again over a period. It should be remembered here in the ordinary usage the word durable is used to denote some thing costly but in economics durable goods refer to those goods which can be used again and again which need not be costly. Durable use goods can also be durable use consumer goods and durable use producer goods.

Eg: Durable use consumer goods include motor car, clothes, jewelry etc.

Durable use producer goods include machinery, factory building, goods transport vehicles etc.

d) Material and non-material goods

Material goods: Material goods are those goods which have physical existence, visible, tangible and concrete like land, building, furniture, egg, meat etc.

Non-material goods: Non-material goods are those goods which do not have physical existence, they are intangible, invisible like good will of a business, patents, service of a veterinarian, doctor etc.

e) Transferable goods and non-transferable goods

Transferable goods: Transferable goods are the goods which can be transferred from one person to another. *Eg.* Machinery, books, land, building, sheep, goat, cow etc.

Non-transferable goods: Non-transferable goods are the goods which cannot be transferred from one person to another. *Eg.* skill and wisdom of a technician, a veterinary doctor, teacher etc.

Consumption

It is defined as the destruction or using up of the utility contained in the matter or the commodities and services to satisfy human wants.

Example: Eating food stuff, wearing clothes, receiving services from a technician, vet, dentist, teacher etc. are all consumption in economics.

When milk, egg or fruits are eaten, the form of these goods get changed and digestible nutrients like sugar, proteins etc. are absorbed later are used as energy or stored in the body. Undigested material gets excreted. But the total matter is present undestroyed in one form or the other. But the original utility present in the milk, egg or fruit is destroyed or used up to satisfy human wants.

Characteristics of consumption

- Using of free goods and services is not considered as consumption in economics. Using up of economic goods commanding some price are considered as consumption in economics.
- By consumption there is no destruction of matter but only utility part is destroyed.
- Utility is not always destroyed in a single act of consumption except in the case of single use goods. Otherwise in durable use goods the utility is destroyed used up in several acts of consumption.
- Mere destruction of utility is not consumption. It should satisfy some human wants to qualify for the term consumption.

Importance of consumption

Consumption is an important phase of all human economic activity.

ie. Production -------distribution---------consumption

It is the beginning and end of all economic activity. Consumption determines the pattern of production, volume of production, level of employment, income and standard of living of people.

Types of consumption

1. **Final consumption or direct consumption:** This refers to those goods which are directly consumed or the consumption is a final act as in the case of consumption of food, clothes etc.
2. **Indirect or productive consumption**: This refers consumption involving goods and services that are used to produce other goods as in the case of raw cotton, machine, tools, fuels etc.
3. **Wasteful or destructive consumption**: When goods are used to satisfy some wants which in reality are wasteful in the long run are considered under wasteful consumption. *Example;* Excessive alcoholic drinks, use of narcotics as a habit, atom bombs etc.

Utility

Utility is defined as the power or capacity of a commodity or service to satisfy some human wants. Food, furniture, clothes, book etc. all have utility. Even poison has its utility as it satisfies some human wants.

Characteristics of utility

1. Utility is different from usefulness: In the ordinary usage utility may mean usefulness. But in economics utility is not usefulness. This can be explained from the fact that poison, alcohol, opium etc. are harmful to human being although they have their own utility as they satisfy human wants.

2. Utility has no ethical or moral significance: A thing may be good or bad, but as long as there is some want satisfying power or capacity in it, the said thing is said to have utility. For example, looking at an indecent picture or a pornographic picture is considered bad by many societies, but many people in such societies buy them and may watch them stealthily. Thus these pictures also satisfy some wants of these people. Therefore even a porno picture has its utility.

3. Utility and satisfaction are different: The difference between utility and satisfaction can be depicted in the following way.

Utility	Satisfaction
a) Want satisfying power in a commodity or service	Satisfaction is what one gets by consuming the commodity or service
b) Utility is the "expected" satisfaction that can be derived when consumed	Satisfaction is what one realises after consuming commodity or service
c) Utility of a thing is the thought of the commodity before it is consumed.	Satisfaction is what one gets after consumption
d) Utility of the source or cause of satisfaction	It is the result of utility

4. Utility is different from pleasure: There are many commodities and services that do not give pleasure when consumed. But their consumption may be highly beneficial for those who consume them. For example consumption of bitter medicines or getting injected with antibiotics etc. are acts of consumption of utility present in these commodities. These consumption are actually inflicting discomfort and even pain. Therefore utility is not always a pleasure.

5. Utility is subjective: Utility of a commodity or service varies from person to person. It is subjective. For example meat has great utility to a non-vegetarian, but has no utility to a strict vegetarian. Similarly music has utility to a person who can hear and love music, but has no utility

to a total deaf. A picture has utility to a person who can see, but has no utility to a blind person.

6. Utility can be objectively measured: For example the price of an egg is rupee one and that of a litre of milk is rupees thirteen then their utilities are rupee one and rupees thirteen respectively.

Forms of utility

There are different forms of utility. They include:

a) Form utility, b) Place utility, c) Time utility,

d) Ownership utility & e) Service utility

a) Form utility: By changing the form of a commodity its utility can be altered. For example raw egg has different utility compared to an egg omelet. Actually utility of raw egg increases when it is converted to an omelet. A log of wood when converted to a piece of furniture the utility of wood increases.

b) Place utility: Depending upon the place, the utility of a commodity also varies. For example a woolen blanket has more utility in a cold place compared to a very hot and humid place. Similarly moving timber from forest to a carpenter's workshop enhances the utility of wood.

c) Time utility: Commodities gain or loose their utility over time. That is to say utility varies due to time. For example when raw meat is preserved in cold storage its utility is enhanced. Raw rice when stored for months gain further utility. Food if not preserved properly, looses its utility upon time(storage). Food grains preserved during the time of plenty gets enhanced utility when the same are used at times of scarcity.

d) Ownership utility: Transferring a book from an illiterate owner to a literate owner, land from a non cultivator to a cultivator, money from a non entrepreneur to an entrepreneur are all good examples which illustrate how ownership changes the utility of various commodities.

e) Service utility: Services rendered by doctors, veterinarians teachers, lawyers etc. all constitute service utility.

Law of diminishing marginal utility

It is one of the important laws of economics. It is a law of consumption. According to Prof. Alfred Marshall the law of diminishing marginal utility states that "the additional benefit which a person derives from a given increase of his stocks of anything diminishes with the growth of the stock he has". If one goes on consuming a particular commodity (i.e, additional or extra utility) derived by him from every successive unit consumed goes on decreasing.

Illustration of the above law

Let us assume that a hungry person consumes milk one cup after another continuously without any time gap. In such a situation his hunger is satisfied to more extent by the consumption of first cup. That means the first cup of milk gives him more utility. By consumption of second cup and successive cups the utility or satisfaction derived is lesser and lesser than the satisfaction derived by the consumption of first cup. That means the marginal or additional utility goes on decreasing although the total utility is on the increase.

The law is applicable only when;

a) the units consumed are identical in all respects ie. size, colour, quality, taste, etc.

b) the units consumed are reasonably large, ie. cups of milk and not spoons or drops of milk.

c) the units must be consumed continuously without any time gap.

c) the person consuming the commodity must be mentally sane and a normal person.

Example B2.1: Raghu consumed milk at different levels of units and the total utility derived from the consumption of particular unit of milk was depicted in the following table:

No. of units of milk consumed (cups of milk)	Total utility derived from the consumption of all the units(total no. of cups of milk)	Marginal utility derived from the consumption of every additional units of milk.
1	40	40 – 00 = 40
2	70	70 – 40 = 30
3	90	90 – 70 = 20
4	100	100 – 90 = 10
5	100	100 – 100 = 0
6	90	90 – 100 = -10
7	70	70 – 90 = -20
8	40	40 – 70 = -30

Note: From the table, it showed that the total utility increases but to some extent, it starts decreasing at that marginal utility becomes negative. It should be remembered here that the law of diminishing utility does not state anything about the rate of diminishing of utility. In the above example for convenience sake the numbers are chosen in an arbitrary manner and hence no significance should be attached to the rate of diminishment of utility.

Some people tend to think that law of diminishing marginal utility is not applicable to acquisition of money, precious materials like, gold, silver, diamonds or for consumption of alcohol etc. But in reality acquisition of more and more of any thing decreases the utility of that thing.

The law of diminishing utility forms the basis for law of demand, basis for progressive taxation and is of practical importance to all the consumers. Based on this only the taxation policy of Governments is formed. Higher income group is always taxed more than the lower income group of people.

When viewed philosophically there is an inherent moral in the law of diminishing utility. While there is need for acquisition of commodities or wealth, but its acquisition beyond certain level to satisfy ones greed really will have negative utility.

Value

Value is defined as the purchasing power of a thing in terms of other things. Actually it refers to other things, a thing can get in exchange.

Eg: 1) If one kilogram rice can fetch three kilograms of ragi, then value of 1 kg of rice = value of 3 kg of ragi.

2) If 1 kg of milk can fetch 10 eggs then the value of 1 kg of milk = the value of 10 eggs

Any commodity or service that has utility, can satisfy human wants, must be scarcely available (and not free in nature), must be measurable and that is capable of being sold or bought (ie, marketable) - all such commodities have value.

Price

The value of a thing when expressed in terms of money is called ***price*** in economics. Price is the amount of money that one has to pay for a thing in the market or the amount of money a thing can get in exchange in the market.

Value and price are not same in the money economy. But in barter economy where goods are exchanged for goods, value and price have the same meaning i.e. they are synonymous.

Wealth

In the ordinary language the term '***wealth***' refers to money, property or riches. But in economics wealth means all those goods which satisfy human wants, which are scarce in relation to demand and which command exchange value or price in the market. In short it means all those economic goods which are bought or sold in the market.

Characteristics of wealth: Commodities to qualify for the term wealth should conform to the following:

Utility: They must have power or capacity to satisfy human wants.

Scarcity: They are scarcely available in nature compared to their demand.

Transferability: Should possess ownership utility i.e. the goods can be transferable from one person to another and can be bought or sold in the market.

External to man: It must be external to man and not intrinsic to human beings. *Example:* Gold, furniture, land, vehicle, stocks, shares, cigarette, services of doctor or veterinarian are all wealth.

Non wealth: Skill and intelligence of persons, good health, love, affection, friendship, degrees, diplomas, free air, water, sunlight, good looks of a person etc are all intrinsic to person and hence do not constitute wealth.

Classification of wealth

Individual wealth: This refers to wealth owned by individual.

Social wealth or collective wealth: Public roads, parks, play grounds , public transports etc. constitute special wealth.

National wealth: Mountains, rivers, land, good climate etc. owned with in the territory of a country is considered as National wealth.

Cosmopolitan wealth: It is the international wealth like huge mountains, rivers etc. that cross the various boundaries of different countries of the world constitute cosmopolitan wealth.

Relationship between wealth and money: All money is wealth but all wealth may not be money.

Relationship between wealth and capital: All types of capital are wealth, but all wealth are not capital. Example: Motor car used for business is capital, but when the motor car is used for personal purposes it is not capital.

Relationship between wealth and income: Wealth yields income. Wealth is the means and income is the end or result of wealth.

Wealth and welfare: Welfare is the wellbeing of a person or a society. Wealth can bring a lot of welfare. Welfare is a state of mind or it is abstract. It differs from individual to individual, from place to place and from time to time. Wealth is just one of the means of providing welfare. But all wealth may not promote welfare. Harmful goods like opium, cigarette, alcohol etc. do not promote welfare. Also wealth acquired with too much of hard work without enjoying the basic needs of a person may not in reality add to the welfare of a person. Only when the wealth is distributed properly in the society, wealth promotes welfare of the society. But if wealth is concentrated among few individuals there is no social welfare.

3

Factors of Production and Their Rewards

Production: The term production refers to creation of or addition of utility to an existing matter or thing to make it more capable of satisfying human wants.

The following are different types of production

a) Agriculture and Livestock production on Land.

b) Production by extraction of things placed by nature.

   Example: Extraction of minerals from earth, wood from forests, fish from seas, rivers etc.

c) Manufacturing type of production:

   Example: Milk powder from milk, TV sets from individual components or conversion of raw materials into some finished products.

d) Production as a result of trade, banking, warehousing, transport, acts of buying, selling etc.

e) Production due to professional services like the services of a veterinarian, dentist, lawyer, teacher etc.

Factors of production: *Land, Labour, Capital* and *Organisation* (Enterprise) are the four factors of production.

Normally land and labour are considered as primary factors of production while capital and organisation are considered secondary factors of production. However, each factor of production is having its own primary or secondary place depending on the type of production activity.

Example: Labour is primary in labour intensive production like beedi manufacturing, capital and organization are primary in heavy industries like BHEL, HMT, etc.

Rewards of production

a) Land is rewarded by ***rent.***

b) Labour is rewarded by ***wages.***

c) Capital is rewarded by ***interest*** &

d) Organisation is rewarded by ***profits.***

Land

In economics land does not mean just an area of surface of earth, but it includes all the materials and forces which nature gives freely to man either on the surface of earth or inside the earth or in water or as free air, sunlight and heat.

Importance of land is for the following reasons

1) Production of Agricultural crops.
2) Raising of livestock.
3) Production of industrialised goods.
4) For extraction of minerals, petroleum, precious metals, water etc.
5) For transport.
6) It influences life style, income, standard of living of people etc. indirectly

Peculiarities of land

1) Free gift of nature, 2) Limited in area, 3) Indestructible, 4) Immobile (not in the astronomic sense), 5) variable in quality from one place of earth to another place 6) Values differ and 7) Subject to Law of diminishing returns.

Productivity of land is influenced by

1. Natural factors like rain fall, minerals, coast line, climate etc.
2. Human factors like hard labour, application of suitable technology etc.
3. Location factors like situation in city, semi urban or rural area.

Reward for land – *Rent*

In the ordinary sense the term rent refers to the periodical payment made by one person to another for using same asset say land, building, machine, vehicle etc. This is actually called contract rent as the payment here is actually based on the contract agreed upon by two parties. Here the rent or contract rent actually comprises of (a) charge for the use of asset, (b) interest on the capital invested on the asset, (c) allowance for depreciation or repair of the asset.

But, rent in the economic sense is called economic rent or pure rent. Originally economic rent was used to refer to the payment made by a tenant to a landlord for the use of land for production. So originally economic rent was referred to the payment made for the land and not to other factors of production. According to Ricardo rent is that portion of the produce of the earth, which is paid to the landlord for the use of original and indestructible powers of the soil.

According to ricardian theory

1) Rent is the payment made to the land used and to any other factors of production.
2) Rent is the amount paid only to the use of land and not towards any other charge where in other facilities are provided on the land.
3) Rent is the surplus over and above the costs of production.

Modern theory of rent

Every factor of production can command rent if its supply is inelastic or limited. Rent arises whenever any factor of production is scarce in relation to demand. Further rent is the surplus or excess payment made for a factor of production over its transfer earning.

Transfer earning refers to the reward that a factor of production can get in the next best alternative use. This is illustrated in the following example:

Let us presume a unit of land commands Rs. 5000/- year when used for cultivation. The same land when used for some other use say commands only Rs. 3000/-, then transfer earning is rupees three thousand (Rs. 3000/-). The surplus over its transfer earning is Rs. 5000 – 3000 = 2000/-. That is the surplus over its transfer earning namely Rs. 2000/- is called rent. Higher demand for land yields higher rent and lower demand leads to lower rent.

Labour

Labour in the ordinary language means physical or manual work done by an unskilled worker. But in economics labour is any exertion of mind or body undergone partly or wholly with a view to securing some good than the pleasure derived directly from work. Labour includes all manual and mental effort undertaken for a reward or a monetary consideration or for production of some wealth. The services rendered by mother to son or by wife to husband out of love and affection is not labour. Services of veterinarian, doctor, dentist, teacher, factory worker etc. all constitute labour.

Some times labour is classified into productive labour and unproductive labour. Productive labour refers to the work that results in some things material or ends in satisfying a want for a price.

Unproductive labour is that labour which employs unlawful activity such as gambling, dacoity, pick pocketing, smuggling etc to satisfy human wants.

Labour is a very important factor of production as it produces wealth and labour itself in the form of human resource constitutes wealth.

Salient features of labour and labourer

1. Labour is inseparable from the person labourer.
2. Labourer sells only his physical labour and not his person.
3. Labour is perishable, as the labour lost for a day is lost for ever and labour cannot be stored.
4. Labourers are human beings and hence they have all the associated human feelings, likes, dislikes, physical limitation etc and hence a labourer cannot work like a machine.
5. Labourers differ in their efficiency, because of differences in their skill, intelligence, physical strength, background, experience etc.
6. Labourers do not wish to move away as far as possible from their native areas unless circumstances force them to do so. This is because of their attachment to their native place, landed property, language, culture, familiar environment, friends and relatives. In other words labourers are less mobile and usually resist change of work place.
7. Quite often when the availability of jobs are less than the supply of labourers, the labourers may have to work for wages much less than what they deserve.
8. Supply of labourers is independent of demand. The supply of labourers depends on a number of factors like rate of growth of population, proportion of working persons, number of working days and working hours, favourable or unfavourable wage structure, presence of gender bias in the social structure, and migration of labourers. Immigration increases supply of labourers in the importing country and emigration decreases supply in the exporting country. Government regulations preventing child labour, placing restrictions on employment of women into certain hard jobs and fixing minimum wages etc. also affect the supply of labourers.

Number and efficiency of labour supply

When we talk of the number of labourers it refers to the quantitative aspect of the labour force which is dependent on the size and growth of population. The efficiency of labour supply refers to the qualitative aspect of labour which is dependent on several factors like racial quality, climate, health, education, training, working condition, equipments available, hours of work, level of wages, management, social security measures, proper division of labour, personal qualities, sound trade unions, political considerations and manpower planning.

When we talk of quantitative aspect of labour which is dependent on size and growth of population, it is desirable that a student of economics must acquaint the theories of population.

There are two theories of population namely

a) Malthusian theory of population developed by Thomas Robert Mathus in 1798 and later modified in 1803.

b) Optimum theory of population put forth by Edwin Cannon in 1805.

Main features of Malthusian theory of population

1. Both population and food production improve.
2. Population increases in quick geometric scale ie. $n, n^2, n^3, n^4, ...n^n$ because sex is universal and permanent.
3. Food production increases in arithmetic progression ie, n, n+1, n+2, n+3,........n+n.
4. Because of the difference in rate of growth of population and food production, population will overtake food supply resulting in starvation of people. There will be famine, epidemics, diseases and other natural disasters resulting in large scale death of people and animals. This brings in some kind of adjustment in population. In other words nature takes its own course in checking population through these ghastly natural happenings. They bring misery to people.
5. As the nature's methods are very harsh, Malthus advocated certain preventive methods to check population by adopting a) postponement of marriage, b) observing celibacy or remaining unmarried, c) practicing moral restraints or self control on sex. Modern contraceptive methods were not known during the days of Malthus and as clergymen and a catholic priest, he was opposed to family planning methods as they were against the religious faith during his days.

However, Malthusian theory had the following criticisms:

a) Population increases but not geometrically.

b) Modern inventions have increased food production more rapidly than arithmetic progression.

c) Malthus did not consider animal food production as animals grow as faster as human beings.

d) Growth of population should not be linked only with food production. Because it is always possible to exchange goods to food if a particular country's economy is good.

e) Preventive checks advocated by Malthus are not practicable in reality.

f) Dr. Edwin Cannan said that a baby comes not only with a mouth and stomach, but also with a pair of hands to work.

In spite of the above criticism, it may be concluded that there is some element of truth in Malthusian theory, because we have been witnessing large scale natural disasters that are occurring in different parts of the world contributing to some extent in the control of population.

Optimum theory population

This theory was put forth by Edwin Cannan in the year 1805. This theory was later further developed by economists like Dalton, Robbins, Car Saunders and others.

Main features of Optimum theory of population:

a) Every country has certain level of natural resources and a certain level of technical knowledge.

b) For a given level of natural resources there will be a level of population for which the per capita income is highest. This is called optimum level of population. If population increases beyond this optimum level it is considered as over population. If the population is below this level then it is considered as under population. Therefore the terms over population and under population are flexible and not absolute. These levels vary with variation in resources, technology, new inventions etc. If there is increase in resources there is change in the optimum level of population. If resources improve and population is less per capita income will fall and if resources are less and population is more then also there is decrease in per capita income.

c) Under population can be checked by encouraging growth of population.

d) Over population can be checked by checking the growth of population through family planning methods etc.

e) Under production can be prevented by increasing the resources.

Reward for labour – wages

In economics the term wage refers to any reward paid to the mental or physical work or labour performed by any category of worker. It may be a factory worker, farm labourer, a doctor, teacher, lawyer or a scientist. However the term wage is misunderstood in the ordinary sense as reward paid to a lower level worker who contributes physical labour. On the other hand the term wage in the strict economic sense includes all types of remuneration like salaries, commissions, fees, service charges etc. received by the workers for their respective mental or physical services rendered.

Wages are of two types. They are (a) Money wage and (b) real wage. Money wage refers to the actual reward received by a worker in terms of money or currency. But real wage refers to all other benefits a worker receives along with money wage. The other benefits that contribute to the real wage include rent free quarters, free canteen facilities, subsidised food, transport, clothing, footwear, free uniform, subsidised or free medical benefits, free education to children, paid holidays, restricted hours of work, incentives for extra work, regularity of service or job, promotional opportunities, good working conditions etc.

Demand for labour and supply or availability of the labour are the two factors that determine the wage pattern.

Capital

Capital is a man made factor of production. Capital does not mean mere cash. It means wealth that is used for producing additional wealth. It refers to all man made wealth or goods which are used for further production of wealth. It includes cash, man made raw materials, tools, implements, machines, vehicles, furniture, buildings etc. which are man made and not free gifts of nature.

Characteristics of capital

1. It is productive in nature as it helps in producing other wealth or goods.
2. As capital is man made, it is a produced means or factor of production.
3. It is a source of income.

4. Capital is separable from its owner and is mobile from one place to another.
5. Capital can be variable as it can be increased or decreased.
6. It is an exhaustible factor as it can be used up in the process of production.
7. Capital includes money that is used for further production and not the money that is used for personal consumption or the money that is hoarded. All money is not capital and all capital is not money.
8. All capital is wealth, but all wealth is not capital. Only the wealth that is used for production is wealth. Example: Building used for factory is capital but the building used for residential purposes is not capital.
9. Capital is a source of income where as income is the result of or contribution of capital.

Significance of capital

a) Capital contributes to modern large scale industrial and agricultural production.

b) Capital increases the productivity of labour as for example in the case of a farmer, the productivity of land improves when the farmer uses a pair of bullocks or a tractor for ploughing the land. Productivity of land can be improved if manure and fertilisers are used.

c) Capital contributes to over all economic development and increases per capita income.

d) Factory buildings etc. can be built by using capital.

e) Capital provides raw materials like sugarcane to sugar factory, milk to milk powder plant, cotton to textile mills etc.

f) Capital helps in the purchase of tools, machines, providing means of transport by way of buildings, roads, ships, railways etc.

g) Provides means of subsistence to factory workers particularly during the period when the factory is yet to make profits.

h) Capital helps in creating employment.

Classification of capital

There are several bases of classification of capital.

On the basis of degree of durability, capital is classified into (a) Fixed capital and (b) 1.Circulating or working capital.

- Fixed capital refers to durable producers' goods like building, machinery furniture etc. which can be used for many years.
- Circulating capital or working capital refers to those goods which can be used only once in that form. Fuel used for production, raw materials used in production etc. are good examples of circulating capital.

2. Based on the scope for alternatives capital is classified into (a) Sunk capital and (b) Floating.
   - Sunk capital refers to that capital which can be used only for specific purpose. There is no alternative use. Railway lines printing machines etc, cannot be used for any thing other than for what they are meant.
   - Floating capital refers to that capital which can be put to alternative uses. Cash, fuel etc. are good examples for floating capital.
3. Based on the type of trade: (a) Production capital and (b) Consumption capital.
   - Production capital – Any goods that are used for further production are also production capital.
   - Capital used for personal consumption is not capital at all. Therefore consumption capital is a misnomer.
4. On the basis of ownership:
   - Individual capital – Capital owned by individual.
   - Social capital or Government capital – owned by society or Governments like Public roads, railways etc.
   - National capital – capital owned by individuals and Government put together constitute National capital.
5. On the basis of transferability:
   - Material capital like building, machinery etc which can be transferred from one person to another.
   - Personal capital like skill, intelligence or experience of workers which cannot be transferred from one person to another.
6. On the basis of expression:
   - Money capital ie. capital expressed in terms of money.
   - Real capital ie. capital expressed in terms of building, machinery etc.

Capital formation

Capital formation or Capital accumulation is the process of increasing the stock of real capital or stock of capital goods of a country during a particular period – say a year. These goods are used for further production.

The economic development of a country depends on its capital formation. Larger capital formation leads to higher investment resulting in greater production, increased rate of employment and better income. The betterment of income naturally leads to better standard of living. Countries like Canada, USA, Great Britain, Japan etc., have higher capital formation.

Steps involved in capital formation

1) Creation of savings by the people.
2) Mobilisation of savings by banks and other financial institutions.
3) Conversion of savings into capital goods by investment of savings in production.

Factors determining capital formation

1) Ability to save which depends on income,
2) Willingness to save influenced by sub factors like:
    a) Love and affection of the family,
    b) Provision for old age,
    c) Provision for emergency,
    d) Social prestige,
    e) To have political influence, and
    f) Social habit.
3) Existence of banks and other financial institutions,
4) Rate of interest,
5) Taxation policy,
6) Opportunities for investment must be able to attract entrepreneurs to come forward for investment, and
7) Political condition.

Reward of capital: Interest

Interest in the ordinary sense means the total reward paid by a borrower to the Lender of capital. This is known as *Gross interest.* This gross interest includes a) the payment for the use of capital in production, b) interest for the risk in lending (bad debts), c) payment for the inconvenience caused to the lender and d) payment for the expenses of the management of loans.

But in Economics, interest is called "*Net interest*" which is the reward paid for the use of capital in production.

Rate of interest depends on the demand and supply of money. That is to say when demand is more than the supply the rate of interest increases and if the demand is less than the supply, the rate of interest decreases.

Organisation or enterprise

Meaning of organisation: The work of bringing together the other three factors of production namely Land, Labour and Capital in proper proportion and making them work harmoniously so as to obtain the best results is called organisation or enterprise. Organisation also includes the work of marketing the goods and bearing the risk of business.

Successful production and successful business depends upon efficient organisation. Further organisation determines the volume of production. It is the efficient organisation that is responsible for modern large scale production.

Entrepreneur: The person who organises business is called an entrepreneur. He brings Land, Labour and Capital together, initiates production, arranges for marketing and bears the risk of business.

Types of business organisations or Business Enterprises

Business organisations are of the following types:

1) Sole proprietorship, 2) Partnership, 3) Joint stock company,

4) Co-operative society and 5) Public sector company.

1. Sole proprietorship

Single owner enterprise is called sole proprietor business or enterprise. Small businesses like running a small livestock unit, petty shop, small hotel, service centre etc., are good examples of sole proprietorship enterprises. In this type of business the proprietor owns, controls and enjoys all the profits of his organisation. Single owner also bears the total risk of the business. In the event of loss the liability is unlimited towards the owner. The creditors can claim the private property and also the total assets of the business in order to make good the credit owed by the owner of the business. The sole proprietorship organisation may cease to exist after the death of the proprietor in case he has no interested heirs towards his business. Thus there are chances of lack of continuity.

2. Partnership organisation

Whenever fairly large sums of capital are required, single owner may not be able to provide in. In such cases more than one person up to a maximum ten persons in case of banking enterprises and up to a maximum of twenty persons in other non banking enterprises can join together and contribute to the capital of the business and share the profits on agreed terms. This is called partnership organisation. Here there are chances of misunderstanding among the partners and there may be no proper control or sometimes one partner may try to cheat the other partner etc., ultimately leading to the collapse of partnership organisation. However if there is good understanding among partners, the partnership business will be a successful enterprise.

Types of partnership: There are two types of partnership namely a) General partnership and b) Limited partnership.

General partnership: In this type the liability of partnership is unlimited. This type is common in India.

Limited partnership: In this type of partnership the liability of some special partners is limited only to the extent of their capital contribution. But the liability is unlimited to one or more of the other partners. Since the limited partner's liability is limited, his rights are also restricted and they cannot take part in the management of the business.

3. Joint stock company

It is a company limited by shares having a permanent paid up or nominal share capital of fixed amount held and transferable as stock and formed on the principle of having in its members only the holders of those shares or stock and no other persons.

A joint stock company has its separate legal existence apart from the members constituting it. A company has perpetuity, limited liability, unlimited membership, particularly in public limited company (minimum is seven). However in a private limited company the maximum membership is fifty (50) excluding the employee members of the company and the minimum is two (2). While the share holders are the owners of the company, the management of the company is entrusted to a board of directors. Shares can be transferred from one holder to another without consulting. Liability is limited only to the personal property of the share- holders. There are a number of statutory regulations to the company.

4. Co-operative societies

A co-operative society is a voluntary organisation formed mainly to promote economic interests of its members. Members have equal rights. A co-operative society has the motto of "each for all and all for each". Example for co-operative society type of organisations include primary milk producers' co-operative society at village level, milk unions at district level and milk federations at state level.

5. Public sector company

Any company undertaken and run by local, state or central government is called public sector undertaking or company. Public sector company is run mainly to bring about rapid economic development and to find huge amount of capital needed for large projects like railways, ship building etc. Bharat Electronics, Hindusthan Machine Tools, Bharat Heavy Electrical Limited, etc. are good examples of public sector organisations.

Role or functions of an entrepreneur

Entrepreneur is the captain of the industry. His functions include,

i) Planning, ii) Starting or execution, iii) Management and supervision, iv) Marketing, v) Innovation and vi) Risk bearing.

i) Planning: The entrepreneur has to plan before hand the product, volume, time, place, technique etc. connected to the business enterprise.

ii) Starting or execution: Entrepreneur has to raise capital, acquire land, construct building, install machinery, buy the raw material, employ the personnel and start the production.

iii) Management and Supervision: After the start of production, entrepreneur must manage to see that right person is given right job, there must be proper division of labour and proper supervision to see that there will be no wastage of resources and ensure proper utilisation of labour force as well as materials in production.

iv) Marketing: Once the products are ready they have to be marketed by adopting best marketing techniques and through proper advertisement. Contact with wholesalers and retailers must be established or the entrepreneur must establish his own retail network.

v) Innovation: Entrepreneur must introduce innovations. He must introduce new products to satisfy the changing needs of the consumers. Introduce new techniques of production. Introduce new raw materials in production and discover new uses.

vi) Risk bearing: The risk concerned with the whole business must be borne by the entrepreneur.

Qualities of a successful entrepreneur:

A successful entrepreneur should possess the following qualities.

i) Knowledge of the trade, ii) Leadership, iii) Power of judgement, iv) Courage, v) Good salesmanship, vi) Foresight, and vii) Intelligence.

Reward of organization – Profit

Reward of organization is profit. In the ordinary language profit of a business is the excess of its total revenue over its total costs. However in economics the term profit refers to the reward or price paid for the services of entrepreneur in production. It is the surplus left over for the entrepreneur from the total income of business after paying to the other factors of production namely land (rent), labour (wages) and capital (interest).

4

Theory of Demand and Supply

Demand is not mere desire for a commodity. It is the effective desire for a commodity, that is to say it is the desire for a commodity backed by adequate purchasing power, willing to spend the purchasing power on the commodity, at a particular price and in a particular unit of time. (say per day, week, month or year).

Demand schedule: The demand schedule shows the relationship between the price and the quantity demanded. The demand schedule may be drawn for an individual or for the whole market. Our demand for an article at one price is different from our demand for the same article at a different price. If the different quantities demanded by us at different prices are tabulated in a list, the list is called the demand schedule.

Eg: Imaginary demand schedule of an individual for eggs per week.

Price per ten eggs	Quantity demanded / week
20	8
18	10
15	12
12	15
10	18

The demand schedule for the whole market can be drawn by adding the quantities demanded by all the buyers at varying prices. The following is the imaginary demand schedule for eggs for the whole market in a particular week.

Price per ten eggs	Quantity demanded by different individual A B C D E	Total quantity demanded
20	8 7 6 9 10	40
18	10 8 7 11 12	48
15	12 10 9 14 15	60
12	15 13 10 16 20	74
10	18 15 12 20 24	89

Governments and business persons are more concerned by the demand schedule of the whole market than the individual demand schedule.

Demand curve

The graphical representation of demand schedule is demand curve. Usually the demand curves slopes downward from left to right which indicates the inverse relationship between price of the commodity and demand for the commodity.

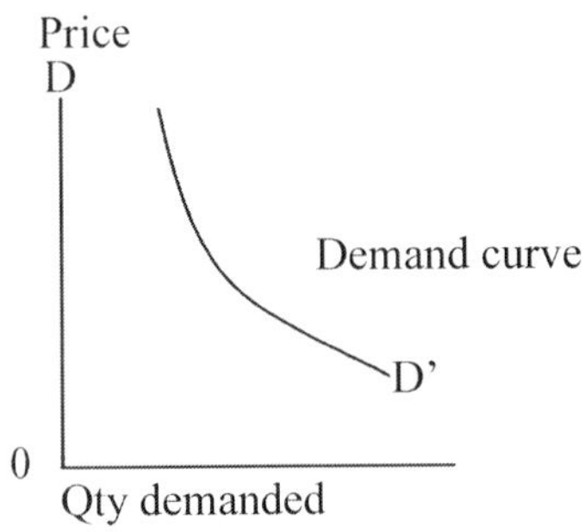

The Law of demand: The law states that the demand for an article varies inversely with its price. Other things being equal, when the price of a commodity falls, the demand for that commodity expands and as the price rises the demand contracts.

The law of demand holds good only under the following conditions:

Consumers' tastes should not change.

Consumers' incomes should not change.

The prices of substitutes remain same.

No new substitutes should have been discovered.

The commodity in question should not be one which confers distinction or honour to a person.

No further changes in price are expected

The law of demand holds good during a short period of time. There may be many factors like change in fashion, custom, season, population etc. which may modify the above conditions. However the above conditions remain fairly constant for a short period of time.

Exceptional demand curve

Instead of sloping downwards, the demand curve may rise upwards whenever there is direct relationship between price and quantity demanded i.e. more quantity would be demanded when the price rises. This trend was first observed by Sir Robert Giffen in 19th Century. Hence this exceptional process is called ***Giffen paradox***. The reasons for such exceptional behaviour may be

- Fear of scarcity of goods in feature
- Possession of a goods conferring distinction in the society.

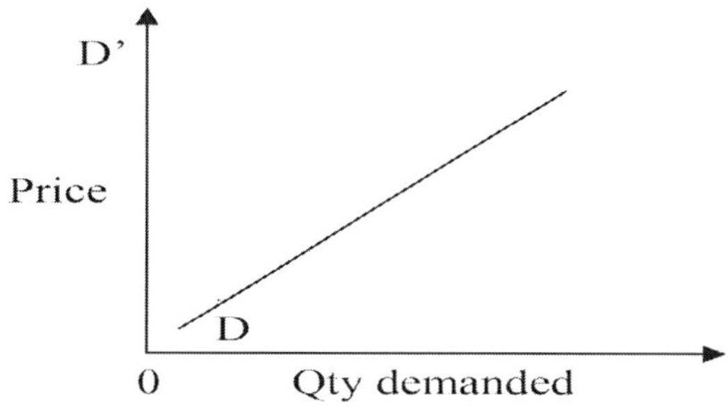

Elasticity of demand

The rate at which the demand varies when the price varies is called elasticity of demand.

If a variation in price of a commodity alters the demand in more proportion than the variation in price, its demand is said to be elastic. But the variation in price causes a less proportionate variation in demand then the demand is said to be inelastic.

The elasticity of commodities vary depending on the nature of the commodities. The demand is elastic in the case of luxuries such as costly motor cars, expensive television sets etc. However the demand is inelastic in the case of necessities like ragi, jowar, ordinary rice etc. The demand is elastic in the case of commodities whose consumption can be postponed or in such commodities which have variety of uses or which have substitutes.

The elasticity of demand is illustrated in the following example.

rice per unit	Percentage variation in price	Demanded units	Percentage variation in demand	Nature of variation in demand	Elastic / Inelastic
10	-	10	-	-	-
15	50	4	60	Negative	Elastic
12	20	9	10	Negative	Inelastic
8	20	11	10	Positive	Inelastic
6	40	15	50	Positive	Elastic

Consider a commodity whose value per unit at normal time is rupees 10 and at that price the total units demanded say is also 10 units. When the price changes to rupees 15/- per unit resulting in say reduction or contraction of demand to four units. In this case there is 50% variation in price and the variation percentage (reduction) in the number demanded is 60, thus the proportion of variation in demand is more in proportion to the variation in price. This is a case of elastic demand. Similarly when the unit price is reduced to Rs. 6/- resulting in expansion of demand to 15 units. The percentage variation in price is 40 resulting in 50% variation in demand. This is again a case of Elastic demand. However when the unit price is altered to rupees 12 or rupees 8, the respective alterations in the total number demanded say are 9 and 11, the variation percentage is 20 resulting in percentage variation in the number demanded to 10. In both the cases the demand is inelastic as the percentage variation in the number of units demanded (10%) is less than the variation in price (20%).

Elasticity of demand

The elasticity of demand is defined as proportionate change in quantity divided by proportionate change in price.

Price elasticity of demand: It is defined as relative responsiveness of quantity demanded of a commodity to the percentage change in it's price.

$$E_d = \frac{\text{\% change in quantity demanded}}{\text{\% change in price}}$$

Income elasticity of demand : It is the responsiveness of change in quantity demanded to change in income.

$$E_d = \frac{\text{\% change in quantity demanded}}{\text{\% change in income}}$$

Luxury goods will have high income elasticity while the necessaries have low income elasticity of demand.

Cross elasticity of demand: It is a measure of responsiveness of demand of a good to a given change in the price of related good.

$$E_{dy} = \frac{\text{Proportionate change in quantity demanded}}{\text{Proportionate change in price of related good}}$$

Magnitude of elasticity

- When the coefficient of elasticity of demand exceeds one, ***the demand is elastic*** ($e>1$).
- When the coefficient of elasticity of demand is less than one, ***the demand is called inelastic*** ($e<1$).
- When the coefficient of elasticity of demand is equal to one, ***the demand is said to be unitary elastic*** ($e=1$).
- When the quantity demanded changes even when the price level remains static, the ***demand is said to be perfectly elastic*** ($e=\alpha$).
- When the change in price does not result in change in quantity demanded, the ***demand is said to be perfectly inelastic*** ($e=0$).

Factors determining the elasticity of demand

- Nature of the commodity – Necessity or comfort.
- Possibility or other wise of postponing the consumption.
- Presence of substitutes.
- The elasticity of demand is always low for such commodities, the prices for which are very high or very low.
- Proportion of income the consumers spend on the commodity – less spent – less elasticity, more spent – more elasticity.
- Multiple uses of a commodity lead to more elasticity where as if the commodity has a single use the elasticity is narrow.
- Elasticity depends on the income of consumers. For higher income group, elasticity of demand for a particular commodity is low. For low income group elasticity of demand for the same commodity is high.

Extension and contraction of demand

Demand changes simply because of a change in price. Though the consumer's demand schedule is fixed, he is solely led by price. He simply goes up and down in the same curve.

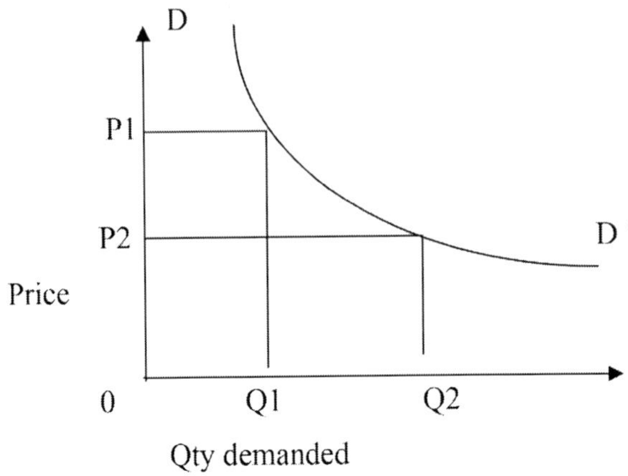

Increase and decrease in demand

The terms increase and decrease in demand are different from the terms extension and contraction of demand. Extension of demand refers to enhancement of demand in relation to reduction in price, where as *increasein demand* refers to real increase in demand due to factors other than price. ie, there is increase in demand to certain commodities irrespective of alternation in price. Similarly contraction of demand refers to reduction in demand in relation to enhancement in price where as *decrease in demand* refers to real decrease in demand due to factors other than price. ie. there is decrease in demand irrespective of variation in price. Some times the terms increase and decrease in demand are referred as *change in demand.*

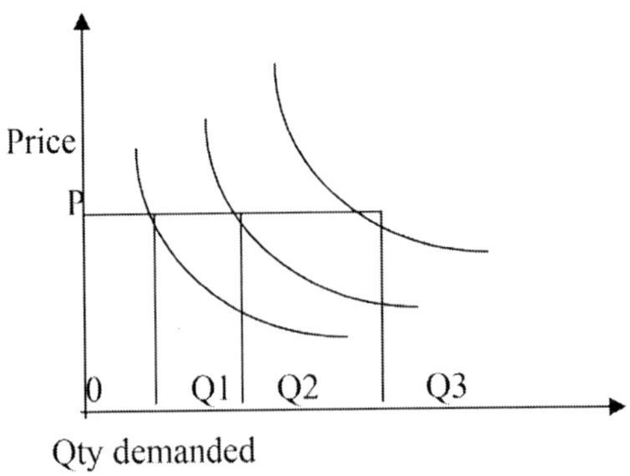

Factors that may effect the increase or decrease in demand:

1. Change in fashion.
2. Change in weather.

3. Change in the quantity of money in circulation.

   Increased money in circulation leads to higher purchasing power which in turn increases the demand. Similarly decrease in the quantity of money in circulation leads to decreased purchasing power resulting in decreased demand for commodities and services.

4. Change in size or composition of population.
5. Change in distribution of wealth: If wealth is more evenly distributed, the demand for necessary commodities will increase.
6. Change in real income of people.
7. Change in habits.
8. Technical progress.

Supply

Meaning of Supply:*Supply* means that quantity of a commodity which the sellers offer for sale at a particular price and at a particular period of time. Supply is different from *Stock*. The stock of a commodity refers to the total quantity of the commodity that exists in the market, while supply is that quantity which is usually offered for sale at a particular price.

Supply schedule is a statement showing varying quantities of a good offered for sale at alternative prices at a given time.

Price of egg (Rs / 100 eggs)	Market supply
280	7,500
240	6,000
175	5,500
150	4,600

Supply curve is the graphical representation of the supply schedule which represent various amount of a good that would be offered for sale at different prices during a particular period of time. Supply curve slopes upward from left to right because, as the price rises the quantity supply increases.

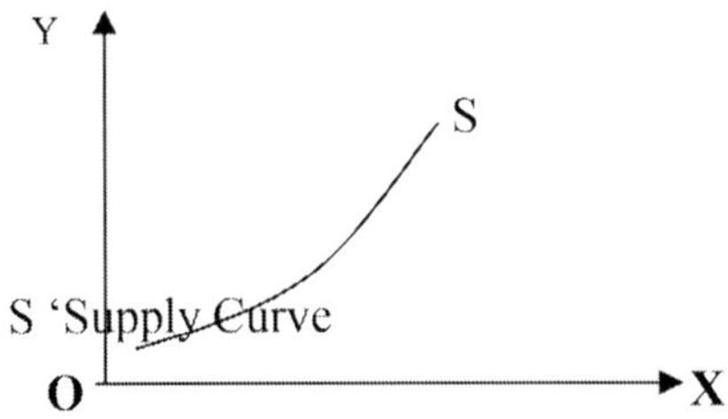

Law of supply: The law states that as the price of a commodity rises, its supply expands and as the price falls, its supply contracts.

The law of supply holds good under the following conditions:

1. The number of manufacturers producing a particular commodity remain constant.
2. The level of technology of production of a commodity remains constant.
3. The production cost remains constant.
4. It is presumed that the supply of a commodity depends purely on its price and not on the prices of other commodities related to it.
5. It is presumed that the seller does not expect any change in the price of the commodities he sells.
6. The natural or geographical factors like rainfall, soil etc. will remain constant.
7. It is presumed that there is no labour trouble affecting the quantity of supply of the commodity.
8. It is presumed that there is no change in the Government policy.
9. It is presumed that there is no change in transport and communications.

Elasticity of Supply

Elasticity of supply refers to the rate at which the supply of a commodity varies when its price varies.

It measures the rate at which the quantity supplied changes due to changes in price.

$$E_{sp} = \frac{\text{Proportionate change in quantity supplied}}{\text{Proportionate change in price}}$$

Supply is said to be *elastic* if a variation in price causes more than proportionate variation in supply and supply is said to be *inelastic* if a variation in price causes a less than proportionate variation in supply.

Types of elasticity of supply

- Perfectly inelastic - $E_{sp} = 0$
- Inelastic - $E_{sp} < 1$
- Unitary elastic - $E_{sp} = 1$
- Elastic - $E_{sp} > 1$
- Perfectly elastic - E_{sp} = Infinite

Example: Supply is elastic to goods like Gold, Silver, Furniture etc.

Supply is inelastic to such goods which are perishable like vegetables, fish, milk etc.

Factors determining elasticity of supply

1. Time factor: Elasticity of supply of a commodity is greater in the long run than in short period.
2. When a firm produces multiple products, the elasticity of supply is more than to a firm producing a single product.
3. Nature of the product: Supply is inelastic to perishable products of Agriculture and livestock. However the supply is elastic to manufactured goods like furniture, machines, consumer appliances etc.
4. If the cost of production rises very fast then the supply is inelastic. But if the cost of production rises slowly the supply is elastic.
5. Size of market: Supply is elastic if the market is wide. But supply is inelastic if the market is narrow.

Extension, contraction, increase and decrease of supply

The terms extension and contraction of supply refer to enhancement and reduction in supply of a commodity in relation to enhancement and reduction in price respectively. The terms increase and decrease of supply refer to real increase and decrease in supply of a commodity irrespective of price. Some times the terms real increase and decrease in supply are referred as *Change in supply.*

Causes for real increase and decrease in supply

- Natural conditions: Timely rainfall and other favourable environmental conditions will bring good supply of Agricultural products irrespective of price.
- Technical progress increases supply.
- If prices of various factors of production decrease the supply increases and vice versa.
- If the means of transport improves the supply increases and vice versa.
- Policy of Government: Lower import duty on goods increases supply and higher import duty decreases supply.

5

Theory of Production

Laws of Production / Laws of returns / Laws of costs

There are three laws of production. They are;

1) Law of increasing returns or Law of decreasing costs.
2) Law of constant returns or Law of constant costs, and
3) Law of decreasing returns or Law of increasing costs.

The Law of increasing returns or decreasing costs:

The law of increasing returns states that as we go on increasing the units of labour and capital in an industry, the total return or total output will go on increasing at an increasing rate more than the proportion of increase in the units of labour and capital and the marginal or additional output also goes on increasing up to certain point ie, up to optimum utilisation of factors of production. Further, as long as the law of increasing returns is in operation the average cost per unit of production will go on decreasing with every additional unit of increase in output.

Note: If the industry is expanded beyond certain point then the law of decreasing returns will become operational.

The law of increasing returns is more applicable to manufacturing industries more than any other type of production like agriculture. In the manufacturing industry it is possible to plan production by improving in machinery, technology etc and maximise production by adding more capital and labour. Nature does not play much role in manufacturing industries.

Illustration of law of increasing returns or decreasing costs

Assumption: The value of each dose unit of labour and capital say is Rs. 50,000/-

Number of doses or units of labour and capital	Total output in tons or total returns	Marginal output per unit or additional output in tons	Average cost per unit of produce ie. per ton.
1	50	50-0 = 50	$\frac{1x\ 50000}{50} = 1000$
2	110	110-50 = 60	$\frac{2\ x\ 50000}{110} = 909.09$
3	190	190-110 = 80	$\frac{3x50000}{190} = 789.47$
4	300	300-190 = 110	$\frac{4x50000}{300} = 666.66$
5	450	450-300 = 150	$\frac{5x50000}{450} = 555.55$

Law of constant returns or law of constant costs

The law of constant returns states that with every additional input of labour and capital the total output will increase only in the same proportion to that of additional input of labour and capital. Further it states that with every additional input of labour and capital the marginal returns or additional returns or additional output will remain constant and the average cost of production per unit of produce will also remain constant. This law is more applicable where the extractive and manufacturing types of production are combined.

Eg: When milk production, which is extractive type of production, is combined with industrial type of production of milk powder, the law of constant returns will be operative.

Another example is the combining of sugar cane production, which is extractive type of production with sugar manufacturing, which is industrial or manufacturing type of production. In this type also the law of constant returns is operative.

In reality this law is rarely operational except during the transitional stage between the stages when the law of increasing returns and law of decreasing returns are operational for a short period during the transitional stage. Any industry when it shows the symptoms of constant returns eventually it is giving a sort of warning signal to the entrepreneur that if he further tries to increase the production by employing additional units of labour and capital, he will be entering into the zone of law of decreasing returns.

Illustration of law of constant returns

Assumption: The value of each dose of capital and labour say is 10,000/- (rupees ten thousand only)

Dose of labour & capital employed in units	Total out put in units	Marginal or additional out put in units	Average cost per unit
1	50	50 - 00 = 50	$\frac{1 \times 10000}{50} = 200$
2	100	100 - 50 = 50	$\frac{2 \times 10000}{100} = 200$
3	150	150-100 = 50	$\frac{3 \times 10000}{150} = 200$
4	200	200-150 = 50	$\frac{4 \times 10000}{200} = 200$
5	250	250-200 = 50	$\frac{5 \times 10000}{250} = 200$

The Law of decreasing returns or increasing costs

The law states that with the employment of every additional unit of labour and capital, there is less than the proportionate increase in return compared to the proportion of input. The cost per unit of production increases every additional unit of capital and labour. Further the total output goes on increasing although in less proportion to the input up to certain stage and later on even the total output goes on decreasing.

This law is illustrated in the following.

Assumption: The value of each dose unit of labour and capital is say Rs. 500/- (Five hundred only)

Number of doses of labour and capital	Total output in units	Marginal or additional output in units	Average cost per unit of produce
1	10	10 –00 = 10	$\frac{1 \times 500}{10} = 50.00$
2	18	18 – 10 = 08	$\frac{2 \times 500}{18} = 55.55$
3	24	24 – 18 = 06	$\frac{3 \times 500}{24} = 62.50$
4	28	28 – 24 = 04	$\frac{4 \times 500}{28} = 71.42$
5	30	30 – 28 = 02	$\frac{5 \times 500}{30} = 83.33$
6	30	30 – 30 = 00	$\frac{6 \times 500}{30} = 100.00$
7	28	28 – 30 = -2	$\frac{7 \times 500}{28} = 125.00$
8	24	24 – 28 = -4	$\frac{8 \times 500}{24} = 166.66$

The law of decreasing returns is more applicable to extractive types of production like livestock production, agriculture production, mining, fishing etc. The law may not be applicable to agriculture production when it is taken on a virgin soil and when improved techniques are used.

Production relationships

Efficient farm management to attain maximum profit requires answers atleast to three questions regarding farming.

They are

1. How to produce?
2. How much to produce? and
3. What to produce?

These answers can be realized from various relationships that operate between inputs and outputs. Hence, it is essential for a farm manager to understand the basic concepts of these relationships.

Factor-product (input-output) relationship (How Much to Produce?)

Level of output of a particular product depends upon the quantities of inputs used for its production. This relation between inputs and outputs can be characterized as a production function. Production function is thus a relationship describing the manner and the extent to which a particular output depends upon the quantities of input used.

Production function can be expressed in 3 forms. i.e., Tabular, Algebraic and Graphical.

a. Tabular form

It can be illustrated as follows

Yield Response data on milk (litres) to concentrate feed (kg) in a farm with 10 dairy cows.

Concentrate feed (kg) (X)	Milk yield (litres) (Y)
0	15
5	20
10	35
15	55
20	75
30	90

b . Algebraic form

Algebraically, Production function can be expressed as $Y=f(x)$,

Where Y- represents dependent variable such as milk and x-represents independent variable such as feed, with 'f' denoting "function of".

If the independent variables are two, the production function can be written as $Y=f(X_1, X_2)$. For a number of independent variables (say 'n' variables) this function can be expanded as $Y=f(X_1, X_2, X_3, X_4, \ldots\ldots X_n)$. Normally, there are more than one independent variable involved in the production of any commodity.

In the case of single variable production function, only one variable is being varied, while others are held constant.

Such a production function can be expressed as follows.

$Y=f(X_1/ X_2, X_3, X_4, \ldots\ldots X_n)$

Here, X_1 is the variable input, and $X_2, X_3, X_4, \ldots\ldots X_n$ are called fixed inputs

c. Graphical form

The same data can be presented in the form of a graph as given below.

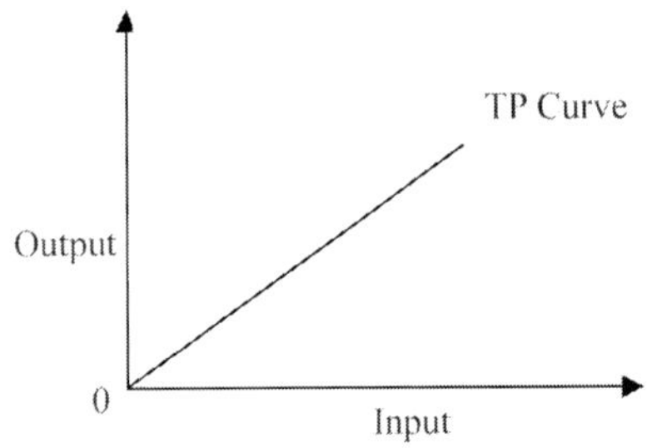

Product concepts

Total Product (TP)

The given amount of output (Y) associated with a particular amount of input (X) is called the total product.

Average Product (AP)

It refers to the average productivity of a resource. It is the ratio of TP to the quantity of input used in producing that amount of product. i.e., AP=Y/X.

Marginal Product (MP)

It refers to the quantity of the additional unit of the input adds to Total Product. Thus the MP can be found by dividing the addition to total output by the addition to total input. i.e.,

MP = $\Delta Y/\Delta X$, where, `Δ' refers to `change'.

MP is the rate of change in TP as the quantity of input changes. MP can also be called as 'slope of the total product curve', because DY/DX measures the slope of TP curve.

Types of production functions (Types of returns)

There can be 3 types of input - output relationships in the production of commodities. The nature of the relationship between a single input and a single output can be either of the following or combination of them.

a. Constant returns production function

In constant returns, each additional unit of the variable input produces an equal amount of additional product. i.e., the amount of product increases by the same magnitude for each additional unit of input. However, this is not a very common relationship in Animal Husbandry but may be possible in other industries.

$$\frac{\Delta Y_1}{\Delta X_1} = \frac{\Delta Y_2}{\Delta X_2} = \frac{\Delta Y_3}{\Delta X_3} = \frac{\Delta Y_n}{\Delta X_n}$$

Example:

X	Y	ΔY	ΔX	MP (ΔY/ ΔX)
0	500	-	-	-
10	550	50	10	5
20	600	50	10	5
30	650	50	10	5
40	700	50	10	5
50	750	50	10	5

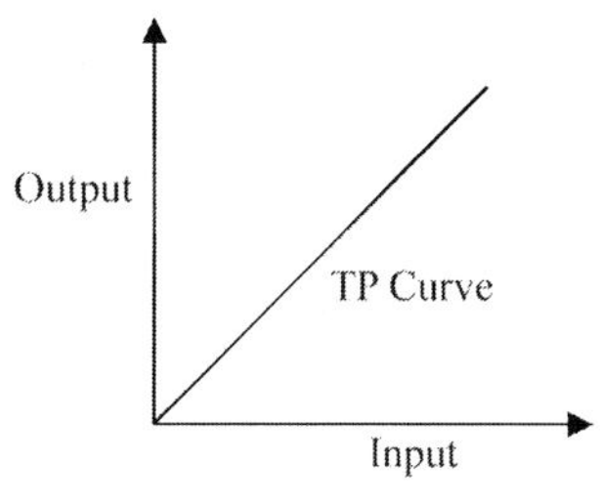

The table and the graph show that every equal increase in the input results in a constant increase in the output and hence, the given production function is known as a constant marginal returns function giving a straight line production curve (TP curve) which is having the same slope throughout its entire range.

b. Increasing returns production function

In this case, every additional or marginal unit of input adds more and more to the total product than the previous unit. i.e., addition to TP is at an increasing rate. In actual practice, the cases of purely increasing returns are rarely available.

Example:

X	Y	ΔX	ΔY	MP (ΔY/ΔX)
10	100	-	-	-
15	125	5	25	5
20	175	5	50	10
25	250	5	75	15
30	350	5	100	20
35	475	5	125	25

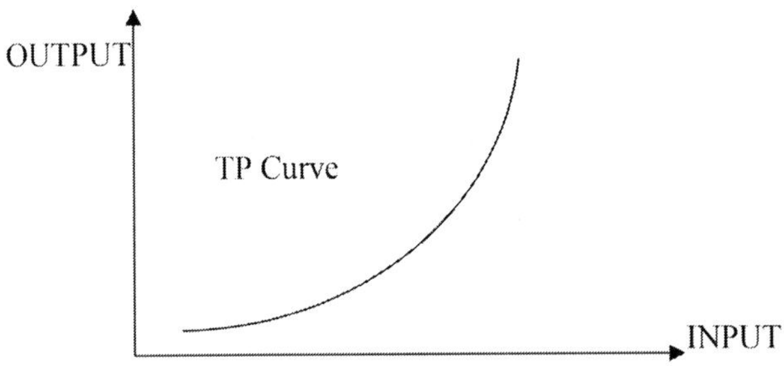

$$\frac{\Delta Y_1}{\Delta X_1} < \frac{\Delta Y_2}{\Delta X_2} < \frac{\Delta Y_3}{\Delta X_3} < \frac{\Delta Y_n}{\Delta X_n}$$

The shape of the curve will go steeper and steeper with the added inputs.

c. Decreasing returns production function

"If increasing amounts of one input are added to a production process while all other inputs are kept constant, the amount of output added per unit of variable input will eventually start decreasing". In this type each additional unit of input add less and less to the total product than the previous unit. Diminishing marginal product exist. This function exists is almost every practical situation in livestock production.

Example:

X	Y	ΔX	ΔX	MP (ΔY/ΔX)
0	50	-	-	-
10	140	10	90	9
20	210	10	70	7
30	260	10	50	5
40	300	10	40	4
50	330	10	30	3
60	350	10	20	1

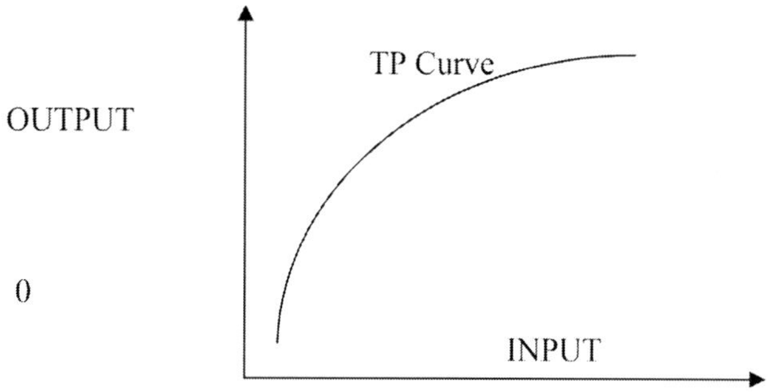

$$\frac{\Delta Y_1}{\Delta X_1} > \frac{\Delta Y_2}{\Delta X_2} > \frac{\Delta Y_3}{\Delta X_3} > \frac{\Delta Y_n}{\Delta X_n}, > \ldots\ldots$$

Elasticity of production

Elasticity of production can be defined as the percentage change in output in response to the percentage change in input.

i.e.,

$$Ep = \frac{\Delta Y/Y \times 100}{\Delta X/X \times 100} = \Delta Y/Y \times X/\Delta X$$

$$= \frac{\Delta Y}{\Delta X} \times \frac{X}{Y}$$

$Ep = \Delta Y/\Delta X \; / \; Y/X = MP \; / \; AP$

A production function with an elasticity of 1 indicate constant returns and the elasticity of more than one and less than one imply increasing and diminishing returns, respectively.

Classical production curve

Region I (Irrational)

Starts from the point of origin up to the point of MPP remain greater than APP (or up to MPP = APP). The APP increases throughout this region indicating that the efficiency of all the units of variable input keeps increasing. As soon as MPP equals APP, it is the end of first zone.

In this region APP keeps increasing and MPP remain greater than AP. Farmer must produce up to the level of input use where the APP is highest (or) if the output has a value, input use once it gives profits should be continued until stage II is reached, because the efficiency of variable input keeps increasing throughout the region I. This is the zone of increasing returns since ep>1 (MP>AP).

Region II (Rational)

This region begins where MPP is decreasing and is less than APP. i.e., the starting point is where MPP=APP and it ends where the MPP becomes 'zero'.

In this region, TPP is increasing MPP keeps decreasing but remains positive and less than APP. The APP is also decreasing. Both APP and MPP are decreasing. This is the zone of diminishing returns, since MP<AP and 0<ep<1.

Though region II is the rational zone, economically optimum point of input use or the most profitable level of input use cannot be determined by using physical production data alone. Cost of input and price of output are necessary to determine the level of production that is most profitable.

Economically optimum point or the maximum profit point of production

In majority of the cases, maximum production does not give maximum profit. As the cost factor plays a vital role in deciding the profitability of the farm-business, it is essential to inject the value information into the technical relationship of production. Economically optimum point of input use can be found out by incorporating the value information into the technical optimality.

Finding the most profitable point of production demands satisfaction of two conditions, viz., 1. Necessary condition, and

2. Sufficient condition

Necessary conditions: It describes a circumstance under which the economically optimum input use can occur. The necessary conditions are

- AP and MP must be decreasing;
- MP < AP; and MP > 0

Sufficient conditions: is satisfied when

a. MVP = MFC or MVP/MFC = 1, and

b. MVP is decreasing. (MVP must intersect MFC from above).

Note: MVP means Marginal Value Product (MPP or MP ´ Py).

MFC means Marginal Factor Cost (price of input)

Optimum point of input use must be some where in this rational zone and the optimum point can be located only when input and output prices are known. It needs to be emphasized that this region of rational production embodies diminishing returns phase.

Region III (Irrational)

Begins where MPP crosses zero point and becomes negative. Negative MPP occurs when so much excessive quantity of the variable input is used that TPP begins to decrease. Since additional quantities of input results in the reduction of total output in this zone, it is not profitable region even if the additional quantities of the resources are available at free of cost. Both MPP and APP are falling and this stage is known as the zone of negative returns. For example, If a farmer operates in this region, it will be irrational because he will incur double loss. i.e., Reduced production and unnecessary additional cost of inputs.

Relationships between Total Product and Marginal Product

Since MP is a measure of rate of change in TP,

- TP will increase at an increasing rate, when MP is on the increase.
- TP will increase at an decreasing rate, when MP decreasing but > 0.
- TP will be maximum, when MP = 0.
- TP will be decreasing, when MP < 0 (negative MP).

Relationship between marginal product and average product

- When MP > AP, AP is increasing.
- When MP = AP, AP is maximum.
- When MP < AP, AP is decreasing.

Classical production curve

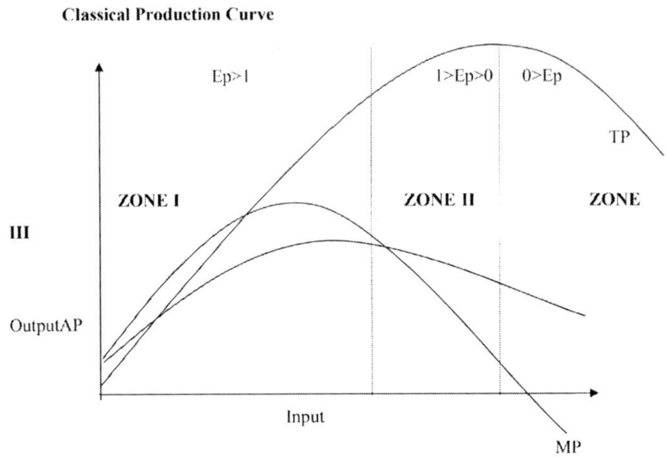

Principle of factor substitution (or) Factor – factor relationship

(How to Produce?)

Factor-product relationship deals with a single input and a single output. However, in actual situations, large number of inputs are being used to produce a good. Thus, farmers often face the problem of choosing the right combination of these inputs.

For example, it is a common problem with the farmers to decide on how much of concentrate and green fodder to be fed to a milch animal to get certain amount of milk or how much of different ingredients of poultry feed to be used for getting a particular level of poultry production. Here, the question is of finding out optimum or least-cost combination of resources in producing a given amount of output.

Cost minimization will not depend only on cost of inputs and price of outputs but also with marginal rate of substitution of factors. Our particular concern is with the possibilities of substituting one factor (X_1) for another factor (X_2) as product level (Y) is held constant. Hence functional relationship becomes Y= f(X_1, X_2,X_3, X_4,……,X_n) where, `Y' is the function of X_1 and X_2 while other inputs are kept constant. More specifically, X_1 = f(X_2). Consider the following table,

Paddy straw (kg) X_1	Concentrate (kg) X_2
2	12
3	8
4	5
7	3
10	2

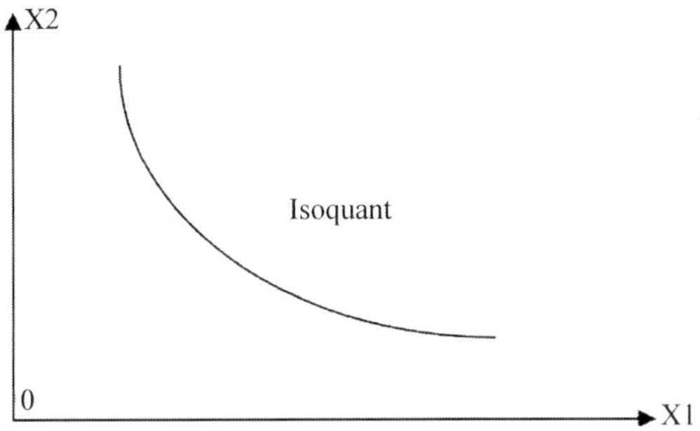

Assume that each combination of X_1 and X_2 in the table produces 10 litres of milk. These different combinations of two inputs can be plotted on a graph as follows:

This curve is known as *Isoquant or Iso-product curve*. An Isoquant shows all possible combinations of two inputs that would produce the same level of output. Similarly, Isoquants may be traced for different levels of output. If a number of Isoquants are drawn on one graph, then the figure is known as *Isoquant map.* Higher Isoquants represent higher level of production or output.

One important concept in Factor-Factor relationship is *Marginal Rate of Factor Substitution (MRFS) or Marginal Rate of Substitution.* MRFS or simply MRS of input X_1 for input X_2 is the number of units of input X_2 which can be replaced by one unit of input X_1 so that the level of output remains the same.

Example

X1	X2	MRFS of X_1 for X_2 $=\Delta X_2/\Delta X_1$
1	12	-
2	8	4
3	5	3
4	3	2
5	2	1

An important feature of MRS (or MRFS) is that MRS generally diminishes. More importantly, MRS (or MRFS) is the slope of the Isoquant.

Types of factor-factor relationships

Fixed proportion combination of inputs (perfect complements)

There are certain inputs that can be combined only in a fixed proportion. An additional amount of one resource or the other will not add to the total product. e.g., Tractor and Driver – Since they combine only in a fixed ratio, Isoquant is `L' shaped showing only one combination, since adding another tractor will normally require another driver too.

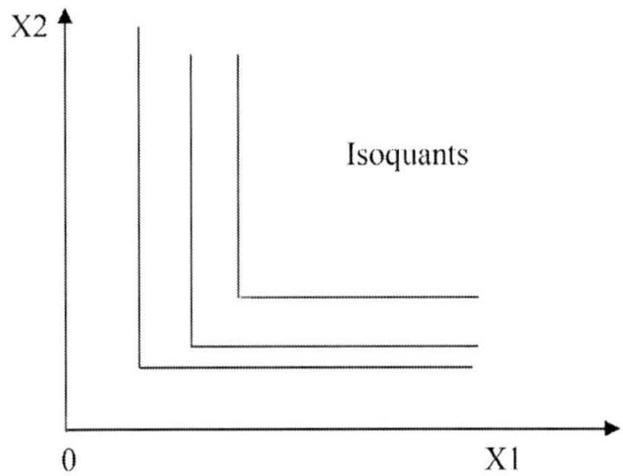

Constant rate of substitution (perfect substitutes)

When the amount of one input changes at a constant rate while it is replaced by another input, then there exists constant rate of substitution. i.e., the slope (MRS) of Isoquant is constant.

Example:

X_1	X_2	MRS
1	10	-
2	8	2
3	6	2
4	4	2
5	2	2

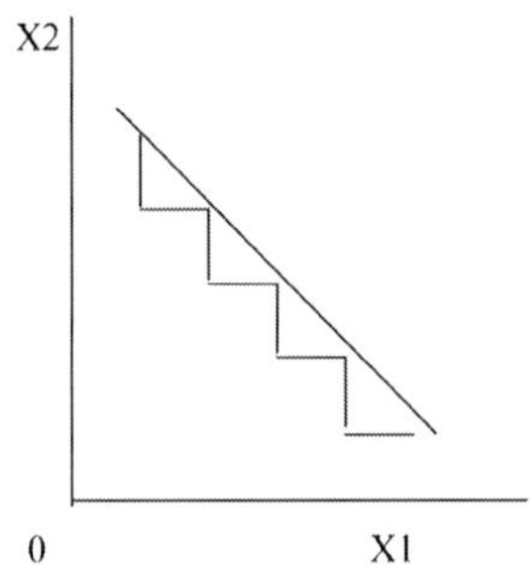

Varying rate of substitution (imperfect substitutes)

There can be increasing or decreasing rate of substitution. In this case, MRS varies over the Isoquant. However, substitution at an increasing rate is uncommon and decreasing rate is more common in livestock production. Slope of Isoquant goes on decreasing in decreasing rate of substitution. In other words, decreasing rate of substitution means that every subsequent increase in the use of one factor replaces less and less of the other (law of diminishing marginal rate of factor substitution).

Example:

X_1	X_2	MRS
0	23	-
1	16	7
2	10	6
3	5	5
4	1	4
5	0	1

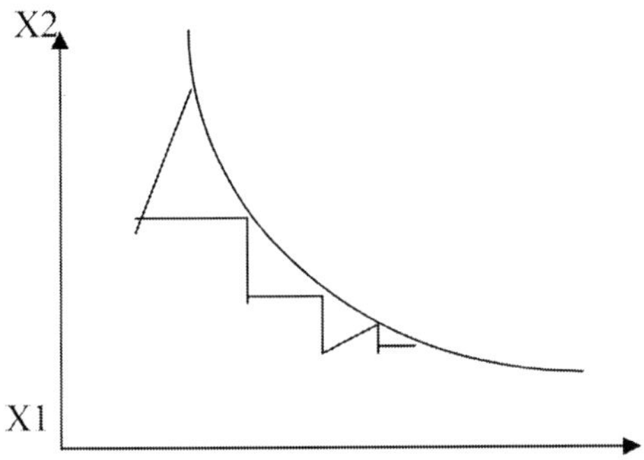

Estimation of least-cost combination of inputs in a production process

Least-cost combination of inputs can be estimated by the following three methods

Tabular method

Compute the total cost of production for various combinations of inputs and find the least-cost of production.

Algebraic method

a. Compute the Marginal Rate of Factor Substitution (MRFS) by dividing the number of units of replaced input by number of units of added input.

$$MRFS = \frac{\text{No. of units of replaced input}}{\text{No. of units of added input}} = \frac{DX_2}{DX_1}$$

b. Calculate the price ratio (i.e)

$$\text{Price Ratio} = \frac{\text{Price/unit of added input}}{\text{Price/unit of replaced input}} = \frac{Px_1}{Px_2}$$

c. Least-cost combination occurs where MRFS = Price Ratio.

$$\frac{\Delta X_2}{DX_1} = \frac{Px_1}{Px_2}$$

Graphical method

Least-cost combination is the point at which Isoquant is tangent to the Iso-cost line (or) Least-cost combination is met when slope of Isoquant (DX_2/DX_1 or MRFS) is equal to the slope of Iso-cost line (Px_1/Px_2 or price ratio).

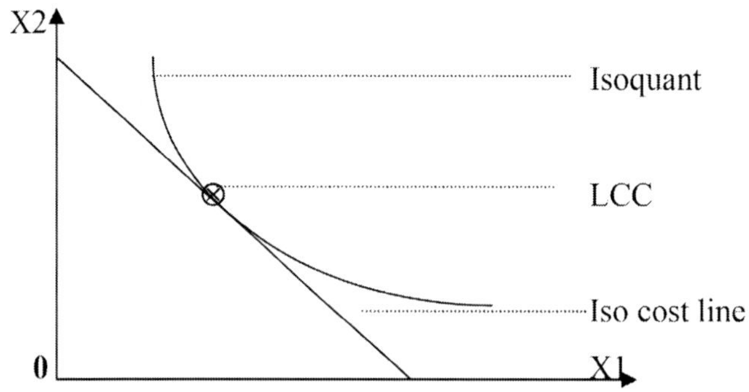

Iso cost line

Iso cost line shows all the input choices that would yield total cost. In other words, it is the locus of combinations of two inputs which would cost same total cost.

Isocline

Iso-cline is line connecting different Isoquants at points where the MRS (MRFS) are equal. `Iso' means equal; `Cline' means slope.

Ridgelines

Ridgelines are special isoclines where MRS (MRFS) is either zero or infinitive. Ridgelines denote the limit of the substitution between inputs. The area bounded by these two ridgelines is of economic relevance and it is the rational zone. Because, beyond the ridgelines any combination of inputs involves greater employment of one or both the inputs to obtain the same level of output.

All ridge lines are isoclines, but not all the isoclines are ridgelines.

Expansion path

Expansion path is also an Isocline, which joins all the least cost combinations. Any farmer, who is aiming to expand his business, will only move on this line.

Product-Product Relationship (or) Principle of Substitution Between Products (or) Enterprise Combination (What to Produce ?)

As the resources at the disposal of farmers are limited and have alternative uses in different production processes, the decision maker is confronted with the problem of what combination of enterprises he should include in his farm plan to maximize profit from his limited resources. For example, the farmer must decide whether to go exclusively for one enterprise or for a combination of enterprises. The decision in this regard depends on the biophysical relationship between enterprises, product prices and the resource base available with the farmer.

Algebraically, the relationship can be written as $Y_1 = f(Y_2)$. It must be noted here that inputs are held constant and try to analyse different levels of combinations of two products that can be produced with available inputs. Studying this relationship will help to achieve the maximum profit efficiently.

Consider the following example, which gives combinations of two products that is cotton and maize that can be produced with the available 10 acres of land.

Cotton (qtls.)	0	8	15	21	26	30	33	35	36	50	75
Maize (qtls.)	120	108	96	84	72	60	48	36	24	12	0

These combinations of two products if plotted on a graph give a curve called **Production Possibility Curve or Iso - Resource Curve** which presents all possible combinations of two products produced with the same resources.

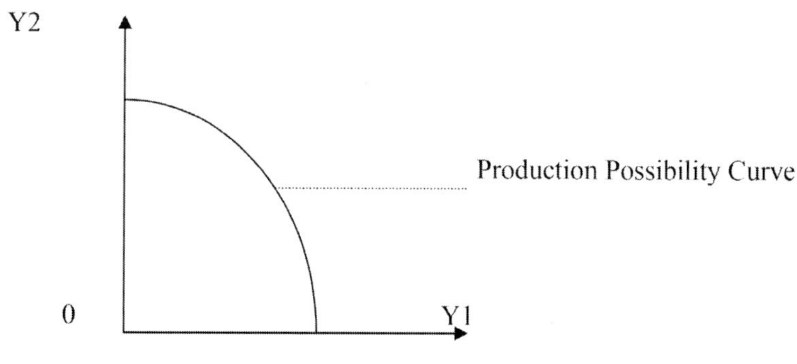

Marginal rate of product transformation (MRPT)

Like MRS in Factor-Factor relationship, here we have **Marginal Rate of Product Transformation** (MRPT). MRPT is defined as the rate of change in the quantity of one output for a one unit increase in the other output with the amount of inputs remaining constant.

MRPT or MRT of Y_1 for Y_2 is the amount of Y_2 replaced by an unit of Y_1 with the resources remaining constant.

$$MRPT = \frac{\text{No. of units of replaced output}}{\text{No. of units of added output}} = \frac{DY_2}{DY_1}$$

MRPT or MRT is the slope of production possibility curve.

Iso-revenue line defines all the possible combinations of the two products that provide same revenue. A line representing any given level of total revenue can be drawn on a graph. e.g., suppose the price of Y_1 is Rs.2/unit and that of other product, Y_2 is Rs.4/unit and the total income or revenue is Rs.100 and how many units of Y_1 and Y_2 to be sold in order to earn Rs.100. Then, selling either 50 units of Y_1 or 25 units of Y_2 will yield the same revenue. Now connecting these two points will give the iso-revenue line. In addition to the above two combinations, there can be many other combinations of Y_1 and Y_2 as found on the iso-revenue line which can yield the same revenue of Rs.100. Changes with price of the products will change the slope of iso-revenue line. Slope of iso-revenue line is nothing but ratio of prices of outputs. i.e., Py_1/Py_2. When Py_1 increases to Rs.5 even 20 units of Y_1 can give the revenue of Rs.100 and hence, the price changes (both increase and decrease) will change the slope of the iso-revenue line.

Types of product-product relationship

Joint products

Joint products result from the same production process. Production of one commodity without other commodity is not possible. e.g., Paddy and paddy straw; Cow and manure; Milk and manure; Mutton and skin, etc.

In such cases, quantity of one product decides the quantity of the other. Product-Product curve for such products will be shown as 'inverted L' shaped.

Complementary products

Complementarity among products exists when increase in one product also increases the quantity of other. e.g., Maize and Berseem.

Supplementary products

This relationship exists when increase or decrease in the level of one product does not affect the production level of other product. e.g., A few poultry birds in the backyard of a dairy farm with 50 cows.

Competitive products

This relationship holds when increase or decrease in the production of one product affects the production of the other product. Competitive products compete for the resources. It means that when two products are competitive some quantity of one product must be given up to increase the level of the other product. Here, there are three types of competition based on the rate of transformation.

a. Constant rate of transformation

b. Increasing rate of transformation

c. Decreasing rate of transformation

While the increasing rate of transformation is common in Animal husbandry the other two are uncommon.

Determination of optimum product combination

There are three methods to find the optimum product combination, which can yield maximum possible profit.

Tabular method

By this method, total revenue for each output combination is computed and then the maximum revenue combination is selected.

Algebraic method

Optimum product combination is found where Marginal Rate of Product Transformation Ratio (MRPT) is equal to Inverse price ratio.

$$MRPT = \frac{Py_1}{Py_2} \text{ (or) } \frac{\Delta Y_2}{\Delta Y_1} = \frac{Py_1}{Py_2} \text{ (or) } Py_1 . \Delta Y_1 = Py_2 . \Delta Y_2$$

Graphical method

The condition for maximum revenue is that the Iso-revenue line should be tangent to Iso - resource or Production possibility curve. i.e., the slope of the Iso-revenue line must be equal to the slope of Production-possibility or Iso-resource curve. No other combinations of products except this combination where the slopes of the two curves are equal will produce maximum return with available resource.

⊗

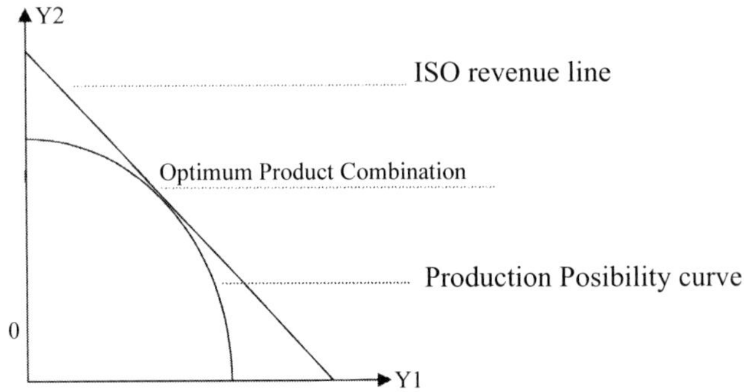

Iso clines, Ridge lines and rxpansion path in product-product relationship

As in the case of input combinations there are iso-clines in output combinations also. ***Isocline*** is a line passing through different production possibility curves at points where MRPT are equal.

Ridge lines pass through the product - product curves where MRPT is either zero or infinitive. The ridge lines are also called as border lines. The area bounded by the ridge lines is called as 'Rational zone' which is of economic relevance.

Expansion path is derived by joining all the points of tangency between the iso-revenue line and production-possibility curves.

Returns to Scale

Returns to scale describes the relationship between output and the scale of inputs when all the inputs are increased in the same proportion.

When all the inputs are increased in the same proportion and the scale of production is expanded, the effect on output would show three stages. The returns to scale would first increase (which happens when increase in output is more than the proportional increase in all the inputs), then, it becomes constant (when the proportions of increases in output and inputs are same) and lastly, it diminishes (when the proportion of output increase is less than that of inputs) This principle is better explained by the following table.

Unit	Scale of production	Total output	Marginal output
1	1 worker + 20 cows	80	80
2	2 worker + 40 cows	170	90
3	3 worker + 60 cows	270	100
4	4 worker + 80 cows	380	110
5	5 worker + 100 cows	490	110
6	6 worker + 120 cows	590	100
7	7 worker + 140 cows	680	90
8	8 worker + 160 cows	760	80

Sources of return to scale

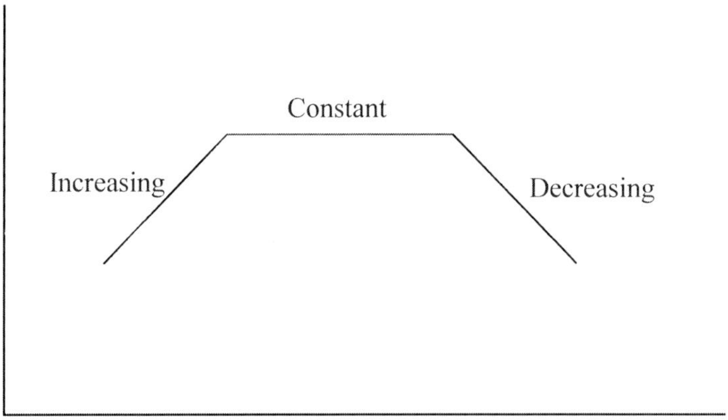

Economies of scale or economies of large scale production

The advantage of large scale production are called the economies of scale. Economies of scale have been classified by Marshall into internal economies and external economies.

Internal economies

Internal economies are those advantages of production which occur as a result of decrease in cost of production as the result of expansion of output. These economies are available to individual firms independently of other farms.

External economies

External economies are the advantages of large scale production which benefit all firms in the industry. Such economies do not accrue to individual firms alone. For e.g., construction of a highway would serve all the farms in the locality.

Concept of short and long run periods

Short run production

In short run, only variable resources are varied in quantity. The supply cannot be fully adjusted based on demand.

Long run production

It is a planning period during which all resources (both fixed and variable) are varied in quantity. The supply can be fully adjusted based on demand.

6

Theory of Cost

Production costs play an important role in the decisions made by the farmers. Cost of production often becomes a policy issue when producers complain that the prices they receive for their product do not cover the cost of production. Cost of production here means the expenses incurred per unit of output. Cost in farming can be divided into categories-fixed and variable.

Fixed cost (or) overhead charges (or) sunk cost

A resources or input is called a fixed resource if its quantity cannot be varied during the production period and in general costs associated with fixed inputs are called fixed costs. Fixed costs have to be incurred even when the production is not undertaken. Eg. taxes, rent, electricity, water charges, insurance, depreciation, labour hired on a year- round basis, interest on investment in equipment and livestock, etc. In short run, some costs are fixed and others can be varied. However in long run, all costs become variable.

Variable costs

An input is a variable input if its quantity can be varied during the period of production and the costs associated with variable inputs are called variable costs. Variable costs vary with the level of production. These costs will not be incurred in the absence of production. Eg. seed tractor, fuel, repairs, feed, fertilizer cost, etc. Labour if hired on daily basis interest on current investment, hired machines and other services are also included in variable costs.

Total costs of production will include both fixed and variable costs.

Cash costs (explicit cost)

Cash costs are incurred when resources are purchased and used immediately in the production process. Cash costs result from purchases of non-durable inputs such as fertilizers, fuel, oil, and casual labour which do not last more than one production process.

Non-cash costs (implicit costs)

Non-cash costs consist of depreciation and payments to resources owned by the farmers. Eg. Depreciation on tractor, equipment, buildings, and payments made to the farmer himself or family labour, management and owned capital.

Opportunity cost of an output is defined to be income it can earn in the next best alternative use. For example, a farmer with 25 kg. concentrate feed, can either feed it to his cows or sell it. If he gives the feed to his cows, the opportunity cost is the amount of money for which the feed can be sold to others .If he sells the feed, the opportunity cost is the amount of extra income, which can be obtained to be the real cost of any input.

Cost function

Production of output requires input, which cost money, and therefore there exist a relationship between output and cost. The total cost curve or cost function represents the functional relationship between output and total cost.

Cost function can be presented *arithmetically* (tabular form), *geometrically* (graphic form) and *algebraically* (equation form).

a) Tabular form

Output	TFC	TVC	TC
0	10	0	10
2	10	2	12
5	10	4	14
9	10	6	16
13	10	8	18
17	10	10	20
22	10	12	22

b) Algebraic form

C = f(Y). Where, C-total cost and Y-output

c) Graphic form

The nature of cost curve depends on the nature of the corresponding production function. Hence, when cost is portrayed on X-axis and the product on Y-axis, the total cost curve will have the same shape as total product curve.

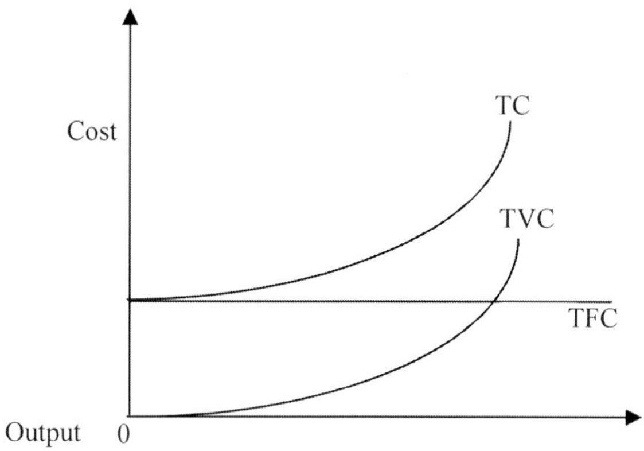

Relationship between TFC, TVC, and TC

TFC - is represented by a straight line parallel to X-axis and TFC - remains unchanged for all output levels in a time period. **TVC**- is zero, when output is zero. It increases as output increases. *The shape of TVC curve depends on the shape of the production function.* **TC** is the sum of TFC and TVC. When no variable output is added, TC is equal to TFC. The TC curve is shaped exactly like the TVCcurve, but is placed above the total variable cost (TVC) curve.

Unit cost curves

Unit costs are Average fixed cost (AFC), Average Variable Cost (AVC), Average Total Cost (ATC) or Average Cost (AC) and Marginal Cost(MC).These unit costs are more important than total costs in decision making process.

Average Fixed Cost is worked out by the total fixed cost by the amount of output. It is fixed cost/unit of output. AFC will vary for each level of output. As output increases AFC continues to decline. When output is zero, AFC = TFC. AFC always slopes downwards regardless of production function.

Average Variable Cost is calculated by the dividing Total Variable Cost by the amount of output. AVC decreases, reaches a minimum and increases thereafter. AVC cannot be computed when output is zero.

AVC = TVC/Output

Average Total Cost can be computed by the dividing Total Cost by the output. ATC, as AVC, first decreases, attains a minimum and increases thereafter. ATC is the cost of producing one unit of output.

ATC = TC/Output

Marginal Cost is the change in total cost in response to a unit increase in output. It is found out by dividing change in total cost (or total variable cost because TFC is not going to change) by change in output.

MC curve decreases first, reaches its minimum point and then raises upwards and passes through AVC and AC (ATC) at their minimum points .In other words, AVC and AC will slope downwards and keep falling as long as MC is below them.

Unit cost curves

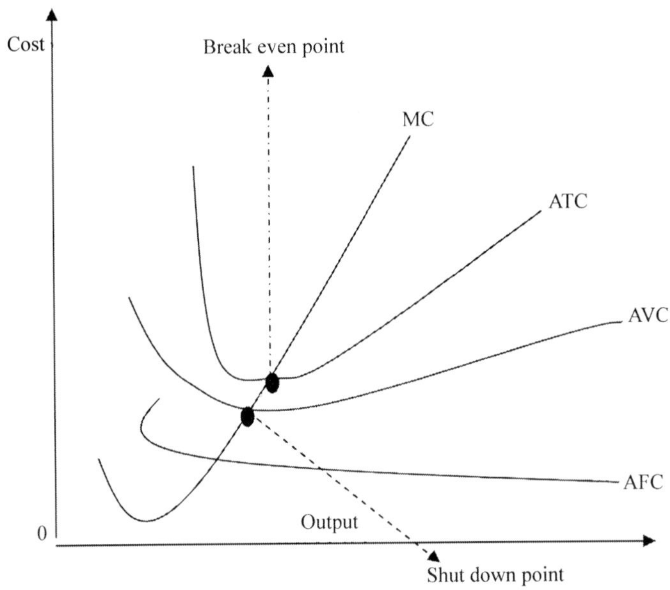

Break-even point is the *minimum of average total cost.* Exactly at this point, the MC will be equal to the ATC and the producer neither gains nor losses anything. Whatever income he gets above this point is his profit. Suppose the farmer is operating below this point he will be incurring loss towards the fixed cost.

In short-run, the farmer will continue to operate even below this profit. e.g., broiler farms.

In the long-run, the producer has to operate above this point to remain in the business.

Shut-Down Point is the minimum point of Average variable cost. Exactly at this point, the MC will be equal to the AVC and the producer will be in a position to meet the expenses towards the variable cost alone. If he operates below this point, he will not be in a position to meet even the variable expenses.

In short run, the producer must be able to operate at least above this point in order to sustain the business.

Long run is a period of time during which the quantities of all factors, both variable and fixed, can be adjusted.

Short run is a period of time, within which the firm can vary its output by varying only the amount of variable factors such as labour and raw materials. Fixed factors such as capital, equipment, top management personnel cannot be varied.

Relationship between Average variable cost and Average product

$AVC = TVC/Y = X \,.\, Px/Y = Px \,.\, X/Y = Px \,.\, 1/AP$

$AVC \; \mu \; 1/AP$

Therefore, AVC is inversely related to AP, i.e., when AP increases, AVC decreases. When AP is maximum, AVC attains its minimum point and when AP decreases, AVC increases. As on a production function, AP measures the efficiency of variable input, for cost curves AVC provides the same measure.

Relationship between marginal cost and marginal product

Marginal Product	*Marginal Cost*
Increasing	Decreasing
At maximum	At minimum
Decreasing	Increasing

Break-even analysis

Break-even analysis determines the level at which the gains and losses are equal. This level of values and quantities is known as the break-even point. Generally, break-even analysis is done by manipulating the most uncertain key factor.

E.g. Determination of timing for culling of dairy cows

The dairy farmer is interested to know at what age the maintenance cost of the cow will be equal to the value of milk from the cow. Break-even point indicates the time at which a farmer should sell the cow. At break-even point, benefits = costs, above break-even point, benefits $>$ costs and below break-even point benefits $<$ costs.

Break-even price

It is the price at which the farm's given level of output, if sold would equable the farmer to at least recover costs.

Break-even output

It is level of production that would enable the farmer to recover costs if the products were sold at the given or prevailing price.

Break-even analysis is a variation of gross margin or partial budget analysis, the same set of data is required. It involves all steps for conducting partial budget analysis. The final step involves calculation of a series of gross margins assuming various values for these critical factors.

Importance of break-even analysis

1. It is used as a measure of risk
2. It yields the minimum or maximum value of the critical factor at which a new technology is expected to become or stop being beneficial to the farmer

Advantages

1. Instead of calculating a fixed value, the result of a budget analysis can be assured in terms of probabilities.
2. If the break-even value is very high or very low, conclusions can be made about the profitability of the change with a high degree of confidence.

The **disadvantages** of Break-even analysis are similar to those of partial budgeting.

The **break-even point** in economics is the point at which cost or expenses and income are equal – there is no net loss or gain, one has "broken even".

The point at which a firm or other economic entity breaks even is equal to its fixed costs divided by its contribution to profit per unit of output, which can be shown by the following formula:-

$$\textbf{Break-even point} = \frac{\text{Fixed costs}}{\text{Contribution per unit output}}$$

The break-even point is also the point on a chart indicating the time when something has broken even, and is a general term for not having gained or lost something in a process.

The contribution per unit can be worked out using

Contribution = Price per unit – Variables costs per unit

Other uses of the term

In nuclear fusion research, the term **break-even** refers to a fusion energy gain factor equal to unity, this is also known as the Lawson criterion.

The notion can also be found in more general phenomena, such as percolation, and is rather similar to the critical threshold. In energy, the *breakeven* point is the point were usable energy gotten from a process exceeds the input energy.

In computer science, the term to a point in the life cycle of a programming language where the language is capable of developing its own compiler or interpreter. This usually marks a transition from a "toy" language usable in the real world.

In medicine, it is a postulated state when the advances of medicine permit every year an increase of one year or more of the life expectancy *of the livings,* therefore leading to a sort of immortality (barring sudden death).

Graphical representation

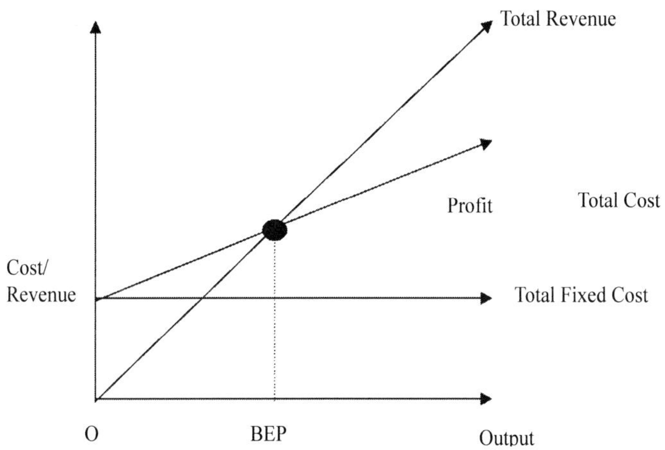

In any business, there is a point where total costs become equal to total revenues and that point is called as Break Even point and the corresponding output is known as Break Even output (BEO). This means that at this point, the business is making neither profit nor loss. Break-even point is the minimum point of average total cost. A farmer must produce atleast this amount of product or out put to cover the total cost of production. Whatever is produced above this point will be the profit for the farmer. The point where the farmer recoups his investment is the Break even point. The investment is in the form of fixed cost and variable cost which constitutes the total cost. When the total cost is equal to total revenue it is Break even point.

There are two approaches to arrive at the Break even point, namely., Linear and Curvilinear approach.

Linear Approach: Here the sale price of output remains constant for all the output sales. Here the total cost curve and the total revenue curve are linear that is these two curves are straight lines, where the total revenue curve cuts the total cost curve at the Break even point and the corresponding output is known as Break even output or break even quantity.

$$\text{Break Even Quantity} = \frac{\text{Total Fixed Cost}}{(\text{Selling price/unit of output}) - (\text{Variable cost/unit of output})}$$

$$\textbf{Break even Price} = \frac{\text{Total Fixed Cost}}{\left\{1 - \dfrac{\text{Variable cost / unit of output}}{\text{Selling price / unit of output}}\right\}}$$

Margin of safety

The margin of safety of a farmer is the difference between its normal capacity and break even output. Margin of safety indicates the shock absorbing capacity of the farmer in terms of risk and uncertainty. In other words it reflects the financial strength of the enterprise.

Margin of safety (Output in units) = Normal capacity – Break even output

Margin of safety in monetary terms = Revenue of the total output - Revenues from Break even output

Percentage of margin of safety

In physical terms = {Break even output/Normal capacity}× 100

In monetary terms = (Revenues from break even output/Revenues of the total output }× 100

Further, the break even analysis is also useful to know the output to be produced to make fixed amount of profits in the business.

Q_t = (TFC + Profit)/(P-V)

P = Selling price/unit of output; V = Variable cost/unit of output

Curvilinear approach: Here the total revenue changes over the period of time, since the some price changes, one output sales to the other. Generally the curvilinear approach is used for perennial crops and also in business where the gestation period is very long.

Exercise: A farmer is having 100 sheep. The Total fixed cost is Rs.100000. The TVC is Rs.60000. The Selling price of a sheep is Rs.2000. Find out the BEP (Physical & Monetary terms) and Margin of safety (Physical & Monetary terms). Find out the percentage of Margin of safety (Physical & Monetary terms). If the farmer wants to have a profit of Rs.20000, how many sheep should he rear.

Answer

When the above formulas applied, the following result was obtained:

Break Even Point (Output in units) = 100000/(2000-(60000/100)) = 71 units (i.e. Farmer should have 71 sheep in farm to be in No profit, No loss condition) Break Even Price (Output in Rs.) = 100000/(1-(600/2000) = Rs. 142857/- (i.e. Farmer should earn amount of Rs.1,42,857/- to be in No profit, No loss condition and earning above this amount is considered as profit)

Margin of safety (Output in units) =Normal capacity–Break even output= 100-71 = 29 units (i.e. Farmer is having 29 sheep above the break even quantity which shows farmer has good shock absorbing capacity in times of risk and uncertainty)

Margin of safety in monetary terms = (100*2000) - 1,42,857 = Rs.57,143/- (i.e. Farmer earns profit of Rs. 57,143/- which shows financial strength of enterprise)

Percentage of margin of safety

In physical terms = (29/100) X 100 = 29%

In monetary terms = (142857/200000) X 100 = 29%

To know the output to be produced to make amount of Rs.20000/- as profits in the business:

Qt = (TFC + Profit)/(P-V) = (100000+20000)/(2000-600) = 86 units

(If the farmer wants to earn profit of Rs.20000/-, then farmer should rear 86 sheep in his farm)

Part C
Livestock Marketing

7

Basic Terms and Importance of Studying Livestock Marketing

Goods and services are created through process of production. After production they have to be transferred or moved from the original producers to the final consumers. This involves the creation of market and the undertaking of number of activities such as buying, assembling, transportation warehousing, risk bearing, financing, selling etc. This constitutes the subject matter of marketing. Hence there is the need for the study of market.

What is market?

Market is derived from the Latin word "Marcatus" meaning trade, merchandise, ware, traffic or place of business. In the ordinary language, market is a place where buyers and sellers meet personally and make their purchases or sales. But in the language of economics, market need not be a place but it may be an area or region meant for potential exchange between a group of buyers and sellers interested in negotiating the terms of purchase and sale of goods and services and such negotiations may be done face to face at a certain place or may be done through other means of communication such as mail, phone, cable, television or through business middle men. Whatever may be the means of communication there will be free exchange or perfect communication between buyers and sellers so that a fairly uniform price prevails for a particular commodity over the whole area at any given time.

Livestock marketing

Livestock and their products are consumed by human beings from the time immemorial. Large number of people are involved in production, trading and consumption of these. Hence there is in existence a process by which producers and buyers of livestock and their products are brought together for negotiations to take place for exchange. This process is termed livestock marketing.

The terms "Egg market", "Milk market", "Meat market", "Wool market", etc. refers to the respective area, zone or place which has the potential for exchange between livestock buyers and sellers negotiating terms of trade in a particular commodity say eggs, milk, meat or wool etc. The size of these markets may be as small as, a small area in a village or may be as large as the whole world.

Importance of the study of livestock marketing

Livestock farmers produce livestock products partly for personal consumption or family consumption, but major portion is produced for sale so that such sales would add to the family income. In India livestock production is in the hands of large number of small farmers, marginal farmers and land less labourers. Only a small number of medium and large-scale farmers are involved in livestock production. However large number of livestock producers carryout their marketing activities either in their local area or transport the same to near by taluk level or district level market places. Quite often these small producers have to carryout distress sale particularly during peak production periods when the demand for the products may be at the low level. Added to this the exploitation of these farmers by unscrupulous middlemen, has always worked against the interest of these farmers, often making livestock production not a profitable enterprise. Some of these problems are considerably eliminated by co-operatives like dairy co-operative societies, poultry marketing societies etc. also have played a significant role in making the livestock production a more profitable enterprise. These co-operative societies have transformed an otherwise unorganised sector into organised sector by taking over procurement, storage, transport, processing and marketing functions from the livestock producers. In these days of globalisation, liberalisation and openness in the economy the marketing process has to be very competitive in order to survive in the global market. This is particularly so in such products like milk, eggs, etc., which are actually produced in excess than the domestic demand necessitating entry into global market. Competition at the global market being so keen, every effort has to be made in the livestock production to maintain the stringent standards of the products while scaling down the production cost to as much minimum as possible. For all this to be practically viable a sound knowledge of production and marketing is required. The subject of livestock marketing aims at providing exactly this knowledge of marketing.

8

Classification of Markets

Classification of market

There are several bases on which markets are classified.

a. On the basis of location

On the basis of the place of location or operation, markets are of the following types:

Village market

A market which is located in a small village, where major transactions take place among the *buyers and sellers of a village*, is called a village market.

Primary markets

- These markets are located in big towns near the centres of production of commodities. In these markets, a major part of the produce is brought for sale by *the producer-farmers themselves.* Transactions in these markets usually take place between the producers/farmers and traders.

Secondary wholesale markets

- These markets are located generally at district headquarters or important trade centres or near railway junctions. Major transactions in commodities take place *between the village traders and wholesalers.* Bulk of the arrivals in these markets is from other markets. Produce in these markets is handled in large quantities. There are, therefore, *specialized marketing agencies* performing different marketing functions such as those of commission agents, brokers, weighmen etc.

Terminal market

- A terminal market is one where the produce is either finally disposed of to the *consumers or processors or assembled for export*. Merchants are well organized and use modern methods of marketing.
- Commodity exchanges exist in these markets which provide facilities to forward trading in specific commodities. Such markets are located either

in metropolitan cities or in sea-ports. Delhi, Mumbai, Chennai, Kolkatta and Cochin are terminal markets for many commodities.

Modern terminal market

- The Department of Agriculture and Cooperation, Ministry of Agriculture, Government of India has taken the initiative to promote modern terminal markets for fruits, vegetables and other perishable commodities in important urban centres of the country to provide the state of the art infrastructures facilities.
- These market are envisaged to operate on a "hub and spoke" format where the terminal market is hub and collection centres are spokes to allow easy access to farmers for marketing their produce.

Seaboard markets

- Markets which are located near the seashore and are meant mainly for the *import and export* of goods are known as seaboard markets. Examples of these markets in India are Mumbai, Chennai, Kolkatta and Cochin.

On the basis of geographical area

Local market

- A village level market. The village markets exist mostly for perishable commodities in small lots. Eg: Vegetable or fruit market, milk or egg market at a shandy level.

Regional market

- Market covering a few taluks or towns forming a market say for food grains etc.

National market

- Area of market is nationwide as in the case of cotton, coffee, tea, cement, etc.National markets are found for durable goods

International or world market

- Here the area of market is the entire world as in the case of gold, silver, diamonds etc. Livestock products like milk powder, egg powder, meat, wool, leather products etc. also have global market.This market exists in the commodities which have a world-wide demand and supply.

On the basis of position of sellers in the market

- Primary market– Primary producers sell their produces to wholesalers.
- Secondary market- Whole salers sell to semi wholesalers or retailers.
- Terminal market- Retailers sell to ultimate consumers.

On the basis of time span

Short-period markets

- Markets which are held only for a day or few hours are called short period markets. Products dealt with in these markets are of a *highly perishable nature*, such as fish, fresh vegetables, and liquid milk. In these markets, the *prices of commodities aregoverned mainly by the extent of demand* rather than the supply of the commodity.

Periodic markets

- These markets congregation of buyers and sellers at specified places either in villages, semi-urban areas and urban areas on specified days and time.
- These markets are held weekly, biweekly, fortnightly or monthly according to local traditions.

Long-period markets

- These markets are held for a longer period than the short period markets. Commodities traded in these markets are *less perishable* and can be stored for some time; these are food grains and oilseeds. *Prices are governed both by the supply and demand forces.*

Secular markets

- These are markets of a *permanent nature*. Commodities traded in these markets are *durable in nature* and can be stored for many years. Examples are markets for *machinery and manufactured goods*.

d. On the basis of volumes of transactions

There are two types of markets on the basis of volume of transactions at a time.

Wholesale market

- A wholesale market is one in which commodities are bought and sold in large lots or in bulk. These markets are generally located in either towns or cities

- Economic activities in and around these markets are so intense that over time the *population tends to get concentrated* around these markets
- These markets occupy an extremely *important link in the marketing chain* of all the commodities including farm products
- Apart from balancing the supply and demand and discovery of the prices of a commodity, these markets and functionaries in them serve as a *link between the production system and consumption system*

Retail markets

- A retail market is one in which commodities are bought by and sold to the consumers as per their requirements. Transactions in these markets take place between retailers and consumers
- Retailers purchase the goods from wholesale market and sell in small lots to the consumers in retail markets. *These markets are very near to the consumers*

e. On the basis of nature of transactions

The markets which are based on the types of transactions in which people are engaged are of two types:

Spot or cash markets

- A market in which goods are exchanged for *money* immediately after the sale is called the spot or cash market

Forward markets

- A market in which the *purchase and sale of a commodity takes place at time t but the exchange of the commodity takes place on some specified date in future i.e., time t+1*. Sometimes even on the specified date in the future (t+1), there may not be any exchange of the commodity. Instead, the differences in the purchase and sale prices are paid or taken.

f. On the basis of number of commodities in which transaction takes place

A market may be general or specialized on the basis of the number of commodities in which transactions are completed.

General markets

- A market in which all types of commodities, such as food grains, oilseeds, fibre crops etc., are bought and sold is known as general market. These markets deal in a large number of commodities

Specialized markets

- A market in which transactions take place only in one or two commodities is known as a specialized market. For every group of commodities, separate markets exist. The examples are food grain markets, vegetable markets, wool market and cotton market

g. On the basis of nature of commodities

On the basis of the type of goods dealt in, market may be classified into the following categories:

Commodity markets

A market which deals in goods and raw materials, such as wheat, barley, cotton, fertilizer, seed, etc., are termed as commodity markets. Specific commodities are bought and sold in these markets. These may either be production goods or consumption goods. In such markets, transactions of specialized commodities take place. e.g. Mumbai cotton market, Punjab wheat market etc.

Produce exchange

- Produce exchanges are the big and well organized markets for raw produce like wheat, cotton, jute etc. and are found in cities or developed industrial centres of a country. One exchange deals in one specialized product. Typical examples of such exchanges are the wheat exchange, Cotton exchange and Jute exchange

Manufactured and semi-manufactured goods market

- In these markets, different types of manufactured and semi-manufactured commodities are bought and sold. E.g. Leather goods market, Kanpur.

Bullion market

- Bullion markets are concerned with the purchase and *sale of gold, silverand other precious stones.* These are highly specialized and well organized markets of the world and are localized in civilized as well as industrially developed centres of a country. Ex: Bombay, Calcutta, Delhi and

Capital markets

Capital market is responsible for meeting the financial requirements of big industrial and commercial concerns. Capital is required at every stage of business which comes from the *money market, stock exchange and foreign exchange.*

Money market

- It includes a number of agencies providing finance to business and industrial concerns. Such markets, on one hand, help the people to invest or deposit their surplus funds either in industrial concerns or in banks and on the other, allow those who are in need of money to take loans through banks for a reasonable remuneration in turn by way of interest

Stock exchange market

- In this market, *shares* are purchased and sold in different parts of the country. Ex. BSE, NSE. These markets are highly specialized and command a very wide area of operation. Main purpose of such markets is *to make investments* in public and private sector undertakings.

Foreign exchange market

- It is a market for buying and selling of *foreign currencies*. It can also be called as an international market concerned with the export and import trade of a country. Mumbai, London, New Delhi are examples of such markets

Services market

- Marketing of services like the transport service, communication service, insurance service, various professional services like hospital service etc. take place.

Labour market

- Human resource service like many staff recruitment agencies which will provide human resource or labour to various employers constitute labour market.

h. On the Basis of Stage of Marketing

On the basis of the stage of marketing, markets may be classified into two categories:

Producing markets

- Those markets which mainly *assemble the commodity for further distribution* to other markets are termed as producing markets. Such markets are located in producing areas. Ex. Uthukkuli Butter Market, Rasipuram Ghee Market.

Consuming markets

- Markets which collect the produce for *final disposal to the consuming population* are called consumer markets. Such markets are generally located in areas where production is inadequate, or in thickly populated urban centres.

i. On the basis of extent of public intervention

Based on the extent of public intervention, markets may be placed in any one of the following two classes:

Regulated markets

- In these markets, business is done in accordance with the rules and regulations framed by the statutory market organization representing different sections involved in markets. The marketing costs in such markets are standardized and practices are regulated.

Unregulated markets

- These are the markets in which business is conducted without any set rules and regulations. Traders frame the rules for the conduct of the business and run the market. These markets suffer from many ills, ranging from unstandardised charges for marketing functions to imperfections in the determination of prices.

j. On the basis of type of population served

On the basis of population served by a market, it can be classified as either urban or rural market

Urban market

- A market which serves mainly the population residing in an urban area is called an urban market. Nature and quantum of demand for agricultural products arising from the urban population is characterized as urban market for farm products.

Rural market

- The word rural market usually refers to the demand originating from the rural population. There is considerable difference in the nature of embedded services required with a farm product between urban and rural demands.

On the basis of competition among producers

Perfect market

- In this type of market there are numerous buyers and sellers and all of them have perfect knowledge of demand, supply and prices.

  Imperfect market: This is a market situation where in the element of competition is present but not in a very intensive manner.

a. Monopoly market: This is a market situation where in there is absolutely no competition among sellers thus creating a monopoly situation. It is situation in which there is only one seller and he *determines the price* of the commodity. Thus, price is generally high. Indian farmer operate in monopoly market when purchasing electricity for irrigation. There *will not be close substitutes* for the product being marketed.

b. Monopsony market: When there is one buyer of a product, the market is termed as monopsony market. Sugarcane farmers face a monopsony market situation.

c. Duopoly market:

d. Oligopoly: It is a market where a small number of firms or sellers market a large amount of the product who can affect the price and pricing policies of the other firm. The product material will have no substitute. E.g. Automobile, TV etc

e. Oligopsony: A few numbers of buyers dominate the market. E.g. Tea and Coffee markets

f. Bilateral monopoly: It is the case of single seller and single buyer. E.g. Defence equipments.

g. Monopolistic competition: As the name implies monopolistic competition has characteristics of both perfect competition and monopoly markets. E.g. Oil industry

9

Concepts of Marketing

According to traditional marketing concept, marketing is a mere physical process or set of activities connected with the exchange of goods or selling. According to traditional concept marketing is sales oriented. According to this concept marketing is more concerned with all those activities or operations which help the flow of goods from the producers or manufacturers to the ultimate consumers or users. From the point of production to consumption, the following steps are involved.

1. Goods have to be gathered and transported there by creating **place utility.**
2. Goods have to be made available to the consumers or users at the time when they are needed by consumers. This is done by storing the commodities in warehouses and cold stores etc. This creates **time utility.**
3. Goods are sold to consumers thereby transferring the ownership or title from the seller to the consumer. This creates **"ownership utility"** or "**possession utility".** The various activities that help in the creation of place, time and possession utilities and help the flow of goods from the centers of production to the centers of consumption or use constitute the subject matter of marketing.

Modern marketing concept

Today marketing is not considered as a mere physical process or set of activities connected with the exchange of goods. On the other hand marketing as a philosophy of business connected with the creation of customers by identifying the needs of the consumers and then organising the business accordingly to meet the needs of consumers. Marketing is consumer oriented in the modern marketing concept.

The following are some of the steps involved in the modern marketing concept.

1. Assess the needs of the consumer.
2. Arrange for the procurement of these materials.

3. Move them from their place of production to the place of consumption
4. Move the goods in quantities that are required by the consumers.
5. Movement of the goods must be made in such a way that the goods are available to the consumer at the right time when he needs.
6. The channels of distribution must be convenient.
7. The price also must be such that the consumer is willing to pay.
8. Effect the transfer of ownership and delivery.
9. Make it possible for more and more people to enjoy the products and services.
10. Consumer must be the king in the modern marketing concept which aims at creating a satisfied customer. Actually marketing precedes and succeeds production ie. marketing begins not after the production of goods but before production starts.

Social marketing concept

While traditional market is sales oriented and modern marketing concept is consumer oriented, the social marketing concept aims at long run public welfare as its main motto. To achieve this, the organisation interested in social marketing makes its management oriented towards generating customer satisfaction and public welfare by applying the theories and techniques of modern marketing to find the solution for social issues or problems such as population control, promotion of education, rural development, improvement of the nutritional standards of masses etc. It is the use of marketing as an instrument for satisfying the needs of the society and achieving the satisfaction of the society as a whole.

Popularizing consumption of milk by organisations like AMUL, KMF, etc. and consumption of eggs by NECC are good examples of social marketing. Another classical example is that of large scale distribution of Nirodh condoms as a measure to control of human population in our country.

Social marketing uses marketing as an instrument to achieve social goals by concentrating on the satisfaction of the society rather than the individual. In this concept the success of the business is judged not on the basis of profit the business makes, but on the impact of the business on the society as a whole.

10

Price Determination Under Perfect Competition

Price determination under perfect competition - It can be called as a market structure characterized by a complete absence of competition or rivalry among the individual firms. The sellers and buyers cannot determine the price, only the Industry decides the price of the goods. It means the forces of supply and demand determine the price of the goods

Perfect competition is defined as a market situation where there are a large number of sellers of a homogeneous product. An individual firm supplies a very small portion of the total output and is not powerful enough to exert an influence on the market price. A single buyer, however large, is not in a position to influence the market price.

Demand under perfect competition

Demand refers to the quantity of a product that consumers are willing to purchase at a particular price, while other factors remain constant. A consumer demands more quantity at lower price and less quantity at higher price. Therefore, the demand varies at different prices. Market demand means the sum of the quantity demanded by individual buyers at different prices.

Supply under perfect competition

Supply refers to quantity of a product that producers are willing to supply at a particular price. Generally, the supply of a product increases at high price and decreases at low price. Similarly, market supply is the sum of quantity supplied by the individual firms in the industry. Each seller and buyer takes the price as determined. Therefore, in a perfectly competitive market, the main problem for a profit-maximizing firm is not to determine the price of its product but to adjust its output to the market price so that profit is maximized.

Equilibrium under Perfect Competition

In perfect competition, the price of a product is determined at a point at which the demand and supply curve intersect each other. This point is known as equilibrium point. At this point, the quantity demanded and supplied is called equilibrium quantity.

Price determination under perfect competition is analyzed under three different time periods

(a) Market Period

(b) Short Run

(c) Long Run

(a) Market period

In a market period, the time span is so short that no firm can increase its output. The total stock of the commodity in the market is limited. The market period may be an hour, a day or a few days or even a few weeks depending upon the nature of the product. For example, in the case of perishable commodities like milk, vegetables, fish, eggs, the period may be a day. Since the supply of perishable commodities is limited by the quantity available or stock in day that neither can be increased nor can be withdrawn for the next period, the whole of it must be sold away on the same day, whatever may be the price.

(b) Pricing in the short run- equilibrium of the firm

Short period is the span of time so short that existing plants cannot be extended and new plants cannot be erected to meet increased demand. However, the time is adequate enough for producers to adjust to some extent their output to the increase in demand by overworking their fixed capacity plants. In the short run, therefore, supply curve is elastic.

The following figure explaining the price determination in short run under perfect competition. At price P, the MC = MR = AR and the MC curve cut the MR curve from below. Therefore at this price each firm is in equilibrium and producing OQ level of output and earning normal profit. If the price is higher ie. At P_1, the firm earns supernormal profit (Since Price is more than ATC) and the output level is Q_1. If the price falls below P (at P_2), the firm incur a loss as the average total cost of production is higher than the price. In short run, the firm at P_2 price, level produce only Q_2 level of output and incur loss. When supernormal profit exists (at price P_1 level), many firms enter into the market and at loss conditions (at price P_2 level), many firms goes out of the business and thus finally the equilibrium attained at normal profit (at price P level).

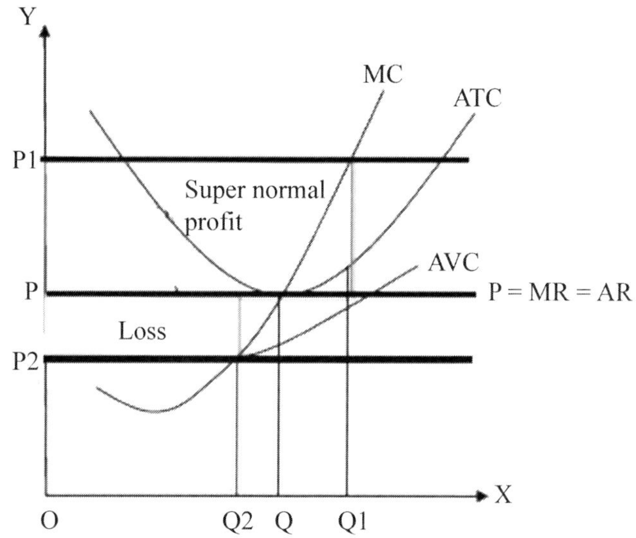

Pricing in the long run

The long run is a period of time long enough to permit changes in the variable as well as in the fixed factors. Thus, in the long run, firms can change their output by increasing their fixed equipment. They can enlarge the old units or replace them by new units or add new units or new units can also enter the industry

Thus, the long run equilibrium will refer to a situation where free and full scope for adjustment has been allowed to economic forces. In the long run, it is the long run average and marginal cost curves, which are relevant for making output decisions. Further, in the long run, average variable cost is of no particular relevance. The average total cost is of determining importance, since in the long run all costs are variable and none fixed.

At short run, firms might gain super normal profit at P_1 price level initially. However, at long run, due to profitability, many firms enter the market which results in increase in supply and with same level of demand. As the result, price will be decreased to P. Thus at long run, all firms will attain equilibrium, where MR=AR=LMC=LAC–SMC=SAC=Price

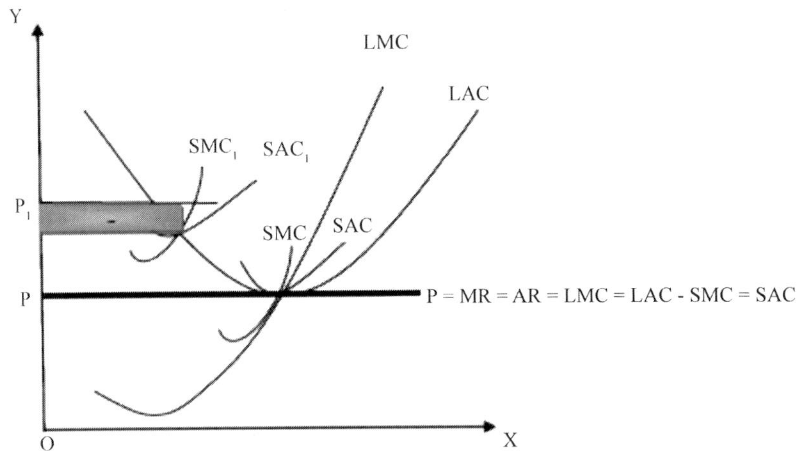

LMC-Long run Marginal Cost
LAC - Long run Average Cost
P - Price
AR - Average Revenue
SMC - Short run Marginal Cost
SAC - Short run Average Cost
MR - Marginal Revenue

Thus, the conditions for long run equilibrium of perfectly competitive firm can be written as: Price = Marginal Cost = Minimum Average Cost.

Market price: The market price is the price at which a certain commodity is transacted at a particular time and place. There are variations in the market price of a commodity even during the course of a day in a market. Hence, it is also termed as the *short-period price*. The factors which influence this price are the level of arrivals of a commodity on a particular day, sudden change in weather, and other related factors.

Normal price: The normal price is an average price telescoped over a period of time, say a season, year or several years. Since the normal price is some sort of an average price it *does not refer to a particular time, place or quality of the commodity*.

11

Marketing Functions

Marketing functions

The process of marketing involve a number of marketing functions. They may be grouped under:

Functions of exchange which include

1) Buying and assembling and
2) Selling.

B. Functions of physical supply which include

1) Transportation and
2) Storage or warehousing.

C. Functions of facilitation which include –

1) Standardization and grading
2) Financing
3) Risk bearing
4) Market information and intelligence.

Functions of exchange

Buying and assembling: Buying refers to buying of goods by manufacturers, middlemen or retailers for resale and not buying of goods by consumers for consumption. Important feature here is that the buying must be at the right time, in right quantity, of right quality, at the right price, from right place or source. Manufacturer buys raw materials. Wholesalers buys ready goods from manufactures. Retailer buys goods from wholesalers. "Goods well bought are half sold" is proverb often talked about in trading circles.

Buying involves several steps. They are

1. Decision regarding the type, quality, quantity, time, source, mode of purchase etc.
2. Preparation of list of goods to be purchased.
3. Selection of suppliers.
4. Negotiations with the supplier regarding term of sale, mode of delivery, terms of payments, concessions if any etc.
5. Placing of purchase orders with the suppliers.
6. Following up of the purchase order to expedite the prompt delivery of the goods ordered.
7. Receipt of goods.
8. Inspection and approval of goods and making of payments for the purchase.

Assembling: The term assembling is used in two different contexts. Assembling refers to bringing individual parts or components of an equipment or a product and joining them together to produce a finished product. However in marketing terminology assembling refers to the process of actually gathering goods which are produced from multiple producers or sources into one central point or place under the control of buyer. This kind of assembling facilitates transport of goods in bulk, ensures continuous supply and reduces transport cost. Assembling helps in the following aspects:

a) Proper handling of products.

b) Storage is made possible in a central point. Storage includes cold storage.

c) Facilitates standardizing and grading.

d) Helps in widening the market.

e) Easy to raise finance by the trader as he can show the bulk material as a source of security to the financing bodies.

f) Manufacturer is relieved of botheration of shortage of raw material.

g) Large or bulk orders can be undertaken by the manufacturer or wholesalers.

Sub-functions of buying

a) Planning of purchase

b) Contactual function

c) Negotiation

d) Contractual function

Planning for purchase

1. Preparation of purchase budget is made based on anticipated volume of sales.
2. Determination of rate of stock turnover.
3. Accounting for changes in fashion, style, taste etc.
4. Accounting for price changes.

a-1. Every year purchase budget is made based on the anticipated or

or expected volume of sales.

a-2. Stock turn over rate: It is the number of times the average inventory or stock that is sold and replaced during a certain period- usually one year.

$$\text{Average inventory} = \frac{\text{Opening stock} + \text{closing stock}}{2}$$

$$\text{Rate of stock turn over} = \frac{\text{Cost of goods sold}}{\text{Average inventory}}$$

Example

Find the stock turnover rate from the following data of a trader dealing with egg trade.

Value of the opening stocks of eggs = Rs. 28,000

Value of the purchases made during the year = Rs. 1,44,000

Value of the closing stock = Rs. 12,000

$$\text{Average inventory} = \frac{\text{Opening stock} + \text{closing stock}}{2}$$

$$= \frac{28{,}000 + 12{,}000}{2} = \frac{40{,}000}{2} = 20{,}000$$

Cost of goods sold =	Opening stock at cost	= Rs. 28,000
	Purchases during the year	= Rs. 1,44,000
		Rs. 1,72,000
	Less closing stock at cost	= Rs. 12,000
	Cost of goods sold	= Rs. 1,60,000

$$\text{Rate of stock turn over} = \frac{\text{Cost of goods sold}}{\text{Average inventory}}$$

$$= \frac{1,60,000}{20,000} = 8$$

Rate of stock of turn over = 8 times.

Purpose of calculating rate of stock turn over is to find out how fast the commodities are moving or how slow they are moving. It reflects on the buying, stocking and selling of goods. Trader plans his buying depending on the fastness or slowness of the stock turn over.

a-3. Accounting for changes in fashion, style, taste etc.

Sudden change in fashion, style, taste etc. will lead to loss in business as the goods in stock may become outdated and goods will be left unsold. To reduce such risks trader has to have sufficient knowledge and vision about the possibility of such changes in fashion, style, taste etc. and plan his buying of the stock accordingly.

a-4. Considerations for effects of change in price

Sudden increase or decrease in price also affects the success of the business. If increase in price is anticipated the trader must go for "forward buying" or buying more quantity of goods than immediately required. If on the other hand sudden decrease in price is anticipated trader must go in for what is called "hand to mouth buying", i.e. buying goods only as much minimal as possible.

b. Contactual function

This refers to the process of searching and determining the sources of supply and maintaining contact with them. In deciding the sources of supply care must be taken to select such suppliers who ensure supply of goods of good quality, charge reasonable price, supply regularly, make timely supply of goods, give better terms like rate of discount, period of credit etc.

Negotiation

It refers to discussion of exchange of ideas that take place between buyers and suppliers regarding terms of purchase, quantity to be bought etc.

d. Contractual function

It refers to actual entering into contract between buyer and supplier to buy and sell goods to effect the transfer of title and delivery of goods. The official order placed by the buyer is binding on both buyer and supplier. If there is any breach in contract the aggrieved party can seek justice in the court of law.

Buying methods

- Concentrated buying- Buying from a single source or very few suppliers.
- Diversified buying - Buying from large number of sources.
- Reciprocal buying.
- Hand to mouth buying.
- Forward buying.
- Speculative buying.

Selling

Selling is the process by which the ownership of the goods and services is transferred from the seller to buyer on terms mutually agreed by the seller and buyer. It also involves not just the transfer of ownership but also actual physical transfer of materials etc. from the seller to buyer and the buyer in turn making payments to the seller on terms agreed mutually.

Sub functions of selling include many decisions with respect to:

a) Proper units of sales

b) Proper package

c) Quantity packed in such a way to cater to different economic sections of consumers.

d) Choosing best marketing channel

e) Proper time and place to approach potential buyers.

f) Making proper advertisement and engaging in many sales promotional activities like announcing discount, incentives etc.

g) Extending post sale services.

Functions of physical supply

a. Transportation: Transportation is a very important marketing function which creates place utility. As livestock products are highly perishable it is imperative that these products have to be transported as quickly as possible from the place of production to the place of processing or consumption. For example fluid milk has to be transported from the procurement center which is usually situated at the village level to a district level processing center. Such transportation may be effected through road, rail or air transport. Often these transport modes are equipped with refrigeration and cold storage facilities to prevent spoilage during transit. Transportation is necessary for providing goods to the consumers in time and also to explore marketing opportunities in far away places.

b. Storage or Warehousing: The term storage or warehousing refers to keeping or holding a product and preserving it for some time. Storage creates time utility. The following are some of the reasons why storage is done.

   - It enhances keeping quality or shelf life of the product particularly appreciable in the case of perishable products like milk, meat, eggs etc.
   - It makes the various products available during all the seasons or for an extended period with in the same season.
   - Storage enhances the quality of certain products like in the case of rice, timber etc. Storage is accomplished by chemical methods or through refrigeration etc.

Facilitating functions

Standardisation and grading: Marketing is accomplished in a better way and in more profitable lines when the products are subjected to certain standards and separation of lots is done on the basis of set standards. This will help in fixing price on what standard the product has.

The term standardisation refers to the process of fixing various qualities or characters to which a particular product should conform. The standardisation is usually done on the basis of weight, colour, consistency, odour; percentage of fat, percentage of solids not fat etc. For example milk has its standards fixed on the basis of percentage of fat and percentage of solids not fat. Karnataka milk federation's most commonly sold fluid milk has 3.5 % fat and 8.5 % SNF. Similarly eggs are standardised on the basis of weight of the eggs. Wool standards are fixed on the basis of colour, fineness, length and curliness or crimp of wool fibre.

Grading refers to the process of separating the products based on the fixed standards. For example poultry eggs weighing 60 grams and above, 53-59 grams, 45-52 grams and 38-44 grams are graded as extra large, large, medium and small eggs respectively.

Financing

It is the process of raising the capital and using the same for carrying out various activities involved in marketing. Finance can be raised as owned capital or borrowed capital. Owned capital as using one's own capital or raising it through shares. Borrowed capital may be through loans from financial institutions or through issue of debentures to public.

Risk bearing

Persons carrying out business, have to bear the risk when ever losses occur. These losses occur due to various reasons. It may be due to sudden fall in the prices or due to destruction of products by way of accidents involving fire, natural calamities like floods, hurricanes, heavy rains etc. Fall in price and changes in consumer demands are called 'market risks' and risks occurring due to natural calamities like rain, flood, fire etc. are called 'physical risks'. Physical risks may also arise due to thefts. Physical risks are covered through goods insurance offered by insurance companies. Market risks may be minimised by intelligent forecasting based on market information, intelligence and wide experience.

Market intelligence

This is the job of collecting, interpreting and disseminating a variety of data necessary for the smooth operation of the marketing process.

Minimization of risks (Speculation and Hedging)

Risk management

Risk management is the process of identifying, assessing and controlling threats to any firms capital and earnings. These threats, or risks, could stem from a wide variety of sources, including financial uncertainty, legal liabilities, strategic management errors, accidents and natural disasters. As a result, a risk management plan increasingly includes companies' processes for identifying and controlling threats to its digital assets, including data, a customer's personally identifiable information and intellectual property. Every business and organization faces the risk of unexpected, harmful events that can cost the company's money or cause it to permanently close. Risk management allows firms to attempt to prepare for the unexpected by minimizing risks and extra costs before they happen.

In the world of finance, risk management refers to the practice of identifying potential risks in advance, analyzing them and taking precautionary steps to reduce/curb the risk. When an entity makes an investment decision, it exposes itself to a number of financial risks. The quantum of such risks depends on the type of financial instrument. These financial risks might be in the form of high inflation, volatility in capital markets, recession, bankruptcy, etc.

So, in order to minimize and control the exposure of investment to such risks, fund managers and investors practice risk management. Not giving due importance to risk management while making investment decisions might wreak havoc on investment in times of financial turmoil in an economy. Different levels of risk come attached with different categories of asset classes.

Marketing risk is the potential for losses and failures of marketing. This includes risks related to pricing, product development, promotion, distribution, branding, customer experience and sales.

Hedging and speculation

Hedging is often confused with speculation. In both cases operators are concerned with unforeseen price changes. They make buying and selling decisions based on their expectations of how the market will move in the future. However, where hedging is essentially a means to avoid or reduce price risk, speculation relies on the risk element. For instance, it would be irrational to carry out a selling hedge if the market were absolutely certain to rise. In the absence of absolute certainty about future market movements, hedging offers an element of protection against price risk, whereas speculation involves deliberately taking a risk on price movements, up or down, in the hope of obtaining a profit.

Speculators are typically sophisticated risk-taking individuals with expertise in the markets in which they are trading and **Hedgers** are individuals who participate in purchasing investments to hedge against one another to obtain the maximum level or profit security price movements. A person who gives an indirect response. One of the principles of speculation involves the opportunity for gain that the investor achieves by agreeing to accept some of the risk passed off by the hedger. In other words, the hedger gives up some opportunity in exchange for reduced risk. The speculator on the other hand acquires opportunity in exchange for taking on risk.

Buyers and sellers of coffee who aim to minimize their price risks in the physical market assume opposite positions, or risks, in the futures market. At any moment there will be a number of buying and a number of selling hedge operations. However, it is unlikely that demand for hedges against buying risks will exactly balance demand for hedges against selling risks. The resulting surplus of buying and selling risks that has not been covered by the usual hedgers is taken up by speculators.

To absorb the vast amounts of futures entering the coffee exchanges, numerous speculators willing to buy one or two lots are required. Likewise, considerable purchasing pressure occurs when traders or roasters hedge to cover their future needs. Prices would increase unless speculators were willing to step in as sellers.

If producers who wish to hedge could always find counterparts who also wished to do so, there would be no need for speculators. However, this situation is unlikely to occur regularly, partly because the periods in which producers carry out hedging operations normally do not coincide with the periods in which consumers try to hedge. The speculator provides the link between these two different periods and interests.

Hedging of livestock

Hedging is one of the marketing tools livestock producers can use to forward price their livestock. Hedging protects against adverse price changes.

Two types of hedgers

There are basically two types of hedgers, one to protect against a price decline (short hedge) and the other to protect against a price rise (long hedge).

This publication will be devoted mainly to discussing short hedges.

• Short hedge

Short hedgers are producers who have livestock that they plan to market in the future but want to protect themselves against potential price declines. Producers become short hedgers if they sell a futures contract (futures contracts that are applicable to the type of livestock they plan to market). A futures contract is a legal agreement to buy or sell a particular commodity asset, or security at a predetermined price at a specified time in the future. Futures contracts are standardized for quality and quantity to facilitate trading on a futures exchange.

- **Long hedge**

Long hedgers are just the opposite of short hedgers. Long hedgers need a product at some future date, do not want to purchase the cash product now, but want to protect themselves against a price rise. Producers become long hedgers if they buy a futures contract (futures contract applicable to the type of feed or feeder livestock they plan to purchase).

An example of a long hedger would be a cattle rearer, planning to buy cattle feed for upcoming three months but wanting to establish a price and protect against a price rise during the next three months. This hedger would buy cattle feed futures to protect against a cash price rise.

Another example of a long hedge by a livestock producer would be buying corn futures to establish a price for corn and protect against a price rise.

Options strategies

If a livestock hedger would like protection against adverse price movements while benefitting from market moves, options provide protection and flexibility.

There are two basic options strategies that a livestock hedger could use.

1. A buyer could have a call option that allows a buyer to establish a maximum or ceiling price for the animals he is buying, while still being able to take advantage of lower prices in the cash market if by any case the opportunity arises.
2. A seller, on the other hand, would have a put option, that allows a livestock seller to establish a minimum or floor price for the stock or meat products he is selling, while still being able to take advantage of higher prices in the cash market, if by any case the opportunities arise.

Speculation

A speculator in the live **cattle** market is an individual who trades the commodities markets with the objective of achieving profits through the successful anticipation of price movements. Speculators are willing to take large risks in the hopes of making quick, large gains. The speculator has no interest in taking delivery of the physical product.

For both livestock buyers and livestock sellers, the following are keys to successful risk management.

1. **Develop a team:** When it comes to risk management, a team approach may work best. This applies to individual operations, family operations or corporate entities. Family or corporate operations may find it easier to

follow this key to success, but an individual can also develop a team by working with friends or family in similar situations.

2. **Consult with advisors:** Advisors may be especially helpful when a livestock hedger is first getting started in the futures and options markets. There are different types of advisors that charge different fees. These include commodity brokers, commodity consultants, universities and state livestock marketing specialists. If a hedger feels they do not have the time or expertise to devote to the important function of risk management, they should feel comfortable getting professional assistance and guidance from those who specialize in this field.
3. **Learn the alternatives**: Whether or not the hedger consults with an advisor, they should learn about all the alternatives for managing the risk associated with purchasing or selling livestock. Even when consulting with an advisor, the hedger should make the final decisions as it is their business that is at risk.
4. **Develop a hedging policy:** A hedging policy could range from a very basic set of rules for the individual or family livestock operation, to a complex legal document for a corporate hedging operation. Regardless, it may be important to have some form of written document to keep decisions within a specific set of trading rules.
5. **Develop a plan:** Whereas a hedging policy is more or less a permanent document with general rules of trading, a plan pertains to a specific time period or for a specific livestock sale or purchase that may occur in the near future. A written plan will help the livestock hedger stick to their risk management goals and objectives. It will include decisions such as which risk management tool to use, pricing objectives and timing. A livestock hedger can develop a different plan for each year, or for each individual purchase or sale due to different market conditions, such as price levels and market volatility.
6. **Get management buy-in**: Management approval comes in different forms depending on the size of the operation. It can range from a simple nod of acceptance by a spouse or other family member, to a signed legal approval on a formal corporate plan. Regardless, if there are others that are impacted by the decisions, they should at least be aware of the risk management plans and sign off on them at some level. Especially with larger livestock operations, it is important that others in management are comfortable with the objectives and the plan to achieve them.

7. **Have the discipline to stay with the plan, but flexibility to adjust**: Depending on changes in the market environment during the course of a hedging plan, this key may require a difficult combination of discipline and flexibility. If there are minor changes in market conditions that appear to be moving against the hedger, he needs discipline to stick with the plan. However, on occasion, due to major unexpected market conditions, it may be appropriate to make adjustments to the initial plan. One of the worse things a hedger can do is to make continuous changes in the plan for every little market hiccup. This could lead to a negative situation called being "whipsawed."
8. **Keep good records:** Record keeping is an often overlooked task requiring a minimal amount of time, but it is essential to good risk management for livestock buyers and sellers. It could be as simple as keeping records on paper, to more advanced computer spreadsheets. Hedgers should keep track of the futures and cash market prices, as well as their local basis. Additionally, they must keep track of the risk management strategies used and the resulting profits and losses. Good records will assist in tax preparation and future risk management plans.
9. **Review the results:** A thorough analysis of the risk management strategies and overall plan is necessary to determine what worked, what didn't work and most importantly, why? Similar to keeping good records, reviewing results—both positive and negative—will help a livestock buyer or seller become a more effective hedger in the future.
10. **Don't look back**: Simply stated, this means to learn from past experiences and realize not all experiences are going to be positive, but not become fixated on the negative. A livestock hedger may actually learn more from a negative experience than a positive one. However, the successful livestock hedger will use past experiences to move forward in a positive manner.

Creation of utilities in marketing process

Making is the process of making a commodity useful, by converting raw material or the goods into a form suitable for consumption, putting it into a place where it can be used, making it ready for use at the right time and placing it in the possession of those who need it. i.e. Marketing is nothing but the creation of utilities. Utilities that are created in the marketing process are Form utility, Time utility, Place utility and Possession utility

1. ***Form utility***: Form utility is added when the processor of the goods (such as milk, paddy and oilseeds) transforms the material into finished

products ready for consumption (such as cheese, rice and edible oil respectively). In doing so, he adds form utility to the raw products, i.e. form utility is created by the processing functions.

2. ***Time utility***: The utility is added when products are stored from the time of production to the time of consumption. Time utility is created by the operations like storage in warehouses and godowns.
3. ***Place utility***: Place utility is added by the transporting system which transfers the gods from one point where it is not needed to another point where it is consumed. Hence, transporting agencies contribute to place utility.
4. ***Possession utility***: Possession utility is added to the product when its ownership is transferred to the final consumer. Thus, all the institutions and agents in the marketing chain which enable transfer of ownership are contributing to possession utility.

12

Market Information

Market information

As defined by Philip Kotler, Marketing information system is continuing & interacting structure of people, equipment & procedure designed to gather, sort, analyze, evaluate, distribute pertinent, timely and accurate information for use by marketing decision makers, to improve their marketing planning, execution and control.

It is the job of collecting, interpreting and disseminating large variety of data which are needed for the smooth operation of marketing processes. In many countries Government agencies undertake this function and sometimes organisations such as chambers of commerce, board of traders etc. perform this function. The Directorate of Economics and Statistics and concerned state marketing departments collect data regarding a) quantity of various products produced in different areas, b) quantities of products held in storage, c) arrivals in various markets, d) prices prevailing in local, regional, national and international markets. The informative data so collected is disseminated through radio, television, news papers, weekly and monthly bulletins. Daily prices are published in most of the news papers. The informative marketing data is also collected through sales executives and from those personnel who are specially appointed as specialists by various trading firms.

In the field of marketing, information is of great importance. Like men, money, machines and materials, information is also a vital input.

Three type of information come out of the systems are

- Recurrent information
- Monitored information
- Requested information

Sources of marketing information

Executive experience: It is the direct counter part of the casual experience that we accumulate from the process of everybody living.

Internal reports: Come from the authorities who work as specialists for the firms.

Marketing research: Studies are conducted using methods of enquiry, observation and experimentation and by using available internal reports.

Marketing models: At a general level, sources may include for example, daily news papers, technical journals, hand books, and reference materials, government publication, corporation annual reports and computer data bases.

Marketing information system (MKIS or MIS)

MKIS should perform the following six functions.

- Assembly -Searching and gathering marketing data
- Processing - Editing , tabulating and summarizing data
- Analysis - Computation (percentages and ratios), combining sales and costs data and other mathematical tasks
- Storage and retrieval - Indexing, filing and locating data
- Evaluation - Determining the accuracy of information
- Dissemination - Routing useful information to appropriate decision makers.

Marketing intelligence: A marketing intelligence system is a set of procedures and sources used by managers to obtain their everyday information about pertinent developments in marketing environment. It is a product of market research and marketing research. In marketing intelligence, marketing managers scan the environment in four ways.

- Undirected viewing
- Conditioned viewing
- Informal search
- Formal search

Marketing managers carry on marketing intelligence mostly on their own by reading books, news papers and trade publications, talking to customers, suppliers and other outsiders and talking with other managers, personals within the company.

Well recognized companies take additional step to improve the quality and quantity of marketing intelligence. First they train and motivate the 'sales force' to spot and report new development. Sales representatives are company's "eyes and ears". They are in an excellent position to pick up information missed by other means. The company must sell its sales force on their importance as intelligence gatherers. The sales force should be provided with easy reports to fill out. Sales representatives should know which type of information to be sent to different manager. Secondly, the company motivates distributors, retailers and other middlemen to pass along important intelligence.

The decision makers in the trading circles make their decisions mostly based on vast data available through direct sources like radio, TV, daily newspapers and other media. But quite often this kind of information is not adequate to make certain intelligent decisions which will have direct bearing on the marketing processes. In such cases the various persons like trade executives, market managers etc. will have to formulate their opinions by scanning through informative data and on the information collected through marketing research. Marketing research is done at industry, retailer and as consumer level to explore the acceptability of the products at various levels. The following are some of the aspects that are explored through such research. They include finding answers to potential market to the products, finding information on product acceptability, brand information, storage life, stock build up, volume of retail sales, finding information on the consumer behaviour etc. It may be concluded that market intelligence is a process of formulating an intelligent marketing strategy based on the vast executive experience, available market information and marketing research.

Marketing opportunities: Every producer or a trader ultimately aims at marketing his product to earn good profits. For profitable marketing to happen there has to be enough environment, consumer base, efficient distribution system, willingness of the consumer to spend for a certain product, encouragement by the state and central governments enough per capita income etc. All these activities which create a potential for profitable marketing constitute marketing opportunities. In this context one can say countries, which have high per capita income like USA, Canada, England etc. have a bigger consumer base. Of late India and China have emerged as the consumer giants and together they may provide one of the biggest marketing opportunities in the world. This is particularly so as these countries once looked down as poor countries are now emerging as consumer giants because of increasing per capita income.

Companies must look internally for strength and weakness and externally to the environment for opportunities and threats. Most opportunities and threats evolves from

- Changes in the demographic, economic, political, legal and cultural environment.
- Change in the competitive environment, such as a technological break through by a computer.
- Events that may or may not be under the company's control such as strike by the work force or a serious fire in an industrial plant.

Finding and evaluating marketing opportunities

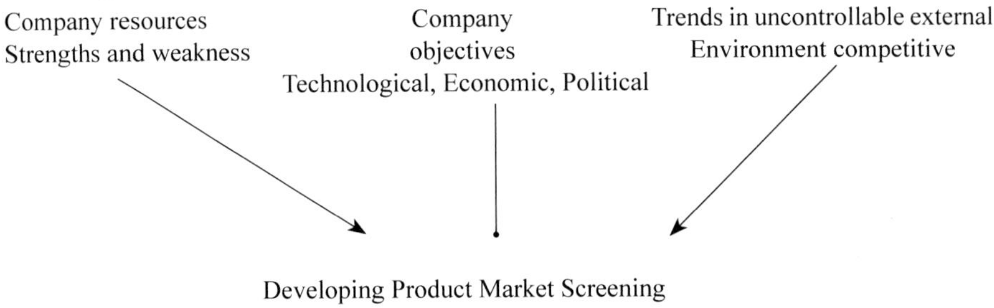

New market opportunities are determined by discovering customer groups with unmet needs. The new market opportunities arise for a variety of reasons in industrialized societies. One is geographical mobility. People live where they did not live before and thus create new markets. The aggressive business firms recognize these new markets and builds new super markets, new discount houses etc. Another source of new market is social mobility. As people become more educated and acquire more sophisticated social environment their interest change frequently resulting in markets for new products.

Yet another cause of new market is psychic mobility, when people change the conception of themselves and their environment along with physical and social mobility.

Indian market is endowed with a traditional yet efficient distribution system spread over the whole of the country down to village level. This system has wholesalers, semi wholesalers, retailers, selling agents, commission agents and brokers. India has one of the best economical distribution system in the world. There is both public distribution system and private distribution system for channelising various commodities to consumers. The ownership of public distribution system is vested with co-operatives, state and central governments, whereas the ownership of private distribution system is vested with private individuals and companies. Now there is good competition between public and private distribution systems, which has resulted in the consumer getting the commodities and services at an advantageous price and quality. The public distribution system particularly takes care of the economically weaker section of the society by giving them certain essential commodities at subsidised rates, thus fulfilling the obligation of social justice. But by and large one can say that in India now exists a free market as most of the restrictions on trading various commodities have been removed due to the government's policy of liberalisation, globalisation and privatisation.

While there is great opportunity for the Indian trader to move the markets in the Indian urban areas, the rural market also has tremendous opportunity. With the advent of TV, Radio and other media entering every nook and corner of the village and with that the advertisements reaching the vast population of the country a wide market for consumer products has been created.

Increase or decrease in marketing opportunities are created due to:

1. changes in population, fluctuations in income of consumers, policy variations of governments, constitutional provisions and cultural practices of a particular area or a country.
2. uncontrolled factors like prolonged strike by factories, accidents in production units, natural calamities etc.
3. geographical mobility of people from one country to another will create new marketing opportunities.
4. life style changes adopted by people as and when their economic and educational standards improve also create new marketing opportunities.

Consumer behaviour

It is defined as "the process where by individuals decide whether, what, when, where, how much and from whom to purchase goods and services".

For successful business an understanding of the consumer needs is the focal point. Hence it becomes inevitable for the business concerns to know the consumer and his behaviour towards buying to understand how buying decisions are taken. It is essential to understand the needs, aspirations, expectations and problems of consumers.

The whole behaviour which ultimately motivates a person to decide to buy something is the consumer behaviour. Consumer behaviour involves both physical and mental activities. Consumer behaviour includes the end user of the products and also the intermediate industrial user who adds further value to a product.

The determinants of consumer behaviour fall under: (A) economic, (B) psychological and (C) sociological factors.

A) The economic determinants include (i) personal income, (ii) family income, (iii) consumer liquid assets, (iv) credit availability to consumer and (v) his living standard.

Personal income referred above is mainly the disposable personal income (DPI) that is available to a consumer for spending in the form of savings after having met the essential spending on food, shelter, clothing and also having payment of taxes, repayment of loans etc. But discretionary personal income (DSPI) refers to that income remaining after having met the expenses on food, shelter and clothing but using the discretion to postpone other expenditure like repayment of loan installments etc.

B) Psychological determinants

i) Knowledge leading to habit. For example the knowledge of the benefits of eating egg a day or drinking a cup of milk a day may lead a person to cultivate the same as a habit.

ii) Motivational forces like desire for security, desire for recognition, desire for affection, adventure or innovation also influence the consumer behaviour.

iii) Sub conscious desires often get surfaced when externally stimulated by an advertisement or recommendation of a product by a friend, neighbour etc.

iv) Mental attitude of a person, differences in personality traits, differences in individual perception influence the consumer behaviour.

C) Sociological aspects that influence the consumer behaviour include

- cultural and traditional practices in a family,
- influence of opinions expressed by reference groups in a society,
- social class and
- caste, religion of the people.

Consumer demand

The term consumer demand refers to the effective desire for a commodity, backed by adequate purchasing power, willingness to invest this purchasing power on the commodity at a particular place, at a particular price in a particular marketing environment by a particular consumer.

Market demand

It is the sum total of the individual demands of all the consumers put together for a particular product, at a particular time, place and at particular price and at varying prices in a market.

Market stagnation

Sometimes during a year there will be periods of reduced economic activity due to various reasons including lack of adequate purchasing power of the consumers. This results in reduction in demand for goods and reduction in production of goods. This in turn reduces demand for labourers and hence their wage rates also. This kind of environment where in there is decline in all aspects of marketing activities is considered as market stagnation.

Market measurement and forecasting

For the business to run on profitable lines the business person must have a fairly clear cut estimate of the current demand for a particular product or service in a given area. In the absence of a realistic estimate for demand the business person may put to hardship because of investments made on huge stocks which may be left unsold. Further under stocking of goods may lead to missing of business opportunities when the demand is higher than the actual stock with the trader. Hence the trader has to undertake market measurement by going through various marketing informative data and also by the past sales experience. He has to estimate the total market demand and also the demand for the product in different areas of the market. The latter helps in selecting a most suitable area where the marketing for a particular product or service can be promoted more aggressively to get higher profit in a shorter time.

Market forecasting is the method of estimating sales volume of a product that a company can expect in a particular future date say in a year or during next 4-5 years. As it is only an estimate it is likely to vary from the actual sales recorded during the forecasting period. This is to be expected as many extraneous unknown factors do operate in influencing sales. This forecasting of sales will enable the producer to plan for the volume of production so as to effect proper sales of the same. Some of the methods by which sales are forecasted are the following:

a) From executive opinion: Executives responsible for company's sales are requested to prepare an estimate of the probable levels of sales on the basis of their experience, market knowledge and other factors.

b) Opinion of company's salesmen and intermediaries who are working at the grass root level are requested to estimate their requirement for the estimating period in respect of the products, territories and customers handled by them.

c) Through market survey: This is done by conducting actual market survey by the company's personnel or by a surveying agency and an estimate of the requirement of the product is arrived at based on the survey findings.

d) On the basis of sales recorded during the previous years.

e) Statistical methods: By using statistical methods it is possible to forecast the market by taking into account the long range trends, cyclical changes, seasonal variations and irregular fluctuations, all based on the previous years sales.

In this there are three different aspects - total market demand, area market demand, and actual sales and market shares.

Estimating total market demand

The total market demand for a product or services is the total volume that would be bought by a defined consumer group in a defined geographic area in a defined time period in a defined marketing environment. Total market is not a fixed number, but a function of the stated conditions.

$Q = n \times q \times p$

Q = Total market demand

n = number of buyers in the market

q = quantity purchased by an average buyer per year

p = price of an average product

Estimating area market demand

Companies face the problem of selecting the best sales territories and allocating their marketing budget optimally among these territories. Therefore, they need to estimate the market potential of different cities, states and countries. Two major methods are available; the market - buildup method, which is used primarily by business goods firms, and the market- factor index method, which is used primarily by consumer goods firms.

Estimating actual sales and market shares

Besides estimating total land area demand, a company will want to know the actual industry sales in its market. Thus, it must identify its competitors and estimate their sales. Another way to estimate sales is to buy reports from marketing research firms that audit total sales and brand sales.

Forecasting future demand

Forecasting is the art of estimating future demand by anticipating what buyers are likely to do under a given set of future conditions. Good forecasting becomes a key factor in company success. Poor forecasting can lead to overly large inventories, costly price mark downs, or lost sales due to items being out of stock. The more unstable the demand, the more the company needs accurate and elaborate forecasting procedures.

Companies commonly use a three- stage procedure to arrive at a sales forecast. First they make an environmental forecast, followed by an industry forecast and followed by a company sales forecast. Companies use several specific techniques to forecast their sales.

All forecasts are built on one of three information bases: what people say, what people do, or what people have done.

13

Marketing of Livestock Products and Defects in Livestock Marketing

Marketing of perishable and non perishable products

Agriculture and livestock products like food grains, vegetables, meat, eggs etc. are highly perishable over time. Under ambient conditions they get spoiled with in a few hours, days or months as the case may be. Livestock products particularly milk is perishable within a few hours if not preserved under refrigeration. Same is the case of meat. Eggs also get spoiled within a few days if not preserved under cold storage. Because of these reasons perishable products pose special marketing problems. Unfortunately in a country like India most of the agriculture and livestock products are produced by large number of small producers and the process of marketing is to a large extent is in the unorganised sector. Fortunately in our country a number of states like Karnataka, Tamilnadu, Maharastra, Gujarath and others, milk is marketed through cooperatives. For example in Karnataka, milk is procured by primary milk producers' cooperative societies, transported, processed and marketed through milk unions located at district level and coordinated at state level by state milk federation that is Karnataka Milk Federation(KMF). Some states also have slightly different marketing organisation for egg marketing also. In the unorganised sector these products go through wholesalers, semi wholesalers, private vendors, retailers and ultimately reach the consumers.

In the case of non perishable goods like TV sets, refrigerators, mixers, grinders and other home appliances there is sufficient time available from the time of production to the time it is used by the ultimate consumer. Mostly these come under industrial products and they go through the producers, wholesalers, semi wholesalers, retailers before they are sold to the ultimate consumer. The manufacturer also gives sufficient guarantee or warranty of the products sold in the case of manufactured non perishable goods.

Defects in livestock marketing

1. **Lack of producer's organization**: The farming community is more or less disorganized at the village level. Except for a few, till now no such organization has developed which may prove a sound basis for strengthening the bargaining power of the farmers. An individual deals in his own product, he sells his surplus produce in the village or at the primary market level with his low bargaining power and hence, he is always at a disadvantage against the organized trading community.

2. Some products particularly eggs are highly fragile.

3. **Forced sale**: In a country like India, majority of subsistence producers are compelled to sell their produce immediately after harvest in order to meet the pressing claims of their lenders even if the prices are not remunerative. Most producers sell their product , repay debts, face a shortage, and fall in debt again . Thus they sell to repay debt only to fall in debt again. Most livestock products are bulky compared to their value and they occupy more space necessitating large marketing space.

4. **Superfluous middlemen:** Since the farmer sells a substantial portion of his surplus produce in the village and nearby markets , there is always intervention of a number of middlemen between him and the consumer and naturally share of the consumer's price received by the producer is reduced.

5. **Malpractices in the market**: Malpractice arise on account of multiplicity of market charges, spurious deductions, unfair weighment and undesirable mode of sale. Weight and scales are manipulated against the seller. There are all kinds of arbitrary deductions for religious and charitable purpose. The burden falls entirely on the seller and he has no effective means to protect himself against such practices. Some quantity is taken away from the producer's produce as sample. This varies from produce to produce. The producers are not paid for this even when no sales are affected.

6. **Absence of grading and standardization and inadequate storage facilities**: Many state governments have not so far prescribed grades and standards for many livestock products. A good number of farmers have little knowledge of grading their produce and usually mix up good and bad quality product into a single lot which secures them a lower price for their produce in the market. There is general inadequacy of good storage facilities both in urban as well as in rural areas. The indigenous methods of storage adopted in village do not adequately protect the produce. As

the result, physical losses go on increasing if the period of storage is lengthened.

7. **Undeveloped modes of transportation**: Without a good transporting system, no individual will have the incentive to produce or to purchase more than minimum. Unless it is reasonably convenient for the farmer to exchange his surplus produce for consumer goods or farm production requisites, he is lacking an important incentive to exploit the full potentials of his animals. Lack of an efficient transport network is the real limiting factor in the attempts to increase livestock production in our Country.

8. **Variability in Output:** The quantity of farm products available depends upon several factors. With the gambling nature, one cannot forecast the quantity of products that would be produced as livestock production is mainly biological depending on weather, rainfall etc for its main inputs like feed, fodder etc.,

9. **Seasonality in production:** Much of farm production is highly seasonal. The production varies from one season of the year to another. Hence, storage facilities must be made ready to hold the product until it is consumed. This seasonality in production thus, raises costs of marketing through demand storage facilities. The seasonal variability in production of items like milk, egg, butter etc is not so acute as it used to be years ago. The widespread use of rapid transportation and refrigeration has tended to reduce the seasonality.

10. **Raw materials**: Farm output which is mainly sold in the farm of raw materials is used subsequently for processing. Sugarcane is to be converted in to sugar, oils seeds in to oil, animals into meat, wool in to cloth before all these are used for consumption. Hence the raw materials produced by the farmers are to be processed at one stage or the other before final consumption.

11. **Perishability**: In relation to other products, agricultural products by nature are perishable. All products ultimately deteriorate in a shorter period of time. Eggs, mutton and milk must move into consumption very quickly, otherwise they would completely lose their value. These perishable products require speedy handling and often-special refrigeration, which raises the cost of marketing.

12. **Others:** The differences in variety, colour, palatability, nutritive value, size, and quality etc. of the products are the other determinants of a good market for these products.

14

Marketing Agencies, Institutions and Channels for Livestock and Livestock Products

In India, we have mostly two types of standards, which govern the sale of foods including milk and milk products.

These are: Legal standards and Quality standards.

Legal standards

Legal standard means the specifications or the requirements which pertain to the law of the Govt. and are set up by the Govt. to meet certain minimum requirements in terms of chemical quality (i.e. composition), bacteriological quality (i.e. hygienic quality), and labelling and packaging requirements.

In our country, legal standards are given under Prevention of Food Adulteration (PFA) Rules, 1954-1955 (which are amended from time to time). Legal standards or PFA standards prescribe the minimum requirements for all types and categories of food. These standards are consistent with the minimum quality that is attainable under Indian conditions by the majority of the farmers, producers, processors, sale agencies etc. Further, any food that does not confirm to the minimum standards laid down by the legal rulers (PFA rules) is said to be adulterated, irrespective whether anything has been added to or removed from the original food.

Quality standards

Quality standards means those specifications which are laid down by the Govt or some expert body constituted by the Govt. for the purpose of producing high quality products. While legal standards are compulsory, the quality standards are not compulsory. They are on voluntary basis.

In our country, we have two types of quality standards

- BIS/ ISI standards
- Agmark standards

Both of these are above the PFA minimum standards. Both of these are useful for producing export quality products.

Major regulations governing livestock products and markets

The livestock products are governed by livestock importation act, Milk and Milk Products Order, Bureau of Indian standards, Prevention of Food Adulteration Act, Essential commodities act and Meat and Food Products order, 1973 (MFPO, 1973). These acts are framed by various organizations that make the stakeholders of livestock products industry to adhere rules both voluntarily as well as compulsorily. Livestock importation act, Milk and Milk Products Order, 1992 (MMPO, 1992) and Meat and Food Products Order, 1973 (MFPO, 1973) are the specific acts governing livestock sector.

Livestock importation act, 1896 controls the import of meat products, eggs and egg powder, milk products and livestock in a manner that such imports do not adversely affect the health of human and animal population of the country. The Milk and Milk products order controls production, distribution and supply of milk products. It also sets sanitary requirements for dairies, machinery and premises and includes quality control, certification, packing, marking and labelling standards for milk and milk products. MMPO 1992, is implemented by the Department of Animal Husbandry, Dairying and Fisheries. While the Ministry of Food and Processing Industries (MoFPI) the regulatory authority for the Meat and Food Products Order, is equally applicable to domestic processors and importers. The major acts MMPO, 1992 and MFPO, 1973 are discussed briefly below.

Milk and Milk Products Order

The main intention of MMPO 1992 is to maintain and increase the supply of liquid milk of desired quality in the interests of the general public and also for regulating the production, processing and distribution of milk and milk Products. Over the years this order had six amendments. The last amendment removed restrictions on setting up of new capacity and to do away with the concept of "Milk shed" while noting that the requirement of registration is for enforcing the prescribed standards of quality and food safety. This modification completely removed the restrictions for domestic investment in dairy sector.

Meat and Food Products Order

For processing of meat products license is issued under Meat and Food Products Order (MFPO, 1973). This act also ensures quality control and hygienic manufacturing conditions. The Ministry of Food Processing Industries (MoFPI) issues licenses to industries in meat sector. This act had been amended in 2005. The revised amendment seeks registration of plants with MoFPI and obtain license for processing and selling of frozen chicken.

The above two acts are controlling various stakeholders in the livestock industry and are responsible for emerging changes

Prevention of Food Adulteration (PFA Act) 1954

The main objectives of PFA Act are:

- To protect the public from harmful and poisonous foods.
- To prevent the sale of substandard food containing harmful substances, and
- To protect the society against unscrupulous and anti-social dealers by eliminating fraudulent practices.

Agriculture produce (Grading and Marking) Act (AGMARK)

Agmark stands for "Agricultural Marking". In order to have a systematic marketing of Agricultural Produce on the basis of well defined quality, Indian Legislature in 1937 passed an act known as "Agriculture Produce (Grading and Marking) Act, 1937. This act is not mandatory. It is permissive in nature. It is one's choice to go for Agmark grading, if one can meet their specifications. Rules under this Act are called "General Grading and Marking Rules, 1937". Rules have been revised in 1988 and are called General Grading & Marking Rules, 1988. Grading of Agricultural items under these rules is called AGMARK GRADING or Agmark certification. Under the Agricultural Produce Act, 1937-grade standards are given for agricultural and allied commodities like cereals, oil seeds, oils, creamery butter, ghee, legumes, eggs etc. Agricultural commodities are categorized into various grades such as, special, good, fair, ordinary etc depending upon the degree of quality (type of composition) in each case. These grades are known as "Agmark Standards" and this way of categorizing or grading the agricultural products in terms of their chemical composition or quality is called "Agmark Grading".

Objectives of AGMARK scheme

- To assure the consumers a product of pre-tested quality & purity.
- To enable the producer of good quality products to have better returns.
- To have a sale of the product in the market with a uniform composition and well defined quality.
- To eliminate the malpractice of adulteration in the movement of the product from producer to consumer.

As told earlier, among the dairy products, only ghee and creamery butter (Table butter or salted butter) are graded under Agmark. Desi or cooking (unsalted or white) butter is not graded under Agmark.

Bureau of indian standards (BIS)

It is a national standards body of India which is responsible for formulating National Standards for various types of articles (both edible & non-edible i.e. food & non-food articles e.g. live stock feed, cattle housing, equipments, dairy products, food additives, food hygiene), testing apparatus and methods etc. The old name of this organization was ISI (*Indian Standards Institution*), which was established in 1947. The new name i.e. BIS came into existence from 1st April, 1987 under the BIS Act 1986.

Objectives and functions of BIS

1. To formulate Indian standards for various articles, processes, methods of test, codes of practices etc and promote their implementation.
2. To promote the Concepts of standardization and Quality control in industries.
3. To coordinate the efforts of producers and users for making improvements in the materials, products, processes and methods.
4. To operate ISI certification scheme.
5. To establish testing laboratories of its own.
6. To operate laboratory recognition scheme to meet the requirements of testing.
7. To offer technical and consultancy services within and outside the country.
8. To have cooperation and coordination with international standard making bodies like ISO.

In India, we had many bodies enforcing standards. This led to lot of confusion for both manufacturers as well as enforcers. In the recent past the concept of globalization or flat word has emerged very strongly, where all the boundaries have been eliminated. However, some barriers to trade with respect to more stringent norms and others have been raised. In this context Indian Standards needed to be harmonized within themselves as well as with the international standards. To eliminate the problems and confusions in the trade of food items including milk, a thought of uniform standards was evolved, which has been culminated in the form of Food Safety and Standards Authority of India.

Food Safety and Standards Act, 2006

An Act to consolidate the laws relating to food and to establish the Food Safety and Standards Authority of India for laying down science based standards for articles of food and to regulate their manufacture, storage, distribution, sale and import, to ensure availability of safe and wholesome food for human consumption and for matters connected therewith or incidental thereto. The FSS act is a bucket for all the older laws, rules and regulations for food safety. The FSS Act is a bucket for all the older laws, rules and regulations for food safety. The FSS Act took 8 older acts into one Umbrella. Prevention of Food Adulteration Act - 1954, Fruit Products Order - 1955, Meat Food Products Order – 1973, Vegetables Oil Products Order - 1947, Edible Oils Packaging Order 1988, Solvent Extracted Oil Order – 1967 and Milk and Milk products Order – 1992.

The Important Functions of FSSAI

- Framing of Regulations to lay down the Standards and guidelines in relation to articles of food and specifying appropriate system of enforcing various standards thus notified.
- Laying down mechanisms and guidelines for accreditation of certification bodies engaged in certification of food safety management system for food businesses.
- Laying down procedure and guidelines for accreditation of laboratories and notification of the accredited laboratories.
- To provide scientific advice and technical support to Central Government and State Governments in the matters of framing the policy and rules in areas which have a direct or indirect bearing of food safety and nutrition.
- Collect and collate data regarding food consumption, incidence and prevalence of biological risk, contaminants in food, residues of various, contaminants in foods products, identification of emerging risks and introduction of rapid alert system.

- Creating an information network across the country so that the public, consumers, Panchayats etc receive rapid, reliable and objective information about food safety and issues of concern.
- Provide training programmes for persons who are involved or intend to get involved in food businesses.
- Contribute to the development of international technical standards for food, sanitary and phyto-sanitary standards.
- Promote general awareness about food safety and food standards.

International Regulations: CODEX, IDF, ISO, FDA, EEC

The different sets of standards arising from the spontaneous and independent development of food laws and standards by different countries inevitably gave rise to trade barriers that were of increasing concern to food traders in the early twentieth century. Trade associations that were formed as a reaction to such barriers pressured governments to harmonize their various food standards so as to facilitate trade in safe foods of a defined quality. The International Dairy Federation (IDF), founded in 1903, was one such association. Its work on standards for milk and milk products later provided a catalyst in the establishment of the Codex Alimentarius Commission and in the setting of its procedures for elaborating standards.

Codex Alimentarius Commission (CAC)

The FAO and the WHO jointly established the Codex Alimentarius Commission (CAC) in 1962 to implement the joint FAO/WHO food Standards Programme. The aim of the commission is to protect the health of consumers by ensuring observance of fair practices in food trade. It promotes co-ordination of work on formulation of food standards undertaken by international governmental and non-governmental organizations. The Codex Alimentarius Commission shall be responsible for making proposals to, and shall be consulted by, the Directors-General of the Food and Agriculture Organization (FAO) and the World Health Organization (WHO) on all matters pertaining to the implementation of the joint FAO/WHO Food Standards Programme. In addition to commodity standards, the Codex Alimentarius includes general standards, which have across-the-board application to all foods and are not product-specific. There are general standards or recommendations for:

- Food labeling;
- Food additives;
- Contaminants;

- Methods of analysis and sampling;
- Food hygiene;
- Nutrition and foods for special dietary uses;
- Food import and export inspection and certification systems;
- Residues of veterinary drugs in foods;
- Pesticide residues in foods.

Adoption of HACCP standards, formulated by CAC, under the sanitary and phytosanitary (SPC) measures has made the HACCP system an instrument of food safety. It has become incumbent on signatory countries of the SPC agreement to implement these standards.

International Dairy Federation (IDF)

IDF is the pre-eminent source of scientific and technical expertise for all stakeholders of the dairy chain. Membership covers 56 countries and is growing. The mission of IDF is to represent the dairy sector worldwide by providing the best global source of scientific expertise and knowledge in support of the development and promotion of quality milk and dairy products to deliver consumers with nutrition, health and well-being.IDF publishes **jointly with the ISO**, standards method of sampling and analysis of milk and milk products.

International Organization for Standardization (ISO)

ISO is a network of the national standards institutes of 158 countries, one member per country, with a Central Secretariat in Geneva, Switzerland, that coordinates the system. ISO is a non-governmental organization that forms a bridge between the public and private sectors. It is the world's largest developer and publisher of International Standards. ISO enables a consensus to be reached on solutions that meet both the requirements of business and the broader needs of society. "International Organization for Standardization" would have different acronyms in different languages e.g. "IOS" in English, "OIN" in French (Organization international de normalization). Its founders decided to give it also a short, all-purpose name. They chose "ISO", derived from the Greek isos, meaning "equal". Whatever the country, whatever the language, the short form of the organization's name is always ISO.

Food and Drug Administration (FDA or USFDA)

FDA is an agency of the United States Department of Health and Human Services. The FDA is responsible for protecting and promoting public health through the regulation and supervision of food safety, tobacco products, dietary supplements, prescription and over-the-counter pharmaceutical drugs (medications), vaccines, biopharmaceuticals, blood transfusions, medical devices, electromagnetic radiation emitting devices (ERED), veterinary products, and cosmetics. The FDA also enforces other laws, which include sanitation requirements on interstate travel and control of disease on products ranging from certain household pets to sperm donation for assisted reproduction. The FDA is formed in 1906 and has its headquarters at White Oak, Maryland. The agency also has 223 field offices and 13 laboratories located throughout the 50 states. In 2008, the FDA started opening offices in foreign countries, including China, India, Costa Rica, Chile, Belgium, and the United Kingdom.

Market intermediaries or Middlemen

Middlemen are those individuals or business concerns specialised in performing the various marketing functions involved in purchase and sale of goods as they are moved from producers to consumers.

Middlemen are classified into

a. Merchant Middlemen

a. Wholesaler

b. Retailer

b. Agent middlemen

a. Broker

b. Commission Agent

c. Speculative middlemen

d. Processor and manufacturers

a. Merchant Middlemen

Take title and therefore own the products they handled.

i. Wholesalers : Sell the commodity to the retailer or other traders but does not sell small quantities to ultimate consumer

ii. Retailer: Buys the products for resale directly to the consumers

Services of wholesalers

- Acts as an intermediate between the producer and the retailers
- Acts as an interpreter of the demand by the consumers and gives guidance to the producer or manufacturer to understand the market

- They keep the prices steady and prevent violent price fluctuation by holding the stock at the time of dull market due to overproduction of commodities and sell stock when market is very bright
- The wholesalers export or import goods and come in contact with the buyers and sellers of foreign countries
- They provide storage facilities for different commodities until they are needed by retailers
- Provides credit both to the retailers and producers

Services of Retailer

- Retailers anticipate the wants of the consumers and supply him the right kind of goods
- Creates time and possession utility
- Perform the services of 'bulk breaking' i.e. dividing larger quantities into small quantity

b. Agent middlemen

Act only as the representative of the clients. They do not take title, therefore, they do not own the product they handle. While the merchant middlemen secured their income from the margin between buying and selling prices, the agent middlemen receives his income in the form of fees and commission.

i. Commission Agents: They are usually granted with broad powers by the sellers. They normally take over the physical handling of the products. They arrange for sale sells the goods in their name, prepare bills, collects the money from the buyer, deduct their fees and remit the balance to the sellers.
ii. Brokers: They usually do not have physical control of the product.

c. Speculative middlemen

They are those who take title to their products with the major purpose of profiting from price movements. The wholesalers and retailers take a minimum risk, where as the speculative middlemen are specialised in taking risk. They often attempt to get profit from short run fluctuations in prices. Speculative middlemen are called as 'scalpers'.

d. Processors and manufacturers

They exist primarily to undertake some action on products to change their form e.g. dairy plant.

Conclusion

We can conclude that the consumer's price could be reduced by reducing the number of intermediaries. To increase the share of consumer's rupee to the producer, the producer and consumer should be brought closer by reducing the number of intermediaries i.e. by shortening the marketing channel.

Distribution

The process of delivering the product to the consumer is termed as distribution. Distribution consists of two interrelated aspects,

- Physical distribution
- Channels of distribution

Physical distribution

It encompasses all the activities involved in the physical flow of products from producers to consumers.

Components of physical distribution

- Transportation
- Storage/warehousing

Transportation

It involves the process of moving the product from one place to other.

Classification of modes of transport for livestock and livestock products

1	Land	Pathways	Head Loads
			Pack animals
		Roads	Bullock carts
			Two wheelers
			Tractors, Trucks & Buses
		Railways	Rail wagon
2	Water	Inland	Canals & Rivers
		Ocean	Ships
3	Air		Aeroplanes

Common means of transportation used for livestock/livestock products

Stage of marketing	Transportation done by	Means of transport used
From the place of production to the village market or railway point / bus stand	Farmer	Head loads Bullock carts Two wheelers Tractor / Trucks
From village market / Railway Station/Bus Stand to primary / Secondary wholesale markets	Traders	Trucks / buses or railway wagons
From retail or wholesale market to consumers	Consumers	Two wheelers Bullock carts Head loads

Problems in transportation of livestock and livestock products

- The means of transportation used are slow moving.
- There are more losses / damages in transportation because of poor packing, overloading of the produce and poor handling.
- The transportation cost per hundred rupees worth of the produce is high because of bulkiness of the produce and prevailing practice of fixing charges on the basis of weight / volume rather than on the basis of its value.

Storage

It involves holding and preserving good from the time they are produced until they are needed for consumption.

Importance of storage

- Protects the quality of perishable and semi-perishable products from deterioration.
- Some of the goods (e.g. woolen garments) have a seasonal demand and to cope with the demand continuous production and storage is necessary.
- Helps in stabilization of prices by adjusting demand and supply.
- Necessary for some periods for the performance of other marketing functions e.g. transportation.
- Storage is necessary for some farm commodities for improvement in their quality e.g. pickles, cheese

Livestock Marketing Channels

Marketing channel

Marketing channel may be defined as a path traced in the direct or indirect transfer of title of a product, as it moves from a producer to ultimate consumer. A channel always includes both the producer and the final customer as well as all agents and merchant middlemen involved in the transfer of title. However, the channel does not include firms such as railway, bank and other institutions which render a marketing service but play no major role in negotiating purchase and sale.

Types of marketing channels

There are two types of marketing channels and they are viz., i) organised marketing channel and ii) Unorganised marketing channel.

Difference between organised and unorganised marketing channels

Organised	Unorganised
Participation of government institution or co-operative union in marketing	Private organisation
Service motive	Profit motive
Consumer price will not have violent fluctuations	Violent price fluctuation in consumer price caused by supply and demand forces

Uniqueness of livestock products

In relation to other products, livestock and poultry products by nature are perishable and all products ultimately deteriorate. Eggs, poultry meat and milk must move into consumption very quickly, otherwise they would completely loss their value. These perishable products require speedy handling and often special refrigeration which of course raised the cost of marketing.

Role of channels

Selection of distribution channels or intermediaries is a managerial decision of developing a set of interdependent organisations involved in the process of marketing a product available to the target consumers, satisfying the demand by supplying goods and services at the right time and place, quantity and price, but they also stimulate demand through the promotional activities of the channels members. In a nutshell, it can be said that channels of distribution serve as a network, which **creates value for the consumerby generating possession, time and place utilities.**

There are a number of middlemen and merchants, including government and co-operative agencies who act as links between the producers and consumers.

Channels of distribution are also the most powerful element among marketing mix elements, successful marketing of a product and consumer satisfaction to a large extent depend on a sound distribution network. A number of utilities are resultant effects of an effective distribution network strategy.

Selection of channel

The channel selection decision is important mainly for two reasons.

i. *Cost involved* in the use of a channel is realised from the price of the product a consumer pays
ii. It has an impact on other marketing decisions like price of commodities and other promotional decisions

An appropriate channel selection strategy based on a *proper market feedback mechanism* can reduce fluctuations in production of commodities as well as consumer dissatisfaction generating from non-availability of product, two most important lacunae of Indian agricultural products marketing system.

In order to achieve the goal of developing well – knit network of channels of distribution for livestock products, producers as well as government agencies and co-operatives should take into consideration the following factors.

i. **Type of the product:** Selling of perishable products like egg and poultry meat requires fast movement of the commodities from producers to the ultimate consumers. Hence a *short channel of distribution* will be effective tool to reach the target consumers
ii. **Nature and extent of the market:** When the consumers are concentrated in limited geographical area and their number is small the producer (farmer) can approach the customer directly
iii. **Cost involved in the process:** Cost is one of the crucial decisions in channel selection process. The possible strategy to come out of this problem before the producer is to go for distributions through middlemen who have their own men, transport and storage facilities for their purpose. This system will involve less financial commitments and prove to be most economic too
iv. **Buying Habits of Consumers:** When a commodity is purchased in bulk, the manufacturer taps the biggest wholesaler. Alternatively, when consumer wants to buy a single unit of large number of commodities he goes to a retailer

Factors affecting marketing channel

Marketing channel for the same commodity may very seasonally and from place to place. Because marketing channel depends on the following factors.

i. Production pattern
ii. Nature and behaviour of the customers
iii. New marketing technology
iv. Changes in the management and Changes in the policies of government and

Marketing channels for meat

i. Producer→ Local village trader→ Wholesale butcher→ Retail butcher→ Consumer
ii. Producer→ Wholesale butcher→ Retail butcher→ Consumer
iii. Producer→ Commission agent→ Wholesale butcher→ Retail butcher→ Consumer
iv. Producer→ Commission agent→ Retail butcher→ Consumer

Marketing Channels for Livestock products

Milk

Unorganized **Organized**

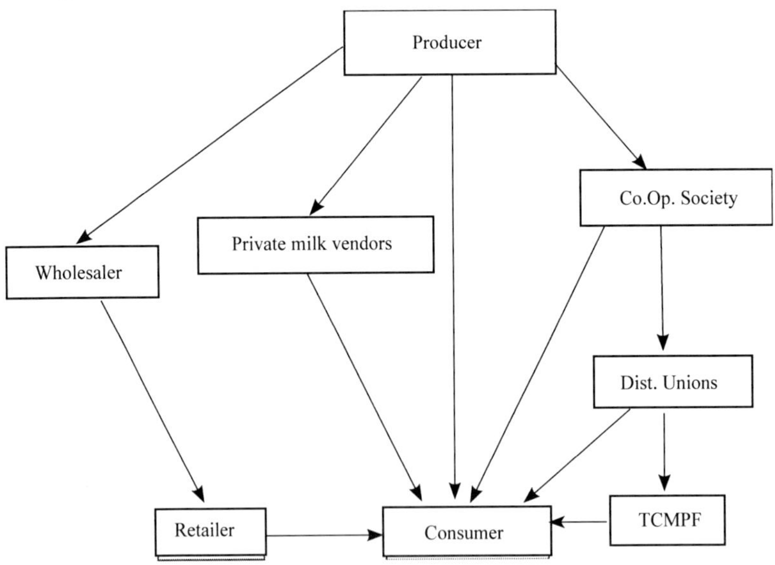

Marketing channels for egg

Egg marketing depends upon several factors like;

- Number of eggs to be marketed Distance of the market
- Availability of labour Transportation facilities
- Other businesses of the producer.

Channels of egg marketing includes

- Village buyers
- Private buyers and assemblers of eggs
- Commission agents
- Wholesale receivers/Co-operatives /auctioneers
- Intermediaries/Egg dealers/Distributors
- Retailers
- Consumers/Individuals/Hotels/Hospitals

Channels of egg marketing

i. Producer→ Trader→ Wholesaler → Retailer → Consumer

ii. Producer→ Wholesaler → Retailer → Consumer

iii. Producer→ Wholesaler → Consumer

iv. Producer→ Retailer → Consumer

Marketing Channels for live animals

- Seller-buyer
- Seller-broker-buyer
- Seller-trader-buyer
- Seller-trader-broker-buyer
- Seller –slaughter stock holder

Marketing channels of poultry

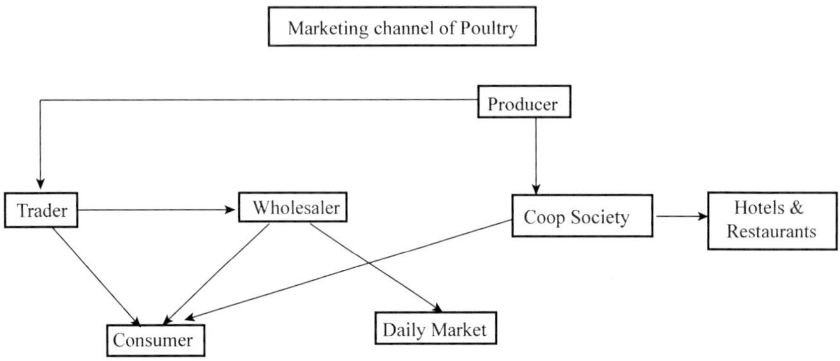

Marketing Channels of Sheep

Channel I (32%)

Producer → Distant wholesaler → Retailer → Consumer

Channel II (42%)

Producer → Village trader → Distant → Wholesaler → Retailer → Consumer

Channel III (13%)

Producer → Local retailer → Consumer

Channel IV (13%)

Producer → Village trader → Retailer → Consumer

Marketing Channels of Fish

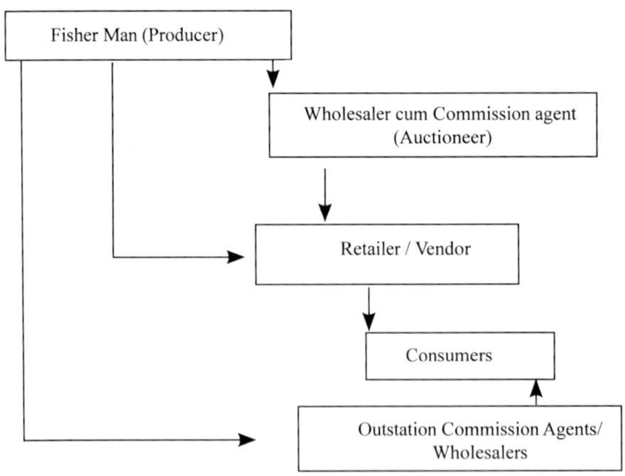

Factors considered in fixing the price in case of

Live animal

- Species
- Breed
- Age
- Body Weight
- Parity
- Pair Set
- Health Status
- Body Conformations-feet, udder, wedges, testicles etc.

Milk

- Volume
- Fat %
- SNF

Egg

- Weight
- Shell thickness
- Albumin Index
- Yolk Index

Meat

- Weight
- Cuttings
- Species
- Quality

Marketing of live animals

Live animals are mostly sold in lots in livestock fairs, periodical markets and daily markets. Each animal is assessed individually by the buyer. Factors affecting the price are size, age, meat, milk yield, breed, sex, quality, locality and season. The Govt. of India established marketing cells in various states to regulate the existing markets and organize co-operative markets to facilitate marketing of products, to make market surveys, to collect and disseminate market news, and to advise better marketing methods and adoption of grading procedures. There is a channel of farmer to middle man to slaughter house in case of meat animals – sheep, goats, pigs and poultry.

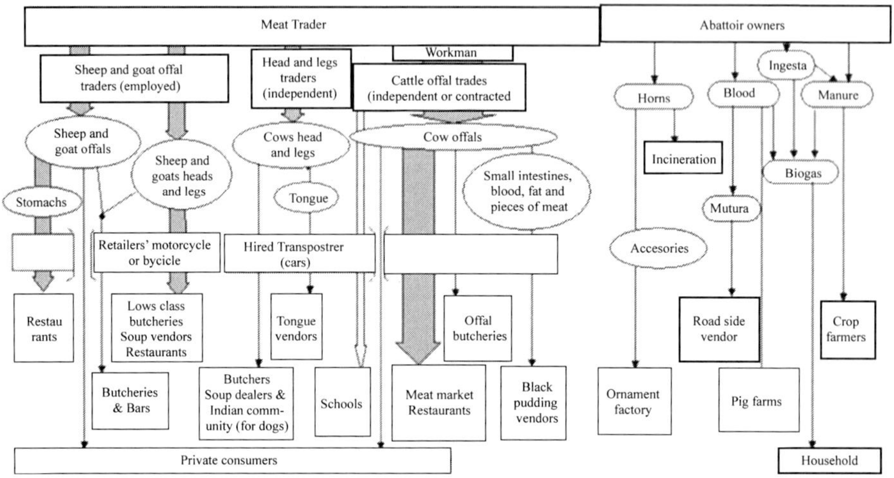
Meat Trader
Abattoir owners
Workman
Sheep and goat offal traders (employed)
Head and legs traders (independent)
Cattle offal trades (independent or contracted
Ingesta
Horns
Blood
Manure
Sheep and goat offals
Sheep and goats heads and legs
Cows head and legs
Cow offals
Incineration
Biogas
Small intestines, blood, fat and pieces of meat
Stomachs
Tongue
Mutura
Retailers' motorcycle or bycicle
Hired Transpostrer (cars)
Accesories
Restau rants
Lows class butcheries Soup vendors Restaurants
Tongue vendors
Offal butcheries
Road side vendor
Crop farmers
Butcheries & Bars
Butchers Soup dealers & Indian comm-unity (for dogs)
Schools
Meat market Restaurants
Black pudding vendors
Ornament factory
Pig farms
Private consumers
Household

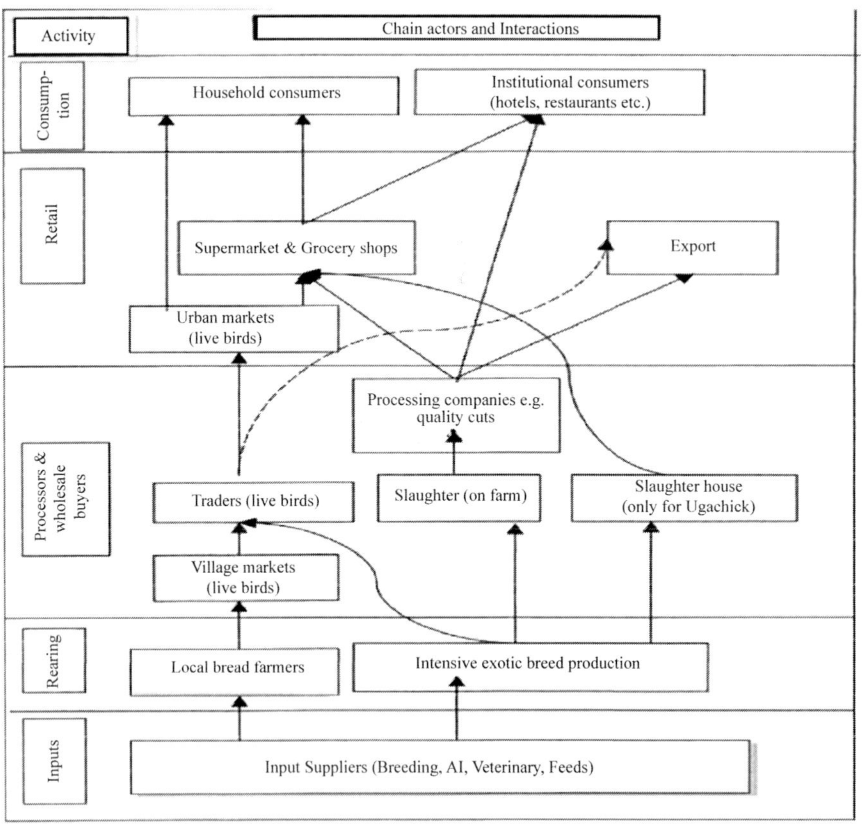
Activity
Chain actors and Interactions
Consump-tion
Household consumers
Institutional consumers (hotels, restaurants etc.)
Retail
Supermarket & Grocery shops
Export
Urban markets (live birds)
Processing companies e.g. quality cuts
Processors & wholesale buyers
Traders (live birds)
Slaughter (on farm)
Slaughter house (only for Ugachick)
Village markets (live birds)
Rearing
Local bread farmers
Intensive exotic breed production
Inputs
Input Suppliers (Breeding, AI, Veterinary, Feeds)

Marketing cost

Marketing cost is the *actual expense required* in bringing goods and services from the producer to the consumer. The difference between the final price paid by the consumer for a commodity and the price received by the primary producer may be taken as the marketing cost. *Marketing cost normally included handling charges, assembling charges, transport and storage costs, processing costs, profit margins to different intermediaries etc.*

Peculiarities of agricultural and livestock production affecting marketing cost

It is a common experience that marketing of agricultural and livestock products is relatively more expensive than marketing of manufactured goods on account of a few peculiar features of crop and livestock production.

a. As production in animal husbandry and agriculture is *scattered over wider areas*, assembly of small lots into sizeable ones is an additional function thereby increasing the marketing cost

b. Agricultural and livestock product *vary so much in their quality* that they have necessarily to be graded so as to confirm to certain well established standards

c. They are usually *bulky, seasonal and perishable* which increase the marketing cost through necessitating functions of transport and storage

The result of the operation of all these factors widen the margin between the price paid by the consumer and that received by the livestock farmer.

Importance of studying marketing cost

a. To know the services rendered by different market functionaries and the remuneration received for their services

b. To identify whether these service are necessary or not and

c. To find out ways and means to reduce the cost thereby increasing marketing efficiency

Marketing Efficiency

Marketing efficiency may be defined as the effectiveness with which a market structure performs its functions. In other words, marketing efficiency can be defined as the maximisation of consumer's satisfaction with the least cost incurred in providing that satisfaction through the system of marketing.

Marketing efficiency can be divided into two components namely operational or technical efficiency and pricing or economic efficiency. *Technical efficiency* pertains to the improvement of the market structure and utilisation of best methods available with maximum effectiveness for performing different marketing functions. E.g. Use of tractors in place of bullock carts for transport, use of telephones in place of manual messengers etc.

Economic efficiency relates to the minimisation of marketing cost through minimising input use in marketing, avoidance of waste, reducing profits to the middlemen etc. The important methods used in the data analysis pertaining to analysing the Economic efficiency of marketing are detailed below.

a. Price spread

This is a term used to describe the difference between consumer and producer price. Normally it is expressed as percentage of consumer price. It is the sum of marketing costs and profit margins of different market intermediaries involved in the marketing. The economic efficiency of a market is generally measured in terms of price spread of the commodity. ***Larger the price spread, greater is the inefficiency in the marketing system.***

Price Spread = Marketing costs + Marketing margin

The example given below will help to understand the concept of price spread.

Milk marketing channel

Producer → Wholesaler → Retailer→ Consumer

Particulars	Rs. Per litre	Per cent
Net price to producer	16.27	71.61
Purchase price of wholesaler	16.27	71.61
Transport charges of wholesaler	0.38	1.67
Storage charges of wholesaler	0.53	2.33
Establishment charges of wholesaler	0.27	1.19
Wastage charges of wholesaler	0.25	1.10
Processing and retailing charges of wholesaler	0.33	1.45
Packing charges of wholesaler	-	-
Labour charges of wholesaler	0.51	2.24
Marketing margin of wholesaler	0.50	2.20
Sale price of wholesaler	19.04	83.80
Purchase price of Retailer	19.04	83.80
Transport charges of Retailer	0.16	0.70
Storage charges of wholesaler	0.09	0.40
Establishment charges of Retailer	0.18	0.79

Particulars	Rs. Per litre	Per cent
Wastage charges of Retailer	0.04	0.18
Processing and retailing charges of Retailer	0.39	1.72
Packing charges of Retailer	0.08	0.35
Labour charges of Retailer	0.46	2.02
Marketing margin of Retailer	2.28	10.04
Purchase price of consumer	22.72	100.00
Gross price spread	6.45	28.39

b. Shepherds' formula

This formula is used to find out the marketing efficiency of a system.

$$\text{Market efficiency} = 100 - \frac{\text{Total cost of marketing}}{\text{Total value of the products marketed}} \times 100$$

Any increase in marketing cost or any decrease in the value of the product marketed would result in increasing marketing inefficiency. Rise in marketing efficiency may result in a rise in revenue to the farmer, a fall in price to the consumer and / or a fall in profit to the middlemen.

Marketing integration in livestock industry

An integrated marketing in Livestock industry covers all aspects of production i.e., from breeding to marketing of the final product. Two kinds of integration exist in marketing:

1. **Vertical integration:** When more than one stage of producing and marketing a livestock product are controlled by the same individual or company.
2. **Horizontal integration:** Two or more companies at one level join together to follow a new marketing opportunity. A completely integrated production and marketing system can also be organized under the management of a growers; wholesale processing co-operative, hence called co-operative integration.

Poultry industry provides dramatic examples of the integration of farm production and marketing activities. Poultry production itself is a highly integrated operation combining specialized breeding, hatchery, grain farming and feed mixing, packing operations and marketing firms.

There are 3 types of production – marketing integration in poultry industry

Owner integration

The integration of production and marketing is controlled by an individual or a single firm. i.e. the facilities for egg production or meat production are under the ownership and the eggs, meat are marketed by him to retailer or consumer.

Contract marketing

Buyer sets minimum standards for the egg or meat to be produced by the producer. Here the egg producer bears price uncertainties in addition to production cost risk. But the quality of egg or meat and the time of delivery are specified and assured.

Contract production

Here the producer is asked to grow the birds or produce eggs for the specific distributor – under closely supervised conditions and for a guaranteed return. i.e. the integrator supplies inputs like chicks, feed, medication, field supervision, etc. and the grower provides the inputs like housing, water, labour, etc. Then the grower returns the bird/egg gets specified returns (5 to 7% per bird) plus incentive for superior feed conversion efficiency.

Marketable livestock commodities

Marketable surplus and marketed surplus

Marketable surplus is defined as the excess of output over sectoral retention and on-farm consumption. Sect oral retention of farm output is primarily for two purposes.

i. for family consumption

ii. for further use in farming operations such as seed, kind wage etc.

Marketable surplus can be expressed as follows

M=Q-C

Where, M-Marketable surplus

Q-Output (old stock + current output)

C-On-farm consumption

Importance of marketable surplus

1. Marketable surplus can make a positive contribution to economic development. Marketable surplus converted into cash put the purchasing power that enables the secondary sectors to sell their goods and services to the primary sector and hence production in secondary sector too increases. Likewise, markets for all the sectors are widened as a result of high marketable surplus in primary sector like animal husbandry.
2. Part of the marketable surplus may be exported or at least marketable surplus would reduce the import leading to saving of foreign exchange.
3. It would also serve as a protection against price inflation.

Marketed surplus

Marketed surplus represents only that portion of the marketable surplus which is actually marketed and placed at the disposal of consuming population. Marketed surplus depends on the availability of storage and transport facilities, cash needs of the farmers, prices prevailing in the market, holding capacity of the farmers etc. Marketed surplus in a given period may be less than, equal to or greater than the marketable surplus of that year depending on the external factors operating in the market economy. Marketed surplus can be equal to marketable surplus especially in the case of big farmers. It is also probable that marketed surplus is more than the marketable surplus which may be so in conditions of higher prices and in condition of farmers being driven to distress sales. A large proportion of the farmers sells out considerable part of their produce at the time of harvest to meet their immediate cash obligations and they purchase back from the markets later when they require the same for consumption.

Factors responsible for marketable and marketed surplus

1. There is no real marketable surplus among the vast majority of our farmers who remain as small farmers and live in only subsistence level. The low productivity and small size of farms also limit the marketable surpluses.
2. As the price of the commodity increases, the farmer will try to dispose as much as possible to earn better income. Hence, price increase increases the marketable surplus.
3. Size of the family
   a. Consumption pattern
   b. Cash requirements of the farmers.

15

Government Interventions and Role in Marketing of Livestock and Livestock Products

Government role in marketing of milk

Ever since independence the dairy sector in India has been regulated. The government projects and programmes in place for enhancing dairy development include subsidies for developing infrastructure for milk processing and testing. The Clean Milk Production Programme is a centrally sponsored scheme that is being implemented by the State Department of Animal Husbandry, Dairying and Fisheries with several objectives: i) the creation and strengthening of necessary infrastructure for the production of quality milk and milk products at the farm level up to the points of consumption; ii) improvement of milking techniques; and iii) training to enhance awareness on the importance of hygienic milk production. Several other rural development initiatives support dairying, such as through the District Rural Development Agency and women's self-help groups. An area of government support that has not been capitalized on so far is the investment in promoting the nutritional aspects of milk, particularly pasteurized milk versus loose milk.

The policy history

Until 1991, the dairying sector was licensed under the Industries Development and Regulation Act (IRDA, 1951). This resulted in preferential treatment given to milk cooperatives that were outside the purview of the legislation. In 1991, the dairy sector was swept up in the move to liberalize the economy. Consequently, the IRDA was replaced by the Milk and Milk Product Order in 1992, which contained the following provisions:

1. The main objective of the MMPO is to maintain and increase the supply of liquid milk of desired quality in the interests of the general public and to regulate the production, processing and distribution of milk and milk products.

2. Any person or dairy plant handling more than 10 000 litres of milk per day or 500 tonnes of milk solid per annum needs to be registered, with the registering authority appointed by the central Government.
3. Every holder of a registration certificate can collect or procure milk only from the milk shed assigned under the registration certificate. The milk shed, is defined as "an area geographically demarcated by the registering authority for the collection of milk or milk product by the holder of a registration certificate".

Amendments were made to MMPO in 2002 to further liberalize the sector and encourage dairy entrepreneurs from the private sector. The milk shed concept was abandoned, allowing for milk supplies to be procured from any area.

Traditionally, the cooperatives have not had much competition from the private sector. In the liberalized environment characterized by open procurement of milk, there is incentive for private players to invest in the sector. Consequently, many agencies, organizations and agents have started buying milk. But a major difference is that they are not backward investing in dairy development activities through the offering of producer services. In the coming years, the lack of involvement in dairy development by the various players is likely to constrain further growth of the industry.

In this environment, dairy farmer organizations and cooperatives will have a strong role to play in supporting dairy development activities. If they were to establish higher prices to farmers, for instance, the private sector and other players would be forced to pay at least that much as well.

Policy and regulatory issues

Agriculture is a state responsibility in India, and the State Department of Animal Husbandry, Dairying and Fisheries, is responsible for the dairy activities. Consequently, the focus of the activities and budgetary allocation is biased towards agriculture rather than livestock.

Enabling environment	
Activities	National sector regulation
Key regulatory actors (ministries)	Department of Animal Husbandry is under the Ministry of Agriculture, hence focus on livestock is underemphasized, particularly in light of the high value of the sector.
Price regulation	Rice setting by cooperatives
Food safety	Regulated through the Milk and Milk Products Order
Informal regulations	Very difficult to control quality in traditional channels
	Huge premium on fat content of milk compared with formal regulations; thus buffalo milk fetches much higher price

Formal sector support	
Domestic sector (national)	Approaches being taken to modernize the sector
Subsidy support	Various subsidies available for milk processing and testing infrastructure
Inward investment promotion	Very little investment on the promotion of health or quality of milk
Provincial/local	
Key regulatory actors (ministries)	State Department of Animal Husbandry, Dairying and Fisheries is the implementing agency at the state level
Informal regulation & transparency	Lack of milk testing equipment and thus transparency, leading to low payments
Formal sector support	Availability of veterinary services; paravets are working with the Department of Animal Husbandry. Dairying and Fisheries
Formal sector support	Availability of services in remote areas through the government
Donor/NGO roles	Donor agencies are very actively involved in livestock sector development

There are several issues related to milk pricing policies that require serious review and reconsideration. The state cooperatives are supposed to base the price paid to farmers on the fat and solid-not-fat (SNF) content of milk.

Also, the cooperative price becomes the benchmark price for other buyers (vendors and private dairy agents) and when it is low, so are the other prices paid. Thus there is no incentive for farmers to sell to the other buyers; only about 15 percent of the milk is sold this way for the marketing of packaged milk and milk products. Policy efforts focus on enforcing testing the quality (in terms of fat and SNF) as the basis for milk pricing. This is already being achieved by ensuring availability of testing machines at all milk collection centres, educating farmers to sell milk only based on testing and setting up policy norms for all players in the sector to collect milk only when it has been tested.

Another important aspect of milk pricing is the huge premium on the fat content compared to the non-fat solid content. Thus buffalo milk fetches a much higher price than cow milk, which has lower fat content. Very soon milk pricing will be based on quality in terms of somatic cell count and this will expand our export potential.

Dairy industry SWOC analysis

Within the framework of the competitiveness drivers and issues, the smallholder dairy sector's strengths, weaknesses, opportunities and challenges have been assessed. The strengths and weaknesses are factors that are directly controllable, while opportunities and challenges derive from the external environment. As evident in Table, there are a large number of weaknesses in the sector, implying considerable scope for interventions. This SWOC analysis entailed matching each of these elements with an appropriate action.

SWOC analysis of performance drivers

Strengths	How to build on them
• Large number of small and marginal farmers involved in dairying • An effective marketing channel helps to meet the demands of the urban consumer • Very large number of animals and huge scope to enhance productivity • Self-sufficiency in medicine production and do not have to rely on exports	• Strengthen economic viability of dairy farms by interventions on the input side as well as ensuring more fair farmer prices • Increase the link between rural production areas and urban markets • Focus on strengthening the indigenous breed to help significantly enhance productivity • Ensure availability of quality medicines by strengthening regulatory framework for quality
Weaknesses	**How to correct them**
• Large share of milk (70–85%) of marketable surplus goes through informal channel where quality is a big concern • Sometimes quality is an issue in the formal channel as well • Very little competition to cooperatives because private sector was not allowed to participate in until recently • Farmers do not share in the benefits of high demand because of poor governance of cooperatives • Milk production is scattered over a large number of farmers producing miniscule quantities • Milk distribution is limited to urban and peri-urban areas • Low milk prices because of lower prices declared by cooperatives, which results in low prices of milk paid by all players • Ad hoc export policies and a ban on exports • Quality of milk and milk products are a barrier to entry to the export market, especially the EU and the USA • Lack of policy focus on strengthening indigenous breeds • Non-existent extension facilities • Farmers' prices are not based on fat measurement, which affects their profitability • Because of low access to credit and risk-taking ability, farmers cannot increase their herd size	• Focus on quality issues even in the informal channel by training traders and by enforcing food quality regulations • Develop infrastructure and training for clean milk production • Support a fair playing field for the private sector • Bring about changes in cooperatives to make them true representatives of farmers instead of functioning as parastatals. • Support to dairying as an enterprise to encourage commercial dairy farming and encourage production and productivity by extension and breed development • Enhance packaged milk distribution in more areas • Strengthen dairy farmer cooperatives to enable farmers to get a higher price for milk • Create rational export policy to enable farmers to take advantage of higher prices • Strictly implement quality regulations and improve infrastructure and training for quality • Strengthen the breed development programmes • Strengthen extension facilities • Create policy regulations to make mandatory testing as a basis for setting milk price • Increase access to credit through dairy farmer organizations and other agencies

Opportunities	How to pursue them
• Increased farmer income by exploiting the high demand • Increased consumer sophistication and awareness of quality reception of quality packaged products (though slowly) • Entry of large corporations in retailing, which can lead to more investment • Immense scope to enhance governance of dairy farmer organizations and thus enable dairy farmers to demand higher prices • Potential for exports due to low cost of production • Overall positive growth environment, which is triggering the Government to enhance infrastructure	• Create policies and activities geared towards enhancing dairy farming activity by increasing, production, productivity and ensuring fair farmer price of milk • Establish enabling policy environment to enhance investment • Create policy support to enhance governance of producer companies • Focus on quality issues that are a barrier to exports • Encourage private sector to increase investment in dairying
Challenges	**How to avert them**
• Large portion of the population does not care about quality issues in milk • Because of high price sensitivity for dairy products, people are not willing to pay for quality • Significant increase in maize prices can increase feed prices • Large informal markets that extend credit are constraining farmers • Low productivity and scattered production leading to high cost of transportation • Emphasis on milk fat and not on SNF content maintaining relatively lower prices of milk	• Initiate consumer education about the negative health impacts of unpackaged products • Develop packaging in small quantities to meet the needs of the poor • Increase milk prices in accordance with feed prices • Support expansion of dairy farmer organizations • Enhance productivity by breed improvement and extension • Enforce price setting of milk based on fat and SNF content to encourage production of cow milk

Source: Meeta Punjabi, Dairy consultant, New Delhi, FAO 2009

Government role in marketing of meat

India has more than 2000 markets where livestock are traded. Livestock markets are under the jurisdiction of the state governments although the direct operation and supervision would generally fall within the purview of the local bodies. State Acts regulate marketing of agricultural produce and the marketing committees are responsible for implementing and enforcing the provisions of the Act. The market for live animals in the country unfortunately has not developed on scientific lines. There are no separate markets for different species of animals. There are no separate enclosures for different species/animals. Brokers facilitate most of the trade. Vertical linkages between the processors/butchers and livestock producers are rare. Wholesale marketing margins amount to about 30% of the consumer price. Market facilities are generally inadequate and if available are poorly maintained. Weighbridges, ramp facilities for loading and unloading, feeding and watering and veterinary facilities are not available. Revenues generated under the act are supposed to be allocated to the markets for operations and improvement but not happening. There is also need to improve retail infrastructure and educate retailers about meat and meat products. Poor infrastructure and cold chain facility are the major stumbling blocks in the path of growth. There is large scope for meat processing in poultry as well as in red meat. The meat processing industry is still nascent. India exports both frozen and fresh chilled meat needs to be improve. The value chain of meat production for the domestic market is very informal. Traders play a very active role in this value chain as intermediary aggregators as livestock owners have limited market access and are isolated from major consumers due to logistical and transport costs. Traders buy animals from various farmers and pool them for further marketing or haul purchased animals to municipal slaughterhouses. During transit of the animals from livestock markets to slaughterhouses health certificates from state veterinarians are also obtained. The animals are either sold to private abattoirs or slaughtered in the municipal slaughterhouse for a nominal fee and supplied to domestic market.

Strengths of Indian meat for export market

- Government of India has laid down standards for export of meat which includes standards for abattoirs, processing plants for various meat products. Registration of abattoirs and meat processing plants is done by the Agricultural and Processed Food Products Export Development Authority (APEDA).
- Government of India accords high priority to quality issues in meat for export. Therefore a stringent regulatory mechanism has been put in place by the Government in the form of mandatory approvals of modern abattoirs for production of meat for export. APEDA is also enforcing HACCP and approves the plants with HACCP accreditation through an interdepartmental panel.
- Animal Health Certificate: According to the current Export and Import Policy of the Government of India, each export consignment is subject to compulsory microbiological and other tests and a comprehensive pre-shipment inspection certificate is issued by a Government laboratory. Each consignment is accompanied by this health certificate. The health certificate also confirms that the livestock have been subjected to ante-mortem inspection followed by post-mortem examination, and that the meat is fit for human consumption.

- India is a member country of the International Organization for Animal Health (OIE), and is mandated to report list "A" and list "B" animal diseases to the OIE at regular intervals
- The country being free from diseases like BSE and Rinderpest has edge over several countries of the world.
- There is little practice of using hormones, antibiotics or any other chemicals to promote growth and fattening of livestock used for export purposes and the Indian meat is considered as nearly organic meat.
- Indian meat is also very competitive in international market and has created a special niche in most of the importing countries.

There is vast scope of Indian Meat Industry in both domestic and international market. Besides implementation of stringent sanitary and phyto - sanitary regulations, the strengthening of livestock and meat markets is essential to boost meat sector in the country. There is a dire need to create awareness among livestock farmers to rear their stock on scientific lines. Extension of proven research on meat animal production must be disseminated as a support to the poor entrepreneurs. The government interventions are also desired to provide platform for marketing of livestock and meat reducing the profit margins of traders so that the farmers get their substantial share. The guidelines for meat safety have been developed but their stringent implementation by Food Safety and Standard Authority of India (FSSAI) especially for domestic markets will win the confidence of consumer and certainly will help in boost the sector.

Other regulations for slaughter and disposal

Some other rules for slaughtering of animals and proper disposal of slaughterhouse waste may be listed as follows:

- No pregnant animal to be slaughtered. The meat animal must be certified healthy and free from disease by a municipal veterinarian before being slaughtered for meat. No cattle under the age of 16 to be killed.
- No animal to be slaughtered except at a municipal or registered slaughterhouse (state muiucipal acts, e.g., Section 415 of the Delhi Municipal Corporation Act, 1957).
- In localities where a municipal slaughterhouse exists, such as Idgah (in Delhi) or Deonar (in Mumbai), it is illegal for animals to be killed anywhere else (state municipal acts, e.g.. Section 407 of the Delhi Municipal Corporation Act).

- Under a notification dated 31st August 1978 by the Ministry of Civil Aviation, it is illegal to slaughter or to deposit slaughterhouse waste within a radius of 10 km from an airport.
- Under the Water Pollution Act, it is illegal for slaughterhouse waste to be deposited into any water resource.
- No person can, in any public place or public street, carry meat exposed to public view (state municipal acts, e.g.. Section 397 of the Delhi Municipal Act).
- Under the ISI, animals must be rested for 24 hours, given abundant water and rendered unconscious before slaughtering.
- All licensed butcher shops are required to follow the ISI code of health and hygiene standards
- The butcher shop must have a proper waste disposal facility. Blood cannot be sent down public drains.

Government role in marketing of egg

(**Source:** National Action Plan for Egg & Poultry-2022 For Doubling Farmers' Income by 2022, Department of Animal Husbandry, Dairying & Fisheries Ministry of Agriculture & Farmers Welfare Government of India)

The egg production in the country has increased from around 83 billion nos. in 2015-16 to 100 billion in 2019 registering a share of about 6.2% to the global production (FAO, 2019). The per capita availability of egg has increased from 61 in 2013-14 to 79 in 2019 (https://www.ceicdata.com). Regarding the World Players in Egg Production, India is currently 3rd in egg production in the world (as per FAO 2014). China holds the first position followed by U.S.A, India, Mexico, Japan.

Relevant Acts promulgated by DADF, GoI

i. The Prevention & Control of Infectious and Contagious Disease in Animals Act, 2009 to regulate disease transmission from one state to other with the objectives:

ii. Indian Veterinary Council Act, 1984 regulates Veterinary Practice and Education

iii. Importation of Livestock and Livestock products are regulated by the Livestock Importation Act, 1898

Other Acts, Rules & Regulation

i. Food Safety & Standards Act, 2006

ii. Quality Control of Food Products of Animal Origin (Export-oriented)

iii. Residue Monitoring Plan (export-oriented)

iv. Agreement on Sanitary and Phyto-sanitary Measures (Global Trade-Oriented)

v. Bureau of Indian Standards (BIS) & ISO 22000:2005

vi. APMC model Act, 2017

vii. The Prevention of Cruelty to Animals Act, 1960

viii. The Export (Quality Control and Inspection) ACT, 1963

16

Trade Performance of Livestock Sector in India

Export and import- an overview

The major thrust of livestock development strategy in India has been on achieving self-sufficiency in livestock products through import substitution. Several initiatives were taken to develop the Indian livestock sector in the past and India emerged as the largest milk producer in the world and it is also one of the largest producers of other livestock commodities. However, the economic policy reforms and economic liberalization triggered in 1991 have widened market opportunities for the livestock sector. The global demand for livestock products is also on the rise. Such developments offer an opportunity for India to increase its livestock exports, especially for products like bovine meat, whose domestic demand is low. With improved domestic production and marketing efficiency, better access to expanding world market, India has the potential to become more competitive and may augment port of livestock products. The export and import details reveal that there has been a steady increase in the value of imports and exports of livestock and livestock products in India.

Trade: (GAIN Report 2019)

The Department of Commerce of the GOI's Ministry of Commerce and Industry uses its foreign trade policy to regulate trade of livestock and livestock products. The Department of Animal Husbandry and Dairying (DAHD), now under a separate Ministry of Fisheries, Animal Husbandry and Dairying (following May 2019 general elections) regulates imports of livestock and livestock products in accordance with provision of Section 3 and Section 3A of the Livestock Importation Act, 1898 in order to prevent entry of exotic diseases though import of such livestock and livestock products. Also, please note that beef is regarded as being separate and distinct from carabeef, or water buffalo meat. India still prohibits the export and import of beef since cattle slaughter is banned in most Indian states due to religious sensitivities.

Imports

The import of live animals is subject to restrictions: an importer must obtain a license from the Director General of Foreign Trade (DGFT). The DGFT issues licenses based on the recommendation of DAHD after examining the proposal and conducting a risk analysis. Similarly, the import of livestock products is governed by an "open general license" (OGL) but subject to a requisite sanitary import permit (SIP), which is issued following performance of a risk analysis (per internationally recognized scientific principles) and receipt of a veterinary certificate certified by an exporting country's competent authority. The SIP is valid from 6 months to a year (Source: DAHD). Sanitary Import Permit (SIP) for Livestock Products The DAHD has constituted a Committee on Risk Analysis under the Chairmanship of Joint Secretary (Trade) with all the Joint Secretaries as its members to consider the applications received for issuance of SIP to import various livestock products After necessary amendment in the notification S.O. 2666 (E) dated 16.10.2014, the Department has launched the website, https://sip.nic.in, for online submission of SIP applications and issuance of SIPs to various firms/organizations engaged in activities of import of livestock products. The procedure for submission of online SIP application along with the relevant information regarding sanitary requirements is also available on the Department's website www.dahd.nic.in. The SIP applications received are examined and a risk analysis is undertaken by the technical experts of the DAHD basis scientific evidence and World Organization for Animal Health (OIE) regulations. The recommendations of the technical experts are considered by the Risk Analysis Committee to either reject the application or issue the SIP. Aggrieved applicants can seek a review of the decision of the Risk Analysis Committee through filing a review/representation request addressed to the Joint Secretary (Trade) (as outlined in DAHD Annual Report 2018-19).

Indian import certification requirements and documentation for livestock and livestock products is updated below and available at the following link trade. Tariffs for selected livestock products are in Table 1 below (updated recently). Also, please find below hyperlinks to certain import procedures and guidelines related to livestock and livestock products:

Exports

All exported meat products must be processed in abattoirs and meat processing plants registered with the Agricultural and Processed Food Products Export Development Authority (APEDA). Export shipments are subject to compulsory microbiological and other testing for the issuance of animal health certificates by the certified GOI agency. India exports only frozen boneless carabeef, which is mostly thawed and resold in wet markets. In addition to direct consumption, some of the carabeef is processed and consumed as sausage, salami, and burgers. Indian carabeef is preferred due to its affordability, leanness, and halal characteristics, which contrast with traditional beef supplies. Per most recent 2019 trade data (Jan-June, value basis), India is the third largest exporter of (boneless) carabeef and beef, after Australia and Brazil, and followed by New Zealand, the Netherlands, and Ireland. The top five destinations for Indian carabeef exports were Vietnam, Malaysia, Egypt, Indonesia, and Iraq (in descending order). Interestingly, exports from Australia and Brazil were destined for developed markets such as the United States, Japan, China, and the UK, while Indian sales were destined for developing countries, which are mostly price sensitive markets

Additionally, the Food Safety and Standards Authority of India (FSSAI) regulates domestic slaughter and meat processing through the regulation entitled Food Safety and Standards Rules and Regulation, 2011 (FSSR). The FSSR also defines standards and regulations for domestic and imported meat products.

Export of egg and poultry / products

i. Major items exported are table eggs, egg powder, hatching eggs, SPF eggs, live birds, and poultry meat. India has exported 6,59,304.15 MT of Poultry products to the world for the worth of Rs. 768.72 crores during the year 2015- 16 (APEDA, 2017). The strength of exports mainly lies in the competitive cost of production, proximity to international markets and successful regaining of freedom from Highly Pathogenic Avian Influenza (HPAI).

ii. Although some efforts have been made to increase Poultry exports from India, the trade is very small in comparison to the global trade. At present the exports are mainly in table eggs, hatching eggs, frozen eggs, egg powder, and to a small extent for live poultry.

iii. Our major markets are Middle East and Asia. Egg powder is also sent to Japan and in EU. Now we have extended exports to many African countries. We have infrastructure to handle egg exports and we also have primary packing materials and the full logistics cold chain to deliver top quality fresh eggs to all our customers.

iv. Total World Trade Poultry Meat Production - around 90 MMT; Trade (Exports- 11 MMT- around 12% of total production) Egg production- around 1400 billion eggs / 70 MMT; Trade around 10%- 7 MMT

Strategy for exports through value-addition

The production of meat and meat products has shown an impressive growth. The total meat production in the country is 7.4 million tonnes, which includes beef, buffalo meat, mutton, goat meat, pork and poultry meat. However, less than one per cent of the total meat is converted into value-added products like sausages, ham bacon, luncheon meat, kababs and meatballs. As per the "Strategy paper for augmenting exports of value-added products" submitted to APEDA in 2015 by IL&FS, the level of exports of meat and meat products from India is $190 million, the major destinations being the countries in the Middle-East and South-East Asia. The above study undertook a trend analysis of 130 product categories including poultry and poultry products over a period of five years 2009- 2014.

The trend analysis comprised of the following five parameters

(a) Compounded Annual Growth Rate for Volume in Metric Tons

(b) Average Volume of Trade in Metric Tons

(c) Compounded Annual Growth Rate for Value in percentage

(d) Average Value of Trade in Metric Tons

(e) Export Value per Metric Ton. The unit used is Rupees Lakhs.

The above analysis enabled identification of the key products which showed a substantial positive growth. Therefore, as a strategy we are targeting nearly 2% coverage of world trade volume for: (a) eggs which is estimated to be around 3 billion eggs (from present around 0.6 billion) (b) meat which is estimated to be around 250 thousand ton eggs (from present around 5.5 thousand tonnes).

GATT

- General Agreement on Tariffs and Trade (typically abbreviated GATT) was the outcome of the failure of negotiating governments to create the (ITO).
- GATT was formed in 1947 and lasted until 1994, when it was replaced by the World Trade Organization during the final round of negotiations in early 1990s.

Introduction

In the early 1990s Government of India introduced major trade policy reforms which favoured increased privatisation and liberalization of all sectors of the economy. Livestock sector was no exception to this. The second related development was India's signing of the Uruguay Round Agreement (URA) of the General Agreement on Tariffs and Trade (GATT) in 1994, which was rechristened as World Trade Organization. The world trade in livestock products, mainly dairy and poultry has been distorted for decades by both domestic and border prices. Most of the developing countries provide heavy export subsidies to increase their exports, which creates unhealthy competition in the world market. No other nation in the world has as much potential as India to emerge as one of the world market leaders for export of milk products. Meeting domestic consumption growth and export demand also poses a challenge for the Indian livestock sector. To capture the demand-led growth opportunities in livestock sector, policy review is required to improve the quality and safety of livestock products food chain from farmer to consumer confirming with international standards.

World trade organisation agreements

The global trade follows the guidelines of the World Trade Organization (WTO). WTO Agreements were signed in 1994, and their implementation started from January 1995. The WTO agreement that directly deals with food and agriculture is the Agreement on Agriculture (AoA). The objective of AoA is to reform trade in the agriculture sector and to make policies more market oriented. Developing countries have hoped that it would open up export market in developed countries by removing trade distortions. But the standards of the food products cannot be ascertained with physical inspection alone. It involves sophisticated instruments and advanced technology. Sometimes, imperfections, presence of toxins or pathogens cannot be detected at earlier stages. Due to this reason, along with AoA, two other agreements namely Sanitary and Phytosanitary measures and Technical Barriers to Trade was introduced aiming to address these concerns.

India has competitive advantage in primary production of many products on one hand, but their exports are constrained by low level of processing, distortions in world trade and stringent food safety norms in the international market. At the same time, there is imminent threat of cheap imports from European Union and America, who heavily protect their livestock industry through subsidies and market support measures. The capacity of India to penetrate world markets depends on its ability to meet increasingly stringent food safety standards imposed in developed countries.

Sanitary and phytosanitary measures (SPS)

Sanitary and Phytosanitary standards are governed and enforced through number of laws and agencies in India. The Prevention of Food Adulteration Act, 1954 is the main law on food safety and food quality, and it takes account of the livestock commodities also. SPS agreement is meant to promote smooth flow of trade between two countries. The SPS agreement interrelates with other WTO agreements and applies only between WTO member countries. It is between nations that agree not to use SPS measures as an unjustified barrier in trade. SPS measures protect human life from risks arising from additives, contaminants, toxins or disease causing organism in their body, plant or animal carried disease. It protects animal or plant life from pests, diseases or disease causing organism and prevent or limit damage to a country from the entry, establishment or spread of pests. The measures followed to protect human and animal health are objectively based on scientific principles. The SPS measures use Codex Alimentarius Commission (CAC) as a basis for decisions to be made regarding food safety. CAC is an intergovernmental body under the joint sponsorship of the Food and Agriculture Organisation and World Health Organisation. TBT agreement covers the aspects of product specification which include size, shape, weight and packing material requirement including labelling and safety handling. It should be noted that SPS measures deal only with agricultural and food sectors while TBT measures refer to all products, food as well as non-food products. WTO has recognised the standards set by Codex Alimentarius Commission and International Office of Epizootics (OIE) as a reference for food safety and animal health in global trade. The focus of codex standards is to ensure quality and food safety for human consumption. The Codex standards include Hazard Analysis and Critical Control Point (HACCP) system and International Organisation of Standardisation to ensure that livestock products are safe for human consumption. The focus of OIE requirements is animal health related concerns.

Value of import and export of livestock and livestock products

(Rs in Lakhs)

Broad groups	2017-18	2018-19
Livestock	5655	6262
Meat and Edible Meat Offal	2999	3179
Dairy and Poultry Products and Honey	30288	22869
Animal Fodder and Feed	355811	447934
Raw hide and skins & Leather	396771	406558
Raw Wool and Animal Hair	222396	267921
All Groups (Total)	1013920	1154722
India's Total Import	30,01,01,573	35,94,67,461

Broad groups	2017-18	2018-19
Livestock	41148	29809
Meat and Edible Meat Offal	2692150	2603392
Dairy and Poultry Products and Honey	235376	377324
Animal Fodder and Feed	940570	1341335
Raw hide and skins & Leather	563669	504837
Raw Wool and Animal Hair	105976	139017
All Groups (Total)	4579890	4995714
India's Total Export	19,55,54,112	23,07,72,619

Sources: Basic Animal Husbandry Statistics, 2019

Export of livestock products

Quantity in MT

Value in Rs. crore

Product	Qty	Rs. in Crore
Buffalo Meat	805048.08	17621.82
Dairy Products	35143.32	1037.17
Natural Honey	42376.94	480.51
Animal Casings	9603.30	322.05
Poultry Products	178308.04	314.29
Sheep/Goat Meat	5163.80	239.00
Processed Meat	472.33	8.01
Other Meat	362.87	6.89
Total	1,076,478.68	20,029.74

Sources: The Agricultural and Processed Food Products Export Development Authority (APEDA)

Import of livestock products

Quantity in MT

Value in Rs. crore

Product	Qty	Rs. in Crore
Dairy Products	16163.40	329.33
Poultry Products	0.00	23.75
Other Meat	345.00	12.71
Processed Meat	123.00	4.86
Sheep/Goat Meat	10.00	0.77
Total		371.42

Sources: The Agricultural and Processed Food Products Export Development Authority (APEDA)

Part D
Livestock Entrepreneurship

17

Entrepreneur and Entrepreneurship

Entrepreneur - Derived from French verb *enterprendre meaning "to undertake"*.

The entrepreneur as a person brings in overall change through, innovation-for the maximum social good. Human values remain sacred and inspire him to serve society. He has firm belief in social betterment and he carries out this responsibility with conviction. In this process, he accelerates personal, economic as well as human- development.

The entrepreneur is a visionary and an integrated man with outstanding leadership qualities. With a desire to excel, he gives top priority to Research and Development. He always works for the well being of the society. More importantly entrepreneurial activities encompass all fields / sectors and foster a spirit of enterprise for the welfare of mankind. **Urges of an Entrepreneur**

An urge to exercise powers over things and objects persists among all human beings. The urge may vary in degree from person to person. This urge is an intrinsic quality of an entrepreneur. Sociologists consider him as a sensitive energizer in the modernization of societies.

The entrepreneur is a critical factor in the socio-economic change. He is the key person who envisages new opportunities, new techniques, new lines of production, new products and coordinates all other activities. The true entrepreneur is one who is endowed with more than average capacities in the task of organizing and coordinating the various other factors of production. He should be a pioneer, a captain of industry. The supply of such entrepreneurship is however quite limited and enterprise in general consists of several grades of organizational skill and capability. The more efficient entrepreneurs receive a surplus reward over and above the managerial wages and this sum constitutes true profit ascribable to superior talent.

New concept of entrepreneur

The term "entrepreneur" has been defined as one who detects and evaluates a new situation in his environment and directs the making of such adjustments in the economic systems, as he deems necessary. He conceives of an industrial enterprise for the purpose, displays considerable initiative, grit and determination in bringing his project to fruition, and in this process, performs one or more of the following:

1. Perceives opportunities for profitable investments
2. Explores the prospects of starting such a manufacturing enterprise
3. Obtains necessary industrial licenses
4. Arranges initial capital
5. Provides personal guarantees to the financial institutions
6. Promises to meet the shortfalls in the capital; and Co
7. Supplies technical know-how.

Entrepreneurship may be defined in various ways, but the four key elements involved in it are:

1. Innovation
2. Risk-taking
3. Vision, and
4. Organizing skill.

All the four elements are inter-related and form a continuous process in business. Entrepreneurial vision encompasses the relentless pursuit for operational excellence, innovative technology and being responsive to the needs of the market place.

Importance of an entrepreneur

The Entrepreneur is one of the most important inputs in the economic development of a country or of regions within the country. Entrepreneurial competence makes all the difference in the rate of economic growth. In India, State and private entrepreneurship co-exist. The small-scale industrial sector and business are left completely to private entrepreneurs. It is in this context that an increasingly important role has been assigned to the identification and promotion of entrepreneurs for this sector.

The need for a broad-based entrepreneurial class in India arises from the need to speed up the process of activating the factors of production, leading to a higher rate of economic growth, dispersal of economic activities, development of backward and tribal areas, creation of employment opportunities, improvement in the standard of living of the weaker sections of the society and involvement of all sections of the society in the process of growth. Several factors go into the making of an entrepreneur. Individuals who initiate, establish, maintain and expand new enterprises constitute the entrepreneurial class. The social-political and economic conditions, the availability of industrial technology and know-how, state of art and culture of business and trading, existence of markets for products and services and the incentives and facilities available for starting an industry or business, all have a bearing on the growth of entrepreneurship. A conducive environment is created through the policies and interest of the government in economic and industrial development.

According to Bahal- Entrepreneurship does the process of change comprise the following three behavioural components.

- The identification, evaluation and exploitation of an opportunity
- The management of new and transformed organisation so as to facilitate production and marketing of new goods and services
- The creation of value through successful exploitation of new idea (i.e innovation)

According to Cole: Entrepreneurship comprises any purposeful activity that initiates, maintain or develop a profit oriented business in interaction with internal situation of the business, or with the economical, political and social circumstances surrounding the business

Importance and scope of livestock entrepreneurship

- Create employment opportunities
- Increase production
- Economic development of national or region
- Disposal of economic activities
- Improving standards of living of weaker sections

18

Entrepreneur

Entrepreneur is a person who takes the responsibility of initiating and establishing an enterprise or an organisation under conditions of uncertainty.

Some of the essential qualities of entrepreneurs are as follows

1. Creativity
2. Passion
3. Motivation
4. Product or service knowledge
5. Ability to network
6. Self-confidence
7. Optimism
8. Vision
9. Goal mindset
10. Risk-taking
11. Persuasiveness
12. Decision-making
13. Tenacity
14. Money management
15. Adaptability

1. Creativity

Becoming an entrepreneur starts with an idea. You need to see opportunities, find innovative ways to do things and bring solutions to the public. To improve your creativity, develop habits that support the creative system. Think about what makes you feel creative, such as music, meeting people, reading or some other activity. Dedicate a specific part of your day to find inspiration for new solutions. During this part of the day, start by doing what inspires you, then let your mind flow. You can make a list of ideas and select some to pursue.

2. Passion

Passion is what drives entrepreneurs. They usually love what they do, and this helps them invest their time in their projects. To become a more passionate entrepreneur, focus on the meaning of your work. Remember that you contribute to finding solutions that will help many people. Knowing that your commitment makes an impact may give you the drive you need to continue when doubt settles in or when the business gets difficult. Passion is what keeps you focused on your objective.

3. Motivation

Motivation is the will to accomplish certain things. Entrepreneurs are driven to make their business a success and push themselves. To increase motivation, you can start by setting small goals. Small goals can help you reach larger ones and encourage you to aim higher. Recognize the work already accomplished and celebrate your results, even minor ones. Also, keep a positive mindset. Turn your mind away from negativity and daily obstacles to focus on what you want to achieve and the positive aspects of your life.

4. Product or service knowledge

Entrepreneurs know what they have to offer and to whom they can sell it. Clearly define the category of products or services you sell and how they provide value to consumers. Also, study your target clients to make sure you answer their needs. This will allow you to improve your offer continuously so you can stay on top of industry trends. To increase the positive impact of this knowledge, you should continually learn about your market, understand what people need and know the features that differentiate you from competitors. Talk with your clients and use their feedback. With this information, you can adjust your position when necessary.

5. Ability to network

The ability to connect with people and to recognize opportunities for partnership is crucial to successful entrepreneurship. Meeting new people might facilitate access to resources or knowledge that your business needs. It allows you to learn from the success of others, promote your services or goods and meet new clients. To improve your networking skills, you must try to build genuine relationships. You likely have a business goal in mind, but approach people with the objective of a human connection, just like making new friends. If you meet someone who could benefit another person in your network, connect them. Not only will you help someone, but they will probably remember you and want to return the favor.

6. Self-confidence

Entrepreneurs believe they can achieve their goals. They may have doubt, but they persevere through it. They are ready to invest the necessary work because they are confident they can create something better than what already exists. Self-confidence is essential because it allows you to feel better and makes it easier to overcome challenges, take risks and be persistent. Therefore, it contributes to your success overall. To improve self-confidence, you can use the technique of visualization. Visualize yourself as the person you want to be and visualize your business at a stage you would be proud of. You can also practice affirmation by saying uplifting statements about your accomplishments. These techniques can help to change the way you see yourself positively.

7. Optimism

Entrepreneurs are dreamers with a plan in place: They see the positive side of the situation and always move forward. Optimism supports creativity, so it helps business leaders finding new ideas for their products or services and increases their chances of success. To develop your optimism, you can consider challenges as opportunities to grow instead of problems that could stop you. Keep the end goal in mind, and don't dwell on past issues.

8. Vision

Entrepreneurs have vision. They see a big picture they wish to accomplish, which fuels their efforts and pushes them to do more. Moreover, vision is what defines the culture and identity of an organization. Not only does it keep entrepreneurs energized, but it allows them to motivate others and keep them working towards the company's success. To improve your entrepreneurship vision, you can implement a daily action plan. Prioritizing your tasks can keep you from feeling overwhelmed and help you stick to your vision. Also, listen to or read uplifting content to fortify your mind and stay focused on your purpose.

9. Goal mindset

Entrepreneurs are goal oriented. They know what they want to achieve, set a goal and work toward that objective. Determination is vital to overcome possible challenges, and it also inspires trust from the people who work with you. To become more goal-oriented, you can start by identifying what you want to accomplish and clarifying your vision of the future. Then, set a goal with a timeline to guide your actions. This will allow you to witness your progression and help keep you committed to your goal.

10. Risk-taking

Entrepreneurs are ready to take risks. They plan for the unknown so they can make calculated decisions that are profitable for them and their business. To increase your risk-taking abilities, you can start considering your journey as a learning process, including the possible failures. You must keep your goal in mind and commit to persevering. It is essential to take some risks to differentiate from your competition and allow your business to succeed. Once you know how you can manage risk and grow from disappointments, you may become more comfortable with challenging yourself.

11. Persuasiveness

Entrepreneurs know their business and how to talk about it to people. They need to persuade others to believe in their idea. To improve your persuasion skills, learn about your listeners and adapt to their personality. You can share a story to reach them on an emotional level and show your passion. If people can relate to your story, it creates a connection that can grow into loyalty, which is essential for your business success. Another tip is to share your accomplishments and rely on facts to support your arguments and convince people.

12. Decision-making

Entrepreneurs need to make quick decisions and take action for the success of their business. To improve your decision-making skills, you can inform yourself to understand better the problems you try to solve. Assess the impact of the decision you need to make, and allow a corresponding amount of time to decide. You can also narrow your options to ease the process of making a decision.

13. Tenacity

Entrepreneurs overcome challenges. They persevere through difficulties and hold on to their goals and dreams. To improve your tenacity, you can write down your goals and read them every day. You can choose role models and remember great figures of history who had to persevere through failure before they achieved success.

14. Money management

Entrepreneurs need to understand the financial situation of their business. Even if they hire a specialist like an accountant, they are the decision-maker and must know their situation to run the business successfully. You can improve your basic money management skills by preparing a budget and committing to it and investing available funds rather than spending them. You can also acquire more financial knowledge by taking classes or training programs.

15. Adaptability

When they start a business, entrepreneurs often need to multitask. Flexibility in your schedule, as well as in your thinking, is crucial to continue growing in challenging situations. To increase your adaptability, you can approach all activities with an open mind and stay ready to change your ways if necessary. Try new methods and welcome new trends to foster your ability to adapt.

Types of entrepreneur

I. According to the type of business

1. **Business Entrepreneur:** Business entrepreneurs are individuals who conceive an idea for a new product or service and-then creates a business to materialize their idea into reality. They tap both production and marketing' resources in their search to develop a new business opportunity.
2. **Trading Entrepreneur:** Trading entrepreneur is one who undertakes trading activities and is not concerned with the manufacturing work. He identifies potential markets, stimulates demand for his product line and creates a desire and interest among buyers to go in for his product.
3. **Industrial Entrepreneur:** Industrial entrepreneur is essentially a manufacturer, who identifies the potential needs of customers and tailors a product or service to meet the marketing needs. He is a product-oriented man who starts in an industrial unit because of the possibility of making some new product.
4. **Corporate Entrepreneur:** Corporate entrepreneur is a person who demonstrates his innovative skill in organizing and managing corporate undertaking. A corporate undertaking is a form of business' organization, which is registered under some statute or Act, which gives it a separate legal entity.
5. **Agricultural Entrepreneur:** Agricultural entrepreneurs are those entrepreneurs who undertake agricultural activities as raising and marketing of crops, fertilisers and other inputs of agriculture.

II. According to the technology use

1. **Technical Entrepreneur:** A technical entrepreneur is essentially compared to a "craftsman." He develops improved quality of goods because of his craftsmanship. He concentrates more on production than marketing.

2. **Non-technical Entrepreneur:** Non-technical entrepreneurs are those who are not concerned with the technical aspects of the product in which they deal. They are concerned only with developing alternative marketing and distribution strategies to promote their business.

3. **Professional Entrepreneur:** Professional entrepreneur is a person who is interested in establishing a business, but does not have interest in managing or operating it once it is established.

III. According to the entrepreneur and motivation

1. **Pure Entrepreneur:** A pure entrepreneur is an individual who is motivated by psychological and economic rewards. He undertakes an entrepreneurial activity for his personal satisfaction in work.

2. **Induced Entrepreneur:** Induced entrepreneur is one who is induced to take up an entrepreneurial task due to the policy measures of the government that provides assistance, Incentives, concessions and necessary overhead, facilities to start a venture.

3. **Motivated Entrepreneur:** New entrepreneurs are motivated by the desire for self-fulfillment. They come into being because of the possibility of making and marketing some new product for the use of consumers. If the product is developed to a saleable stage, the entrepreneur is further motivated by reward in terms of profit.

4. **Spontaneous Entrepreneur:** These entrepreneurs start their business their by Entrepreneur. They are persons with initiative, boldness and confidence in their ability, which activate, them, underage entrepreneurial activity. Such entrepreneurs have a strong conviction and confidence in their inborn ability.

Clarence Danhof classifies entrepreneurs into four types

1. **Innovative:** This category of entrepreneurs is characterized by innovativeness. Innovative entrepreneurs refer to those who introduce new combinations of factors of production. This category of entrepreneurs visualizes the opportunity and introduces novel ideas, combinations into the production process. They may develop new ideas, concepts, application of new technology, and find new market.

2. **Imitative:** This set of entrepreneurs adopts and imitate the innovations and business policies introduced by the innovative entrepreneurs. They are also referred to as adoptive entrepreneurs. These types of entrepreneurs imitate the entrepreneurs and follow similar entrepreneurial pursuit. They imitate the technology and methods that are found successful. Usually in developing economies and LDCs, this class of entrepreneurs is very useful as because the entrepreneurs of these countries find it difficult to bear the high cost involved in the process of innovation. Imitative entrepreneurs significantly contribute in the growth of enterprise in developing countries.

3. **Fabian:** These categories of entrepreneurs usually imitate other innovations only when they are certain that failure to do so would be detrimental for their business. They are very much doubtful and skeptic in their approach towards adopting new technology or trade. This set of entrepreneurs is not dynamic and adaptive. They are often cautious about their moves.

4. **Drone:** Drone entrepreneurs refer to the type of entrepreneurs who are very traditional, orthodox and conservative in outlook. They are very keen in retaining their traditional business and traditional machinery or systems of the business. They are contented with their existing technology of production despite of changes in the business environment and society. Drone entrepreneurs are usually reluctant to adopt the changes.

Arthur Harrison. Cole Classification

Actually, Arthur H. Cole had divided the history of American entrepreneurship into three stages of entrepreneurial thought process – Empirical stage (from scratch to 1860), Rational stage (1860-1890) and Cognitive stage (from 1890 onwards).

1. **Empirical**: This category of entrepreneurs rarely introduce anything radical, innovative or revolutionary. They are guided by the principle of rule of thumb.

2. **Rational**: The rational entrepreneurs have the information and are aware about the business environment. They understand the prevailing economic conditions and are ready to introduce modifications when necessary.

3. **Cognitive**: Cognitive entrepreneurs are sophisticated. They have experts to advise them and acts upon accordingly. They introduce changes

whenever necessary. These changes may completely break from the existing scheme of enterprise.

Basis of ownership

1. **Private**: Private entrepreneur is motivated by profit and it would not enter those sectors of the economy in which prospects of monetary rewards are not very bright.
2. **Public** Entrepreneurship: In the undeveloped countries Government will take the initiative to start an enterprise where capital requirements are very high and returns are less with longer pay backperiod .

Based on the scale of enterprise

1. **Small Scale**: This classification is very popular in the developing countries. In India, small scale enterprise is defined as an industrial undertaking in which the investment in fixed assets in farm buildings/ animals/plant and machinery does not exceed Rs. 10 million. Small entrepreneurs do not possess the necessary talents and resources to imitate large scale production and introduce revolutionary technological changes.
2. **Large Scale**: In the developed countries large scale enterprises are in greater numbers. They posses the necessary financial and managerial capabilities to initiate and introduce new technical changes. The result is that the developed countries are able to develop and sustain a high level of technical progress.(Layer farms in India have now become large scale investment).

Based on stages of eevelopment

1. **First Generation Entrepreneur:** First generation entrepreneur are those entrepreneurs who do not possess any entrepreneurial background. They start an industrial unit by means of their own innovative skills.
2. **Second Generation Entrepreneur:** Second generation entrepreneur are those entrepreneurs who inherit the family business firms and pass it from one generation to another.
3. **Classical Entrepreneur:** A classical entrepreneur is a stereotype entrepreneur whose aim is to maximize his economic returns at a level consistent with the survival of the unit but with or without an element of growth.

Difference Between Entrepreneur and Manager:

Basis for Comparison	Entrepreneur	Manager
Meaning	Entrepreneur refers to a person who creates an enterprise, by taking financial risk in order to get profit.	Manager is an individual who takes the responsibility of controlling and administering the organization.
Focus	Business startup	Ongoing operations
Primary motivation	Achievement	Power
Approach to task	Informal	Formal
Status	Owner	Employee
Reward	Profit	Salary
Decision making	Intuitive	Calculative
Driving force	Creativity and Innovation	Preserving status quo
Risk orientation	Risk taker	Risk averse

19

Theories and Forms of Entrepreneurship

Theories of entrepreneurship

1. An economic theory
2. Leibensteon's X-efficiency theory
3. Dynamic entrepreneurship innovation theory
4. Harvard School theory
5. Theory of high achievement
6. Theory of change
7. Theory of profit
8. Theory of adjustment of price
9. Theory of market
10. Theory of social change
11. Theory of entrepreneurial supply
12. Theory of personal resourcefulness
13. Theory of cultural values

1. An economic theory

Mark Casson- emphasised that the demand for entrepreneurship stems from the need to adjust to change, and that the supply of entrepreneurship is limited firstly, by the scarcity of the requisite personal quality, and secondly, by the difficulty of identifying them when they are available. He suggested that there are four main qualities which are crucial for successful entrepreneur – main one is imagination

2. Leibensteon's X-efficiency theory

X-efficiency is the degree of inefficiency in the use of resources within the firm: it measures the extent to which the firm fails to realise its productive potential.

- Leibensteon identified two main role of entrepreneur. First role- input completion, which involve making available inputs that improves the efficiency of existing production methods or facilitate the introduction of new ones
- Second one- gap filling, is closing asking to the arbitrage function emphasised by Kirzner. Leibensteon provides a vivid description of gap filling, visualising the economy as a net made up of notes and pathways.

3. Dynamic entrepreneurship innovation theory

Schumpetet considered entrepreneurship as the catalyst that disrupts the stationary circular flow of economy and thereby initiates and sustains the process of development.

Embarking upon 'new combinations' of factors of production- which he succinctly terms innovation – the entrepreneur activates the economy to new level of development.

Five functions of this innovation are

- Introduction of new goods
- Introduction of new method of production
- Opening of new markets
- Conquest of new source of supply of raw material
- Carrying out of new organisation of any industry

4. Harvard school theory

- Entrepreneurship comprises any purposeful activity that initiate, maintain or develop a profit- oriented business in interaction with the internal situation of the business or with economic, political and social circumstances surrounding the business.

Emphasis on two activities

- Organisation or coordination activities
- Sensitivity to the environmental characteristics that affect decision making

5. Theory of high achievement

McClelland identified two characteristics of entrepreneurship, namely, doing things in a better way and 'decision-making under uncertainty'.

He stressed the need for achievement or achievement orientation as the most directly relevant factor for explaining economic behaviour. This motive is defined as the tendency to strive for success in situations involving an evaluation of ones performance in relation some standard of excellence.

6. Theory of change

- Young's theory is a theory of change based on society's incorporation of reactive subgroups. A group become reactive when the following three conditions coincide:
- When a group experiences low social status
- When denied access to important social networks
- When the group has a better institutional resources than other groups in the society at the same level

7. Theory of profit

Knight identifies the entrepreneur as a recipient of pure profit

- Pure profit, according to him, with regard to the entrepreneur, is bearing the cost of uncertainty.
- Argue that business uncertainty can be reduced through 'consolidation'
- Consolidation is to uncertainty what insurance to risk: it is a method of reducing total uncertainty by pooling individual instances.

8. Theory of adjustment of price

- Kirzner- the adjustment of price is the main role of entrepreneur. If wrong price prevails in the market, then an opportunity for profit is created somewhere in the market if a frustrated buyer or seller is willing to pay higher or lower price respectively.
- If different prices prevail in the same market, there is a scope for profitable arbitrage between two segments of market.

9. Theory of market

- Hayek's pointed the absence of entrepreneurs in neo-classical economics is intimately associated with the assumption of market equilibrium.

- This equilibrium is equal to availability of complete market information
- For him, the empirical content of economics is related to the process of adjustment towards an equilibrium
- This process involves the acquisition and communication of knowledge.
- Markets help the people to communicate their discoveries to others and learn of discoveries, their by moving towards a sale of equilibrium.

10. Theory of social change

- Everett Hagen, in his work 'theory of social change: how economic growth begins., mediates on the its psychological explanation. His creative personality is an individual characterised by a high need for achievement, order and autonomy. He views the entrepreneur as a creative problem solver interested in things in the practical and technological realm, and driven by a duty to achieve.
- He considers the withdrawal of status, of respect, as the trigger mechanism for changes in personality formation.

11. Theory of entrepreneurial supply

- This theory was proposed by John Kunkal
- This behaviour model is concerned with the overtly expressed activities of individuals and their relation to fast and present, and surrounding social structure and physical conditions
- His theory is based upon experimental psychology, identifying social variables as the determinants of entrepreneurial supply

12. Theory of personal resourcefulness

- The root of entrepreneurial process can be traced to the initiative taken by some individual to go beyond the existing way of life. The emphasis is on initiative (innovation) rather than reaction, although events in the environment may have been provided the trigger for the person to express initiation
- The personal resourcefulness in this contest is the belief in one's own capability of initiating actions directed towards creation and growth of enterprises.
- Such initiating process requires cognitive mediated self regulation of internal feelings and emotions, thought and actions.

13. Theory of cultural values

- According to Thomas Cochran's theory cultural values, role expectations and social sanctions are key elements of entrepreneurship.
- The performance of entrepreneur will generally influenced by:
- His attitude towards his occupation
- The role expectations held by sanctioning group
- The operational requirements of the job

The Schools of entrepreneurial thought

Macro view

- The macro view of entrepreneurship emphasize on external factors that are beyond the control of the individual entrepreneur.
- In macro view there are three schools of entrepreneurial thought
  - The environmental school of thought,
  - The financial/capital school of thought, and
  - The displacement school of thought.

The Environmental school of thought

- This school of thought says that external factors/forces affect the development of potential entrepreneur's lifestyle. These can be either positive or negative forces in the molding of entrepreneurial desires.
- Here, the focus is on institutions, values, and mores that, grouped together, form a sociopolitical environmental framework that strongly influences the development of entrepreneurs.

The Financial/capital school of thought

- This school of thought emphasis on the capital seeking process where the search for seed and growth capital, venture capital process, financial management is the important focus for the entrepreneur's development.

The Displacement school of thought

- The displacement school of thought focuses on the negative side of group phenomena. It holds that the group hinders a person from advancing or eliminates certain critical factors needed for that person to advance.

- Individual will be forced into an entrepreneurial pursuit unless they are prevented or displaced from doing other activities.
- Three major types of displacement (Political, Cultural and Economic) illustrate this school of thought.
    - Political: This type of displacement is caused by factors ranging from an entire political regime that rejects free enterprise, to government regulations and policies that limit or redirect certain industries.
    - Cultural: This type of displacement deals with social groups precluded from professional fields. Ethnic background, religion, race and gender are all examples of factors that figure in the minority experience.
    - Economic: This type of displacement is concerned with the economic variations of recession and depression.

Micro View

- The micro view of entrepreneurship examines the factors that are specific to entrepreneurship and are part of the internal locus of control. The potential entrepreneur has the ability, or control, to direct or adjust the outcome of each major influence.
- In macro view there are three schools of entrepreneurial thought
    - The Entrepreneurial Trait or Personality Trait School of Thought,
    - The Venture Opportunity School of Thought, and
    - The Strategic Formulation School of Thought.

The Entrepreneurial Trait or Personality Trait School of Thought. The school of thought identifies particular traits that propel people to start ventures. These include: achievement need, creativity, determination and technical knowledge, among others.

The Venture Opportunity School of Thought. Focuses on the opportunity aspect of venture development. The search for ideas, development of concepts and the implementation of venture opportunities are important areas in this thought. Creativity and market awareness are viewed as essential. Developing the right idea at the right time for the right market niche is the key to entrepreneurial success. It is based on the corridor principle: new pathways or opportunities will arise that lead entrepreneurs in different directions. The ability to recognize these opportunities when they arise and to implement the necessary steps for action are key factors. Preparation meeting opportunity equals luck is the underlying issue.

The Strategic Formulation School of Thought. This emphasizes the planning process in successful venture development. Unique markets, unique products, unique peopleor unique resources are vital. It involves: a) Unique markets – Mountain versus mountain gap strategies i.e. identifying major market segments as well as markets that arise from larger markets, b) Unique people. Great chef strategies which refers to the skills or special talents of one or more individuals around whom the venture is built,c) Unique products – Better widget strategies, which refers to innovations that encompass new or existing markets and, d) Unique resources. Water well strategies,

20

Basic Requirements for Entrepreneurship Initiatives in Livestock & Allied Sectors

Introduction

The process of setting up a business is preceded by the decision to choose entrepreneurship as a career and identification of promising business ideas upon a careful examination of the entrepreneurial opportunities. Generation of ideas is not enough; the business ideas must stand the scrutiny from techno-economic, financial and legal perspectives. That is, after the initial screening of the ideas that do not seem promising prima facie, you should conduct an in-depth examination of the chosen three-four before settling for the one where you would like to exert your time, money and energies. You should prepare a business plan that will serve as the road map for effective venturing, whether you may require institutional funding (in which case it is necessary to do so) or not. Setting up of new business enterprises is a very challenging task; you are likely to encounter many problems en route. It's advisable to be aware of these problems.

Project feasibility study

Feasibility literally means whether some idea will work or not. It knows beforehand whether there exists a sizeable market for the proposed product/ service, what would be the investment requirements and where to get the funding from, whether and wherefrom the necessary technical know-how to convert the idea into a tangible product may be available, and so on. In other words, feasibility study involves an examination of the operations, financial, HR and marketing aspects of a business on ex ante (Before the venture comes into existence) basis. Thus, you may simultaneously read this lesson and the lessons on marketing, finance etc. to have a better idea of the issues involved. What we present hereunder is a brief outline of the issues impinging upon the various aspects of the feasibility of the proposed project.

By now, you would have understood that feasibility is a multivariate concept; that is, a project has to be viable not only in technical terms but also in economic and commercial terms too. Moreover, there always is a possibility that a project that is technically possible may not be economically viable. For instance, you can construct a dust free factory in Rajasthan, but it is more economically sensible to do so in Chandigarh/ Bangalore. So even as we take up the various aspects of feasibility one- by-one, it must not mislead into believing that there is a sequence and that there are no interdependencies.

Steps to obtain subsidy for any livestock projects are as follows

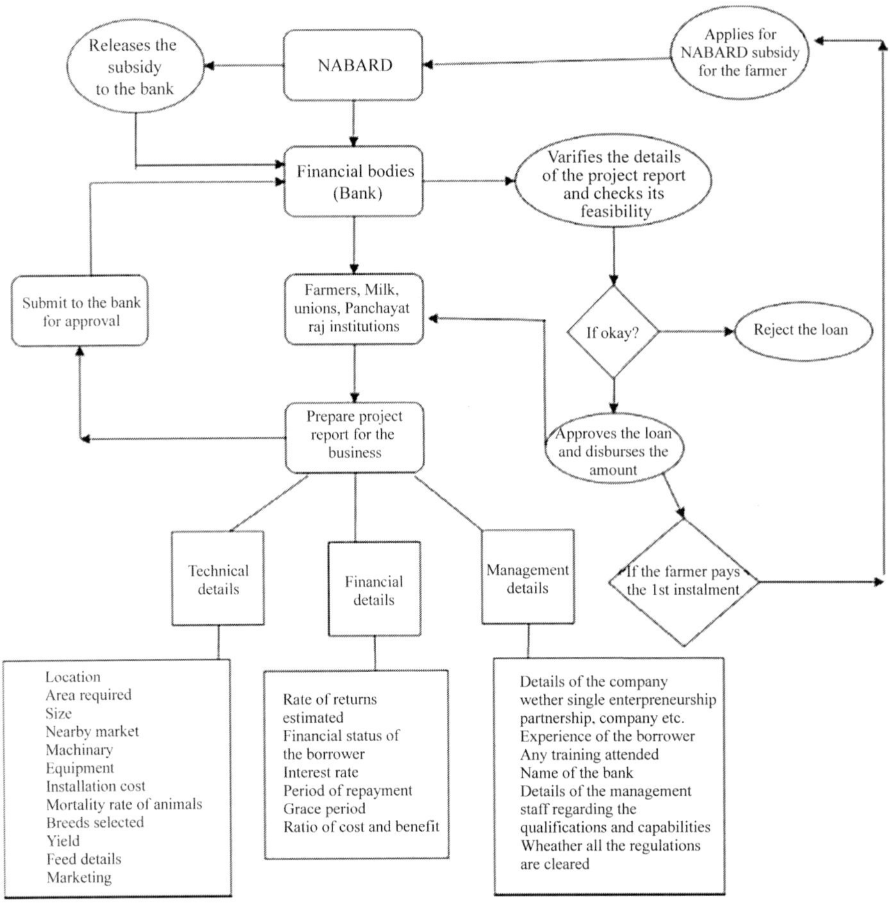

Market analysis

Market, whether a place or not, is the arena for interaction among buyers and sellers. From seller's point of view, market analysis is primarily concerned with the aggregate demand of the proposed product/service in future and the market share expected to be captured. Success of the proposed project clearly hinges on the continuing support of the customers. However, it is very difficult to identify the market for one's product/service. After all, the whole universe cannot be your market. You have to carefully segment the market according to some criteria such as geographic scope, demographic and psychological profile of the potential customers etc. It is a study of knowing who all comprise your customers, for this you require information on:

- Consumption trends
- Past and present supply position
- Production possibilities and constraints
- Imports and Exports Competition
- Cost structure
- Elasticity of demand
- Consumer behaviour, intentions, motivations, attitudes, preferences and requirements Distribution channels and marketing policies in use
- Administrative, technical and legal constraints impinging on the marketing of the Product.

Financial feasibility

The objective of financial analysis is to ascertain whether the proposed project will be financially viable in the sense of being able to meet the burden of servicing debt and whether the proposed project will satisfy the return expectations of those who provide the capital. While conducting a financial appraisal certain aspects has to be looked into like:

- Investment outlay and cost of project
- Means of financing
- Projected profitability
- Break- even point
- Cash flows of the project
- Investment worthiness judged in terms of various criteria of merit
- Projected financial position

Technical feasibility

The issues involved in the assessment of technical analysis of the proposed project may be classified into those pertaining to inputs, throughputs and outputs.

Input Analysis: Input analysis is mainly concerned with the identification, quantification and evaluation of project inputs, that is, machinery and materials. You have to ensure that the right kind and quality of inputs would be available at the right time and cost throughout the life of the project. You have to enter into long-term contracts with the potential suppliers; in many cases you have to cultivate your supply sources. When Macdonald entered India, they developed sustainable sources of supply of potatoes, lettuce and other ingredients for their burgers. The activities involved in developing and retaining supply sources are referred to as supply chain management.

Throughput Analysis: It refers to the production/operations that you would perform on the inputs to add value. Usually, the inputs received would undergo a process of transformation in several stages of manufacture. Where to locate the facility, what would be the sequence, what would be the layout, what would be the quality control measures, etc. are the issues that you would learn in greater details in subsequent lessons.

Output Analysis: this involves product specification in terms of physical features- colour, weight, length, breadth, height; functional features; chemical-material properties; as well as standards to be complied with such as BIS, ISI, and ISO etc.

Economic analysis

Economics is the study of costs- and- benefits. In regard to the feasibility of the study the entrepreneur is concerned whether the capital cost as well as the cost of the product is justifiable vis-à-vis the price at which it will sell at the market place. For example, technically, silver can be extracted from silver bromide, (a chemical used for processing the X-ray and photo films); but, the cost of extraction is so high that it would not be economically feasible to do so.

Likewise, until recently cost of harnessing solar power was prohibitively high. This cost-benefit analysis goes into financial calculations for profitability analysis that we discussed under financial analysis. At this stage it is also useful to distinguish between the economic and commercial feasibility; whereas economic feasibility leads one to the unit cost of the product, commercial feasibility informs whether enough units would sell.

Apart from the cost-benefit analysis as above, which we also refer to as private cost- benefit analysis, it is also useful to do what is known as social- cost-benefit- analysis (SCBA). For example, the entrepreneur may be getting subsidized electricity in which case private cost would be less than social cost. Likewise, exporting units earn precious foreign exchange resulting into social benefits being more than private earnings. Many a time, a project that is worthy on SCBA may find greater favour with the support agencies.

Feasibility indicators

Benefit-cost analysis

Benefit-cost analysis (BCA) is a technique for evaluating a project or investment by comparing the economic benefits with the economic costs of the activity. Benefit-cost analysis has several objectives. First, BCA can be used to evaluate the economic merit of a project. Second the results from a series of benefit-cost analyses can be used to compare competing projects. BCA can be used to assess business decisions, to examine the worth of public investments, or to assess the wisdom of using natural resources or altering environmental conditions. Ultimately, BCA aims to examine potential actions with the objective of increasing social welfare.

Regardless of the aim, all benefit-cost analyses have several properties in common. A BCA begins with a problem to be solved. For example, a community may have the goal of alleviating congestion on roads in an area. Various projects that might solve the particular problem are then identified. As an example, alternative projects to alleviate road congestion in an area might include a new highway, a public bus system, or a light rail system. The costs and benefits of these projects would be identified, calculated, and compared. Decisions are typically not made solely on the basis of BCA, but BCA is useful and sometimes required by law. Without a doubt, results from a BCA can be used to raise the level of public debate surrounding a project.

Benefit cost analysis examples

1. Society must decide whether to open-up an old-growth forest for logging. Logging would provide a variety of benefits, but will also entail costs. The products and employment generated by logging are benefits. Some of the costs of cutting the old-growth forest include the cost of cutting, the loss of wildlife habitat, damages to local streams due to runoff, and the loss of an opportunity to cut the forest sometime in the future.

2 An agency must decide whether to impose regulations to conserve a biologically important wetland. Conserving the wetland has

environmental benefits. The wetland provides habitat for a variety of animals, including waterfowl. The wetland ultimately provides benefits to hunters and bird-watchers. The wetland also provides benefits because it helps to maintain water quality and reduces flooding in neighbouring areas. However, land that would be conserved could be used in a different way, say for agriculture or a shopping mall. This loss in use is an opportunity cost. Landowners may also incur some direct costs in protecting wetlands on their property or some opportunity costs associated with not using these areas in another way. BCA can be used to compare the benefits and costs of imposing the regulation.

Time and discounting

The example used above ignores the issue of time. In comparing the benefits and costs of the project we didn't really consider when those benefits and costs occurred. But in many cases the timing of benefits and costs is an important aspect of the project under consideration. For this reason, dealing adequately with the timing of benefits and costs becomes a crucial part of the BCA. For example, what if the cost of constructing the project is incurred this year, but the benefits of using the project are not felt until next year, after the project is completed. In this case will next year's benefits outweigh this year's costs? To deal with this kind of question, benefit-cost analysis uses a concept known as discounting.

Discounting is a technique that converts all benefits and costs into their value in the present. Discounting is based on the premise that a rupee received today is worth more than a rupee received in the future. This bias toward the present arises because by placing a rupee in a safe investment today, you can increase its value to more than a rupee tomorrow. Another way of saying this is that a rupee received in the future is not worth as much as that same rupee received in the present. That is, the future value of the rupee is discounted. Discounting is the opposite of compounding. Not surprisingly, the rate at which a future value is discounted is closely related to the rate at which present values are compounded, namely the interest rate. As we know from compounding, if the interest rate is 5%, then a rupee placed in the bank today will be worth ` 1.05 a year from now. This means that if the interest rate is 5%, `1.05 to be received next year is worth only `1.00 today.

Whenever the benefits and costs used in a benefit-cost analysis occur in the future, it is important to discount these future values to account for their present value. If the interest rate is *r*, then the following formula can be used to find the present value (*PV*) of an amount (*Pt*) received at some time *t* in the future:

$PV= P_t / (1+r)^t$

To apply the formula, remember:

PV is the present value of the amount invested;

P_t is the rupee value of the future amount in time t;

r is the discount rate; and

t is the year in which P_t is realized.

Benefit cost measures

Several variations on the basic benefit-cost rule can be used to compare the benefits and costs of investments, projects, or decisions.

1. Net Present Value
2. Benefit cost ratio
3. Internal Rate of Return

Net Present Value

The net present value (NPV) is the current value of all project net benefits. Net benefits are simply the sum of benefits minus costs. The sum is discounted at the discount rate. Using this method, if the project has a NPV greater than zero then it appears to be a good candidate for implementation. The formula used to calculate the NPV is:

$$NPV = \sum_{t=1}^{T} \frac{(\text{Benefit}_t - \text{Cost}_t)}{(1+r)^t}$$

Benefit Cost ratio

The benefit-cost ratio (BCR) is calculated as the NPV of benefits divided by the NPV of costs:

$$BCR = \frac{\sum_{t-1}^{t} \frac{B_t}{(1+r)^t}}{\sum_{t-1}^{t} \frac{C_t}{(1+r)^t}}$$

Where: B_t is the benefit in time t and C_t is the cost in time t. If the BCR exceeds one, then the project might be a good candidate for acceptance.

Internal rate of return

The internal rate of return (IRR) is the maximum interest that could be paid for the project resources, leaving enough money to cover investment and operating costs, which would still allow the investor to break even. In other words, the IRR is the discount rate for which the present value of total benefits equals the present value of total costs:

PV(BEnefits) - PV(Costs) = 0

In general, the IRR should be greater than the discount rate for a project to be accepted.

Example: Cash flow statement and financial statement of Goat Project

Cash Flow Statement

Particulars	I year	II year	III year	IV year	V year	VI year
Cash Inflow						
From Sale of Male Lambs	0	252000	563850	272250	255150	563850
From sale of Female Lambs	0	162000	473850	182250	165150	473850
From sale of culled Ewes	0	50000	50000	50000	50000	50000
From sale of manures	6300	9660	13818	9930	9702	13818
From Residual value						262500
Total Cash Inflow	6300	473660	1101518	514430	480002	1364018
Outflow						
Cost of feeding						
a.Ewes	36000	36000	36000	36000	36000	36000
b.Ram	1800	1800	1800	1800	1800	1800
c. Lambs	12600	14400	27000	12600	14400	27000
Insurance cost	32850	32850	32850	32850	32850	32850
Veterinary aid	30240	30240	30240	30240	30240	30240
Total Outflow	113490	115290	127890	113490	115290	127890
Net Cash Inflow	-107190	358370	973628	400940	364712	1236128

Financial Analysis of the Project

Particulars	I year	II year	III year	IV year	V year	VI year
Capital Investment	1112000					
Working Capital	113490	115290	127890	113490	115290	127890
Total Cost	1225490	115290	127890	113490	115290	127890
Total Benefit	6300	473660	1101518	514430	480002	1364018
Net Cash Flow	-1219190	358370	973628	400940	364712	1236128
DCF at 20%	0.833	0.694	0.579	0.482	0.402	0.335

Particulars	I year	II year	III year	IV year	V year	VI year
Disc. Benefit	5250	328931	637453	248085	192902	456807
Disc.cost	1021242	80063	74010	54731	46332	42830
NPV at 20% DCF	-1015992	248868	563442	193355	146570	413977
DCF at 25%	0.800	0.640	0.512	0.410	0.328	0.262
Disc. Benefit	5040	303142	563977	210711	157287	357569
Disc.cost	980392	73786	65480	46486	37778	33526
NVP at 25% DCV	-975352	229357	498498	164225	119509	324044
NPV at 20%	**550219**			**B:C ratio at 20%**		**1.417**
NPV at 25%	**360280**			**B:C ratio at 25%**		**1.291**
	IRR	**40%**				

When NPV and BCR are positive and IRR more than opportunity cost, then the project said to be approved for loan.

21

Avenues of Livestock Entrepreneurship

Livestock farms

The veterinarians can start their own livestock farms with their vast technical knowledge; they can infuse scientific management techniques in their own farms. In the WTO (World Trade Organisation) era, GMP (Good Manufacturing Practices) and SPS (Sanitory and Phytosanitory) measures are of great importance for export of livestock commodities, as the emphasis in international trade is on quality and food safety. If veterinarians start their own scientifically managed livestock enterprise, they can exploit this opportunity. Further, practicing proven scientific management techniques will improve productivity of animals that would lead to overall quantitative and qualitative improvement of livestock sector.

Feed manufacturer

The veterinary graduates can start their own feed mill units for various livestock and poultry species. Commercial feed availability for various unconventional poultry species such as Quail, Emu, Ostrich, etc. are far less than the demand. Manufacturing feed for these species is a niche business as their energy requirement is different from the existing commercially available broiler or layer feed.

Fodder supplier

The main constraint which hampers the growth of livestock production is the inadequacy of nutritious fodder. As there is more than 60% fodder deficit in India, veterinarians can combine together, purchase fertile land and produce quality fodder and supply them to the nearby livestock farmers. They can also start seed / fodder banks in the potential areas.

Farm Equipments Manufacturer / dealer

Number of farm equipments are needed for livestock farms. For example, in case of dairy farms, chaff cutter, milking machine, feeding manager, etc. are needed. Poultry farmers need debeaker, vaccinator, automatic feeder, waterer, etc. Demand for farm equipments increases with the wide adoptation of intensive livestock and poultry farming system. The veterinarians can either start on their own or they can act as dealer for these equipments.

Dog breeder

Dog breeding is an ever green field with potential opportunities in urban areas. Dogs with good pedigree record fetches good price and the veterinarians can readily exploit this opportunity. Combining dog breeding with veterinary consultancy services offer excellent earning opportunity.

Hatchery

Though starting a hatchery requires higher investment, it offers good return.

Pet Animal / Large Animal/ Mobile Clinic

It is the widely practiced by the veterinarians which offer them good earnings in both rural as well as urban areas.

Livestock products processor

Value addition to the livestock products such as milk, egg, meat, and fish have huge profit potential. Value of the products get increased many folds during processing, and thereby provide excellent returns. Veterinarians can start milk parlour, where they can sell processed milk and milk products like flavoured milk, goa, ice cream, etc. or meat centre where fried chicken, chicken 65, mutton khima, etc. could be sold. Marketing of these value added products could be done in their own brand name and they can start chain of parlours / hotels later.

Farm consultant

Livestock farm consultant is a lucrative avenue. Veterinarians with skill and knowledge can earn well in specialized dairy farms, stud farms, breeder farms, hatchery, sheep / goat farms. After some years of experience in managing the farms, they can start their own farms independently or with partnerships.

Contract farming

Contract farming is a emerging system where the livestock farmers are given all the inputs such as chicks/animals, feed, medicines, technical inputs, etc. Farmers have to rear the chicks/animals and the integrator will take care of the marketing activities. Veterinarians can join together and venture into contract farming. Being technical savvy would help them in getting loans, maintaining farm business and marketing the products.

Leather industry

Leather industry is so far unexplored by the Veterinarians. It offers great profit potential. The skin and hide from animals are usually purchased by the intermediaries in the villages at a throw away prices and are sold to the processors at a huge margin. The processors add value to the raw skin and make products and export / sell them at a very high price. The veterinarians can perform the role of this intermediaries.

Agents for by products utilization

The livestock feed manufacturers and pharmaceuticals require several ingredients such as bone meal, fish meal, blood meal etc. which they are getting from the agents at contract basis. Here, veterinarians can make interventions. They can make a tie-up and could meet the requirements of feed manufacturers at a reasonable price and also can earn money.

Veterinary pharmaceutical industry

It is also a lucrative opportunity but needs huge investment. After working some years in the pharmaceutical industry and learning experience, veterinarians can initially start a small one with fewer drugs which can be expanded later to the needs of local farmers. From thereon, they can grow slowly.

22

Livestock Entrepreneurship Training and Development Programmes

National institute for entrepreneurship and small business

Development (NIESBUD)

The National Institute for Entrepreneurship and Small Business Development (NIESBUD) was established in 1983 by the Ministry of Industry (now Ministry of Small Scale Industries), Govt. of India, as an apex body for coordinating and overseeing the activities of various institutions/ agencies engaged in Entrepreneurship Development Particularly in the area of small industry and small business. The Institute which is registered as a society under Govt. of India Societies Act (XXI of 1860). The policy, direction and guidance to the Institute are provided by its Governing Council whose Chairman is the Minister of SSI.

Entrepreneurship development institute of India

The Entrepreneurship Development Institute of India (EDI), an autonomous body and not-for-profit institution, set up in 1983, is sponsored by apex financial institutions, namely the IDBI Bank Ltd, IFCI Ltd. ICICI Ltd and State Bank of India (SBI). The Institute is registered under the Societies Registration Act 1860 and the Public Trust Act 1950. The EDI has been selected as a member of the Economic and Social Commission for Asia and the Pacific (ESCAP) network of Centres of Excellence for HRD Research and Training. EDI as a member of the Network will have interactive access to information on other 123 member institutions via Internet. EDI will also be invited to collaborate with ESCAP in the development and delivery of a series of ESCAP HRD courses to train social development personnel working to alleviate poverty in the region.

Indian institute of entrepreneurship

With an aim to undertake training, research and consultancy activities in the small industry sector focusing on entrepreneurship development, the Indian Institute of Entrepreneurship (IIE) was established in the year 1993 at Guwahati by the erstwhile Ministry of Industry (now Ministry of Small Scale Industry), Government of India as an autonomous national institute. The policy direction and guidance is provided to the Institute by its Board of Management whose Chairman is the Secretary to the Government of India, Ministry of Small Scale Industries.

Ministry of small scale industries

Ministry of Small Scale Industries is the nodal Ministry for formulation of policy, promotion, development and protection of small scale industries in India. The Ministry of Small Scale Industries (SSI) designs and implements the policies through its field organizations for the promotion and growth of small scale industries. The Ministry also performs the functions of policy advocacy on behalf of small scale industries (SSI) sector with other Ministries/ Departments.

Small Industries Development Organisation (SIDO)

SIDO was established in 1954 on the basis of the recommendations of the Ford Foundation. Over the years, it has seen its role evolve into an agency for advocacy, hand holding and facilitation for the small industries sector. It has over 60 offices and 21 autonomous bodies under its management. These autonomous bodies include Tool Rooms, Training Institutions and Project-cum-Process Development Centres. SIDO provides a wide spectrum of services to the small industries sector. These include facilities for testing, training for entrepreneurship development, preparation of project and product profiles, technical and managerial consultancy, assistance for exports, pollution and energy audits, etc. SIDO provides economic information services and advises Government in policy formulation for the promotion and development of SSIs.

The National Small Industries Corporation Limited (NSIC)

The National Small Industries Corporation Ltd., an ISO 9001:2000 Company, was established in 1955 by the Government of India with a view to promote, aid and foster the growth of Small Industries in the country. NSIC continues to remain at the forefront of industrial development throughout the country, with it's various programs and projects, to assist the small scale sector in the country. The Corporation provides integrated Technology, Marketing and Financial support to Small Scale Sector.

National Institute for Small Industry Extension Training (NISIET)

The NISIET, since its inception in 1960 by the Government of India, has taken gigantic strides to become the premier institution for the promotion, development and modernization of the SME (Small and Medium Scale

Enterprises) sector. An autonomous arm of the Ministry of Small Scale Industries (SSI), the Institute strives to achieve its avowed objectives through a gamut of operations ranging from training, consultancy, research and education, to extension and information services.

Small Industries Development Bank of India (SIDBI)

Small Industries Development Bank of India (SIDBI) was established in April 1990 under an Act of Indian Parliament as the principal financial institution for promotion, financing , development of industry in the small scale sector and co-ordinating the functions of other institutions engaged in similar activities. Since its inception, SIDBI has been assisting the entire spectrum of SSI Sector including the tiny, village and cottage industries through suitable schemes tailored to meet the requirement of setting up of new projects, expansion, diversification, modernisation and rehabilitation of existing units.

Rural Self Employment Training Institutes

RSETIs are Rural Self Employment Training Institutes, an initiative of Ministry of Rural Development (MoRD) to have dedicated infrastructure in each district of the country to impart training and skill upgradation of rural youth geared towards entrepreneurship development. RSETIs are managed by banks with active co-operation from the Government of India and State Governments.

Objectives of the RSETI's

- Rural BPL youth will be identified and trained for self-employment.
- The trainings offered will be demand driven.
- Area in which training will be provided to the trainee will be decided after assessment the candidate's aptitude.
- Hand holding support will be provided for assured credit linkage with banks.
- Escort services will be provided for at least for two years soon to ensure sustainability of micro enterprise trainees.
- The trainees will be provided intensive short-term residential self-employment training programmes with free food and accommodation.

The Khadi and Village Industries Commission (KVIC)

The Khadi and Village Industries Commission (KVIC) is a statutory body created by an Act of Parliament (No.61 of 1956 and as amended by Act No. 12

of 1987). Established in April 1957, it took over the work of the former All India Khadi and Village Industries Board. The broad objectives that the KVIC has set before it are: The social objective of providing employment, The economic objective of producing saleable articles, and The wider objective of creating self-reliance amongst the poor and building up of a strong rural community spirit. The KVIC is charged with the planning, promotion, organisation and implementation of programs for the development of khadi and other village industries in the rural areas in coordination with other agencies engaged in rural development wherever necessary.

Trainer's training programmes

Enterprise Launching and Management

EMT Accreditation Programmes

Barefoot Managers

Self-Employment / PMRY

Project Formulation & Appraisal

Planning &Organising EDPs

Small business promoter's programmes

Entrepreneurship Orientation for Weaker Sections/DWACRA Functionaries

Grassroot Management Training

Women Empowerment through Enterprise Development

Orientation Programmes for Voluntary Organisations

Small Business Development

Micro-Enterprise for Women/SC/ST/Weaker Section

TRYSEM/ISB Beneficiaries

23

Essential Criteria for Development of Entrepreneurship in Livestock and Allied Sectors

Entrepreneurship theory has been evolving over the last 20 years and is ever growing. It is defined as a verifiable and logically coherent formulation of relationships, or underlying principles that either explain entrepreneurship, predict entrepreneurial activity or provide normative guidance (prescribing the right action in particular circumstance). Entreprenuership is interdisciplinary and contains various approaches that would increase one's understanding of it. One way to examine these theories is with a 'schools of thought' approach that divides entrepreneurship into specific activities. These activities may be within a 'macro view or a micro view', but all address the conceptual nature of entrepreneurship.

Development of entrepreneurship

Creativity: Creativity and innovation are often used to mean the same thing, but each has a unique connotation. Creativity is the ability to bring something new into existence. Ideas usually evolve through a creative process whereby imaginative people bring them into existence, nurture them, and develop them successfully. The creative process for an idea contains five stages – germination, preparation, incubation, illumination, and verification.

Germination: The manner in which an idea is germinated is a mystery. Most ideas can be traced to an individual's interest in or curiosity about a specific problem or area of study.

Preparation: After germination, creative people start on a conscious search for answers. It may be a problem to solve - such as the determination of people like Bharat Ratna C. Subramaniam and Dr. M.S. Swaminathan to make India self sufficient in food and to help the Indian farmers resulted in Green Revolution. If it is an idea for a new product or service, then market research is the business equivalent.

Incubation: Incubation is a stage of mulling it over while the subconscious intellect assumes control of the creative process and may take time depending upon the problem, individual, etc. This is a crucial aspect of creativity because when we consciously focus on a problem, we behave rationally to attempt to find systematic resolutions.

Illumination: It is the fourth stage which occurs when the idea resurfaces as a realistic creation. It may be triggered by an opportune incident, as in the case of Alexander Flemming's discovery of Penicillin. This stage is critical for entrepreneurs because ideas, by themselves, have little meaning unless and otherwise they are converted into reality. It is the recognition of idea as being feasible solution.

Verification: It is a stage of development that refines knowledge into application. This is often tedious and requires perseverance by an individual committed to finding a way to harvest the practical results of his or her creation. An idea may be good and useful, but if it lacks applicability, it could not be executed.

Innovation: Entrepreneurs innovate and is the specific instrument of entrepreneurship which differentiates them from others. It is the act that endows resources with a new capacity to create wealth and in fact creates a resource. Successful entrepreneurs, whoever they may be or whatever their aim may be, try to create value and to make a contribution. Still successful Entrepreneurs aim high and not content simply to improve on what already exists, or to modify it. They try to create new and different values and it is the most important function of an entrepreneur, according to Joseph Schumpter and is the core attribute of an entrepreneur. For an innovator, the market is never too saturated. The entire world progress based on innovation only.

Once entrepreneurship is decided upon, there are three main routes an entrepreneur may follow:

- **Starting a new livstock business**
    - The entrepreneur can begin from scratch on all his own ideas, as there are no existing problems or concerns from a previous owner. He has the freedom to start the business in his own way. However, the risk is higher and he has to devote time, effort, and money—especially for start-up expenses such as equipment, a building, etc.
- **Purchasing an existing livestock business**
    - Advantages of purchasing an existing business include smaller start-up costs and building on the existing goodwill or loyalty of established

customers. This option is good if the entrepreneur does not have a great deal of business experience. Disadvantages might include inheriting existing problems such as poor location, stiff competition, fluctuating market, equipment problems, and poor reputation.

- **Taking over a family livestock business**
  - In this situation, an entrepreneur has the support and training available from the family members, creating trust and togetherness that bonds the business as one entity. Maintaining separate family and business relationships is the biggest obstacle to overcome, making it difficult to get away from the business. Personality conflicts, different interests, changed values, and burnout are a few reasons that family-owned businesses don't survive to the second generation. A person who grows up in the family business may be ready to spread his or her wings and explore new career aspirations.

Types of business ownership

- Liability, taxes, and financing options will be the deciding factors when choosing the appropriate business structure for an entrepreneurial venture. Whether the business is organized as a partnership or as a corporation could affect the management process, ability to receive a loan and the type and cost of benefits the business can offer.

Sole proprietorship

- *Sole proprietorship* is the easiest, oldest, and most popular form of business to create. Sole proprietorship usually involves one person owning and operating a business; the owner and business is the same person. The owner is the only one responsible for the activities of the business. This form of business is usually a service business that is handled and operated by one person. Eg. Veterinary Consultants, Auditors.
- The factors associated with the sole proprietorship, along with their advantages and disadvantages, are as follows:
  - Profits are taxed as income to the owner personally.
  - Tax rate is lower than the corporate tax rate.
  - Owner has complete control of the business.
  - There is unlimited liability for company debts.
  - Little reporting is required, and government regulation is minimal.

Sole Proprietorship	
Advantages	Disadvantages
• easy and inexpensive to create • one owner has complete authority over the business • taxes are not separate from the owner's; usually at a lower rate • no certificate of incorporation • no bylaws, minutes, stock shares • all profits go to owner • higher flexibility	• full liability for debts, etc. • higher risk of losing personal assets, such as car, home, etc. • personal responsibility for workers' injuries • no one to take over if owner becomes sick • difficult to obtain finances for business • requires more money invested by owner • temptation to mix business money with personal money • only as successful as the skills, abilities, and talents of the owner • business dies when owner dies

Normally, farmers are sole proprietors. They operate their farming businesses as the owner or boss of the working operation. Any other business owner who operates under the status of "self-employed" also falls within this category of sole proprietor, such as the local electrician, plumber, and mechanic. Farmers do not have to apply for government certificates or status because they are assuming full responsibility for the business.

- The sole proprietorship is the oldest, simplest, and most common form of business entity. It is a business owned by a single individual. For tax and legal liability purpose, the owner and the business are one and the same. The proprietorship is not taxed as separate entity. The earnings of the business are taxed at the individual level, whether or not they are actually in cash. There is no vehicle for sheltering income. For liability purposes, the individual and the business are also one and the same. Thus, legal claimants can pursue the personal property of the proprietor and not simply the assets used in the business.

Partnership

- *Partnership* involves two or more persons who unite in the operation and management of a business venture. This type of partnership may be established for legal or tax purposes. The prospect of becoming a partner in a business can be an incentive to new employees. Most effective partnership arrangements include professional service businesses, such as accounting and law firms.
- Some aspects associated with the partnership form of business are as follows:

- Business is subject to little government regulation.
- Business is relatively easier to establish.
- Formal partnership agreement is highly recommended to address possible conflicts that could arise in future.
- Each partner is liable for all debts.
- All profits are taxed as income to the partners according to the percentage of ownership.
- Business name must be registered with the Registrar of Companies.

- A clearly written agreement containing the partnership terms is essential.
- Have a clear and realistic agreement that anticipates future incidents.
- Include a buy-sell agreement in which terms are provided for the departure of one or more partners from death, disability, retirement, or resignation.
- Consider carrying life insurance on each partner, so the partnership can pay the remaining partner's estate for the value of his or her interest in the business.

Partnership	
Advantages	Disadvantages
• share ideas and skills among partners • secure investment capital more easily • tax rates lower than corporation • more flexibility of ownership and income	• personality conflicts and relationship strains • liable for each other's actions • difficulty in obtaining financing • a partner's bankruptcy may affect the other partners • can't sell business unless all partners agree

Private limited company

Private limited company is a one

- Has a minimum paid-up share capital of Rs.1 Lakh or such higher capital as may be prescribed; and
- By its Articles Association:
  - Restricts the right of transfer of its share;
  - Limits the number of its members to 50 which will not include:-
- Members who are employees of the company; and
- Members who are ex-employees of the company and were members

while in such employment and who have continued to be members after ceasing to be employees;

- Prohibits any invitation to the public to subscribe for any shares or debentures of the company; and
- Prohibits any invitation or acceptance of deposits from persons other than its members, directors or their relatives.

Public limited company

- The Company defined under section 3(1)(iv) of the Companies Act, 1956 is a public company which-
  - Is not a private company;
  - Has a minimum paid-up capital of Rs. 5 lakhs or such higher capital as may be prescribed;
  - Is a private company but subsidiary of a public company.

Private companies deemed to be public companies

- Certain private companies are deemed to be public companies by virtue of section 43 A, viz.-
  - When 25% or more of its paid-up share capital is held by one or more body corporate;
  - When its average annual turnover (during the last 3 years) exceeds Rs. 25 crores;
  - When it holds 25% or more of the paid-up share capital of Public Company; or
  - When it accepts or renews deposits from the public after making an invitation by an advertisement.

Corporation

- A *corporation* is a business that is chartered or registered by the state and that operates separately from the owner or owners. The advantages and disadvantages of this business form are as follows:

Corporation	
Advantages	Disadvantages
• easier to raise money/capital (issuing shares of stocks) • limited liability of owners, only owing for what is invested • better status for employees (pensions/ retirement, dividends) • easier to change ownership	• expensive to set up and organize • profits taxed twice • extensive record keeping and paperwork

Limited Liability Corporations are the most recent form of business, combining the best of both worlds (partnerships and corporations).

- *Advantages*
    - Limited liability of corporation members
    - Not liable for company's debts
    - Tax advantages of a partnership
    - Shareholders only taxed once
    - Popular among professionals (doctors, lawyers, etc.)
    - Owners risk only their investment
    - Personal assets not at risk
- *Corporations* are legal entities comprised of persons who have obtained a charter legally recognizing the corporation as a separate entity that has its own rights, privileges, and liabilities that are separate from the individuals that form the corporation. The Corporation can own assets, borrow money, and perform business functions without directly involving the owners.
    - Most complex form of business corporation
    - Comprised of three groups of people: shareholders, directors, officers
    - Subject to more regulations than sole proprietorships and partnerships
    - Earnings subject to double taxation (the corporation is taxed and shareholder dividends are taxed)
    - Limited liability
    - Not a total protection from lawsuits
- The largest businesses in India, such as Venkateswara Hatcheries Ltd., Suguna Chicken, TCS and Infosys are examples of Corporations.

They encompass such a wide array of businesses and involve so many investors and stockholders that their liability and security are ensured.

Skills Required for Development of Entrepreneurship

1. Management skills
2. Inter-personal skills
3. Business acumen
4. Business communication

Management skills

Planning, organizing, staffing, directing, coordinating, reporting

Inter-personal skills/ communication

Verbal Communication: Verbal communication means such a communication that takes place by means of a language or words". It includes the following contents.

a. Oral communication (Speaking & listening)
b. Written communication (writing & reading)

1. **Speaking:** In order to send message in business, speaking plays a vital role. Giving instruction, conducting interviews, attending meetings, sending orders through telephone calls are very common in today's business.
2. **Writing:** It is used when a complex message is sent. Placing order through letters, informing employees through circulars, sending reports and memos, filling different government forms, keeping records in writing are some examples of this aspect of verbal communication.
3. **Listening:** - People in business spend more time in obtaining information then transmitting it. Listening is the most important way to receive information: information regarding order of employers, instruction, rules and regulation, customer trend etc, are obtained through listening. But in listening, people generally forget 75% of the message after few days.
4. **Reading:** Reading reports, memos, policies, circulars, and different business statements are essential for an organization: Reading involves understanding and interpreting the material.

Non Verbal Communication: It means communication without the use of language or words. It includes appearance, body language, silence, etc. Its explanation is as follows;

1. **Facial Expressions:** Face and eyes are helpful means of nonverbal communication. They reveal hidden emotions such as anger, confusion, enthusiasm, fear, joy etc.
2. **Gestures, postures & movement:** Postures means the language primarily composed of hand and fingers. Communication of deaf people and signal given by traffic constable are the example of posture. Gestures and body movement also indicate many things. Shaking hand with firmness indicates a warm relationship, moving back and forth reveals nervousness.

Importance of non-verbal communication

1. **Reliability:** Non verbal communication is more reliable then verbal communication. Words can be controlled more easily but it's difficult to hide facial expressions like sadness, gladness, joy etc. So, non-verbal communication is regarded as a more reliable means for transmitting message.
2. **Support to verbal communication:** Body language and appearance support the verbal communication. A wave of hand, smile etc might be very useful to explain and understand a particular point of view.
3. **Quickness:** A denial or acceptance expressed by moving head saves lot of time. So, it is important in this respect that non-verbal communication transmits the message quickly.

Function of non-verbal communication

There are following six functions of it.

(1) To provide information either consciously or unconsciously.

(2) To regulate the flow of conversation.

(3) To express emotion

(4) To qualify, complement, contradict or expand verbal message.

(5) To control or influence others.

(6) To facilitates specific tasks, such as teaching a person.

Business acumen

Business acumen is keenness and quickness in understanding and dealing with a business situation in a manner that is likely to lead to a good outcome.

Business acumen characteristics

- See big picture of an organisation- how the key elements of a business related to each other, work together to produce profitable growth, and relate to the job do each day
- Understands important company communication and data, including financial statements
- Use knowledge to make good decisions
- Understands how his actions and decisions impact key company measures and the objectives of your company
- Effectively communicate ideas to other employees, managers, executives and the public
- Have a acute perception of the dimensions of business issues
- Can make sense out of complexity and an uncertain future
- Are mindful of the implications of a choice for the affected parties
- Are decisive
- Are flexible if further change is warranted in the future
- Understands how their actions and their behaviour impact their financial decisions- making and how this in turn affects financial outcomes at the unit and the corporate level.

Business communication

Communication is defined as "The flow of material information perception, understanding and imagination among various parties". Business includes those organizations, which are engaged in the production and distribution of goods and services to earn profit. Therefore Business communication means, "Flow of information, perception etc. either within a business organization or outside the organization among different parties serving communication function of an organisation".

Elements of the process of communication

Communication is the exchange of ideas between two minds. This process of exchanging idea is based on following five factors.

1. **Sender:** Sender is the person who initiates the process of communication. He generates an idea in his mind regarding production invention, innovation, request, order, enquiry etc. So, he is the first factor of communication process and his function is to generate an idea. Therefore, it is necessary that the idea should be clear, and convertible into message. For this purpose, the sender needs to apply his knowledge and imaginative power.
2. **Message:** The idea in the mind of sender is transformed into words that is called message. The sender decides on the length, style, organization and tone of the message. The message may be presented in many ways, depending on the subject, purpose, audience, personal style, mood and cultural background.
3. **Media:** The media of transmission of message are electronic media as T.V., radio, computer and print media as newspapers, letter, magazine etc. media play a very important role in helping the receiver's understand the message. A wrongly chosen medium can interrupt the process of communication, Selection of medium depends upon message, audience, urgency and situation.
4. **Receiver:** Receiver is the person who gets the message from the sender, decodes it, understands it and interprets it.
5. **Feed Back:** Having understood the message, the receiver responds to the sender in yes or no or asks further questions. This process is called feedback.

Organizational communication

A business Organization is a group of people associated to earn profit. Various kinds of activities have to be performed by the people of an organization so as to earn profit. These activities need an effective and systematic communication. Without efficient communication, one cannot even imagine to do work and hence will be unable to earn profit. Since the aim of business organization is to earn profit, the organization will die without profit and this death is a result of the absence of communication. This is why communication is called life blood of a business organization.

Communication inside an organization

Different employees and officials in an organization need to communicate to each other.

This internal communication with its importance is shown in the following way:

1. **Setting goals and Objectives:** Mostly, the organizations have a variety of formal and informal objectives to accomplish. These objectives may be financial results, product quality, market dominance, employees satisfaction, or service to customers. So the communication enables all the persons in an organization to work towards a common purpose.
2. **Making and implementing decision:** In order to achieve the objective, people in a business organization collect facts and evaluate alternatives, and they do so by reading, asking questions, talking or by plain thinking. These thoughts are put into a written form. Once a decision has been made, it has to be implemented which requires communication.
3. **Appraisal:** Having implemented the decision, management needs to determine whether the desired outcome is being achieved. Statistics on such factors as cost, sales, market share, productivity and inventory levels are compiled. This is done through computers, manual papers, memos or reports.
4. **Manufacturing the products:** Getting an idea for a new product out of someone's head, pushing it through the production process and finally getting the product also require communication. Designing the plan regarding product, introducing the workers, purchasing raw material, marketing and distributing the product all require effective communication.
5. **Interaction between employer & employee:** Employees are informed about policies and decisions of employers through circulars, reports, notices etc. Employers also get in touch with employees through application, complaint etc. So, communication plays a vital role in the interaction of employer and employee.

External communication

1. **Hiring the employees:** If a company wants to hire someone, it advertises the vacancy, receives applications, calls the candidates, takes the interview and then offers job to the successful candidates. The whole process requires communication.
2. **Dealing with customers:** Sales letters and brochures, advertisements, personal sales calls, and formal proposals are all used to stimulate the customer's interest. Communication also plays a part in such customer

related functions as credit checking, billing, and handling complaints and questions.

3. **Negotiating with suppliers and financiers:** To obtain necessary supplies and services, companies develop written specification that outlines their requirement. Similarly, to arrange finance, they negotiate with lenders and fill out loan applications.
4. **Informing the investors:** Balance sheet, income statement, and ratio analysis are used to inform the investors regarding performance of business.
5. **Interacting with Govt.:** Government agencies make certain rules to regulate the economy. These rules are communicated to organizations through various papers. These organizations try to fulfil, these requirement like filling taxation form and other documents.

Management / interpersonal skill & business communication

- One type of communication travels from individual to individual in face-to-face and group settings. Such flows are termed interpersonal communications, and the forms vary from direct verbal orders to casual, nonverbal expression. Interpersonal communication is the primary means of managerial communication.
- The problems that can arise when managers attempt to communicate with other people can be traced to perceptual and interpersonal style differences. Each manager perceives the world based on his background, experiences, personality, frame of reference, and attitude.

Interpersonal styles

- Interpersonal styles differ among individuals, and understanding these differences is important for managerial and organizational performance. Interpersonal style refers to the way in which an individual prefers to relate to others.

Interpersonal styles and communication

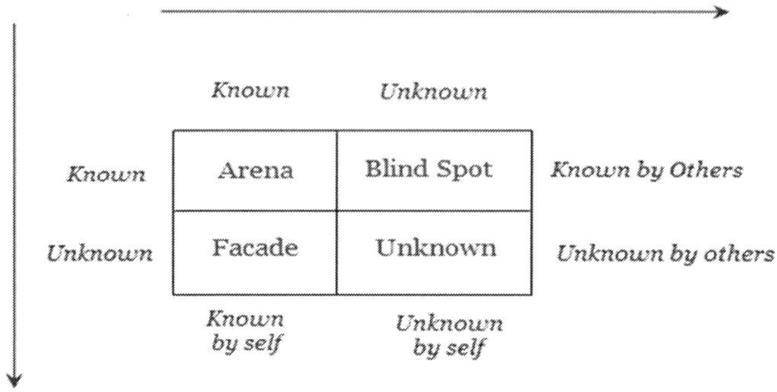

- *The arena:* The region most conducive to effective interpersonal relationships and communications is termed the arena. Here, all the information necessary to carry on effective communication is known to both the sender (self) and the receivers (others).
- *The blind spot:* When relevant information is known to others but not to the sender (self), a blind spot result. In this context, a person (self) is at a disadvantage when communicating with others because he cannot know the others' feelings, sentiments, and perceptions. Consequently, interpersonal relationships and communications suffer. The greater the blind spot, the smaller the arena, and vice versa.
- *The facade:* When information is known to the self but unknown to others, the person (self) may resort to superficial communications; that is, he may present a façade. A façade is a false front. The façade area is particularly damaging when a subordinate "knows" and an immediate supervisor "does not know." The façade, like the blind spot, diminishes the arena and reduces the possibility of effective communication.
- *The unknown:* If neither party knows the relevant feelings, sentiments, and information, each party is functioning in the unknown region. Such a situation often is stated as "I can't understand them, and they don't understand me." In this predicament, interpersonal communications are sure to suffer.

Exposure and feedback

- Interpersonal communication problems are the results of unsound relationships. An individual can improve unsound relationships by adopting two strategies-exposure and feedback.
- *Exposure:* Increasing the arena area by reducing the façade area requires

that one be open and honest in sharing information with others. The unwillingness of companies to discuss salary matters is an example of inadequate exposure.

- *Feedback:* When the self does not know or understand, more effective communications can be developed through feedback from those who do know. Thus, the blind spot can be reduced with a corresponding increase in the arena.

24

Financial Credit & Its Management General: Principles and Practices

Sources of agriculture/ Livestock finance

Finance for agriculture can be obtained from formal and informal sources

Formal sources

Credit co-operatives

Commercial banks

Government

Regional Rural Banks

Informal sources

Money lender

Friends and relatives

Traders

Landlords

3 R's OF CREDIT

To estimate the rationality of a loan, it is essential to know credit analysis.

The considerations involved in credit analysis generally fall into three groups:

Returns

Repayment capacity

Risk bearing ability

These are popularly known as the three R's of credit.

Returns

This R of credit has great significance for the creditor as well as the borrower.

It requires that both the borrower and the financier should be satisfied with the returns from credit.

The problem of determining the profitable use of capital is a part of decision making and it involves selection of enterprises, determining the most economically optimum production techniques and determining the size of each enterprise.

Repayment capacity

It is the test of economic feasibility.

It determines the amount the farmer will be able to spare for repayment of loan.

It is generally acceptable that if an investment is profitable, the loan can be repaid without any difficulty.

Risk bearing ability

Risk bearing ability implies the capacity to cope with an unexpected low income and unpredictable expenses and losses due to the vagaries of nature and other hazards such as diseases and price fluctuations.

3 C's OF CREDIT

They are character, capacity and capital.

Character implies the borrower's moral qualities, such as honesty, integrity and sense of responsibility which all influence the risk bearing ability and repayment.

Capacity signifies the potential of the borrower to repay the loan, when it is due and depends upon his income.

Capital reflects the net worth of the borrower (assets minus liabilities) which also reflects his repayment and risk bearing ability.

Methods of Repayment of Loans

Three methods are commonly used.

Straight end repayment or lump sum repayment

The entire loan is paid on the expiry of the term but the interest on the loan is paid each year.

Partial repayment or variable repayment

A part of the loan together with a part of the interest on the loan is paid up every year.

Amortization method

Amortized even repayment

An equal amount is repaid every year. This includes a larger proportion of the principal and a smaller amount of interest in each succeeding installment of payment. The method of payment is suitable when income is likely to flow at a constant rate throughout the period. The annual installment is arrived at through the formula given.

$$1 = B\frac{i}{1-(1+i)^{n}}$$

Where,

I = Annual installment in Rs.

B = Principal amount borrowed in Rs.

n = Loan period in year.

i = Annual interest rate in fraction.

Amortized decreasing repayment

The amount of the principal remains constant and the share of interest declines with every installment of repayment. Thus, the annual payment becomes smaller every succeeding year.

Financial statement

Some of the financial statements useful to know the financial structure and position of any livestock enterprise are listed below:

Balance Sheet

Profit and Loss Statement

Cash Flow Statement

Balance sheet

A balance sheet is a summary statement of all the assets and liabilities of a business at a given point of time. To be precise, it presents the net value of assets and liabilities in a concise form at a given time and is usually prepared towards the end of the financial year. Balance sheet is also known as Net Worth statement. In a typical Balance sheet, the assets are listed on the left hand side and liabilities are listed on the right hand side.Apart from this, at the bottom of right hand side of balance sheet Net worth or Equity is mentioned.Generally the left hand side values are equal or balances the right hand side values and hence this statement is called as Balance sheet.

Asset

An Asset may be defined as a property which a farmer/firm owns. A Liability is the amount of money owed by the farmer/firm to others. On the basis of liquidity, assets/liabilities are classified into:

Current assets

The assets which are used up in one production cycle and which can be easily converted into cash.

Eg. Cash on hand, accounts receivable, market securities, inventories etc.,

Medium term assets

The assets which are used up in production process for more than one year and upto 5 years.

Eg. Animals, equipments etc.,

Fixed assets

The assets which are used up in production process over a long period and which cannot be easily converted into cash.

Eg. Land, buildings, machinery etc.,

Current liabilities

They refer to short time commitments of the business/farmer which has to be repaid within the current year.

Eg. Accounts payable, taxes payable, interest payable.

Working/Medium term loans

They refer to commitments of the business farmer which could be deferred at present but the due falls in the next season and their time period ranges from 1 – 5 years.

Eg. Medium term loans for Animals or small machinery such as chaff cutter loans etc.,

Deferred liabilities

They refer to long term loans and other such commitments which could be repaid over a period of 5-15 years.

Eg. Long term loans for land, feed mill, hatchery etc.

Net worth/equity

It is the difference between the total assets and total liabilities in the business.

The most liquid current asset is cash in hand and the least liquid current asset is inventory.Eg. Milk can.

The most liquid current liability is money at call and the least liquid asset is long term loans.

Test Ratios

The balance sheet is analysed by estimating various ratios to understand the exact financial position and stability of the farm business.

Current ratio

Current Ratio = Total current assets/ Total current liabilities

Current ratio indicates the capacity of the farmer to meet immediate financial obligations (liquidity). A ratio of more than one indicates a favourable position of the farm business.

Intermediate or working ratio

Intermediate Ratio =Total current assets+Total intermediate assets/ Total current liabilities+ Total intermediate liabilities. Working ratio indicates the liquidity position of the farm business over an intermediate period of time, ranging from 2 to five years. Here, there is time for the farmer to build up the farm business to improve his liquidity position. The ratio should be more than one.

Net capital ratio

Net Capital Ratio= Total assets/ Total current liabilities.

NCR indicates the solvency position of the farmers and more than one indicates that the funds of the institutional agencies are safe. A consistently increasing ratio over the years reveal the sound financial growth of the farm business.

Acid test ratio or quick ratio

Acid test ratio or Quick ratio= Cash receipts+Accounts receivable+marketable securities available in more than one year/ Total current liabilities. Indicates adequacy of cash and income surpluses to cover all current liabilities during the period of one to two years.

Current liability ratio

Current liability Ratio = Current liabilities/Owner's equity which indicates the farmer's immediate financial obligations against the net worth and a ratio of less than one indicates a healthy performance of the farm business.

Debt-equity ratio (Leverage Ratio)

Debt-equity Ratio = Total debts/Owner's equity which reflects the capacity of the farmer to meet the long term commitments also.

Equity-value Ratio

Equity-value Ratio = Owner's equity/Value of assets.

Highlights the productivity gained by the farmer in relation to the assets.

Assets (What you Owe) Current Assets	Liabilities (What you Owe Current Assets
1) Cash or assets which can readily be turned into cash within 12 months. 2) Examples: Cash in Checking or Savings Account, Seed and other Supplies on hand, Accounts Receivable, Crops in Storage, Livestock Held for Sale (steers, pigs).	1) Obligations which must be paid within 12 months. 2) Examples. Principal payments due in 12 months, Accounts Payable, Taxes Due.
Non-Current Assets 1) Intermediate Assets (1 to 10 year life) Examples: Machinery and Equipment Vehicles, Breeding Livestock. 2) Long Term Assets (>10 year life) Land, Buildings and Improvement, Residence and Rental Property.	Non-Current Liabilities 1) Intermediate Liab. Examples: Principal on Intermediate Loans. 2) Long Term Liabilities Examples: Remaining Principal due on Long Term Loans

Profit and loss statement (Income Statement)

Profit and Loss statement is an important financial statement employed to assess the performance of farm business. It shows the operational efficiency of the farm business in terms of receipts, expenses, profits and losses. Generally it is prepared by the entire farm for one agricultural year.

However, it may also be prepared over a period of time. So, we can know the trend in receipts and expenses which indicates the success or failure of a farm business. Thus it contains basically three important items, namely., Receipts, Expenses and Net income.

Income statement

Receipts: They include returns from all the enterprises in the farm. It also includes the appreciation in the value of assets, gifts, many other types of receipts etc. However the returns from the sale of capital assets such as land, buildings, machinery, etc. are not counted as receipts.

Expenses: All the expenses and the variable inputs are taken as operational expenses which includes the interests on working capital. The fixed expenses include, depreciation, interests on fixed capital, rental value of owned land, land revenue, etc. The amount spent on the purchase of any capital asset does not come under expenses.

Net Income: It is calculated in three different ways.

Net Cash Income: This is worked out by reducing total cash expenses from the total cash receipts.

Net Operating Income: It is calculated by reducing the total operational expenses from the gross income.

Net Farm Income: It is worked out by deducting total fixed expenses from the net operating income.Of the three types of net incomes, net farm income is the best measure and is most frequently used for assessing the performance of farm business.

Cash flow statement

This is also known as cash flow summary or cash flow budget or flow of funds statement. Cash flow statement is a summary of cash inflows and cash outflows of a business organization in a particular period, say a season or a year. It is usually prepared for the future, hence the name cash flow budget. The merit of this particular statement is that, it helps to assess the time at which the funds are required for farming and other allied enterprises, sources from which these can be raised, the purpose for which the loan is required, the need of sale and purchase of capital assets, the time and quantum of repayment, etc. Cash flow statement is prepared at the beginning of the agricultural year and checked every quarterly.

For convenience, quarterly checks are made

Cash receipts

Cash Balance

Total Operating Sales

Total Capital Sales

Non-farm income

Borrowings

Total

Cash expenses

Operating Expenses

Capital Investment

Family Living Expenses

Payment of Previous year's Debts

Payment of ST Loans and Installments on Investment Loans

Total

Cash Balance is the difference between Cash Receipts and Cash Expenses

The Cash Flow Statement

Cash Inflows	Cash Outflows
Beginning Balance	Cash Farm Expenses
+ Cash Farm Income	+ Capital Purchases
+ Non Farm Income	+ Family Living Draw
+ Capital Asset Sales	+ Income Taxes Paid
+ New Monies Borrowed	+ Principal Payments
	+ Ending Balance

Cash Inflows - Cash Outflows = 0

CASH FLOW RATIO

$$\text{GOAL} = \frac{\text{Cash Inflows}}{\text{Cash Outflows}} = \text{Greater than } 1.1$$

Advantages of cash flow budget

It is a summary of all the financial matters of the farmer in a comprehensive report.

This helps to estimate the total credit needs (Short term, Medium term and Long term) of the farmer along with time and quantum; to plan the repayment schedule, in making purchases and sales at the appropriate time thereby helping to minimize the credit dependence, so that the farmers can keep limits to avoid wastages to keep ready input requirements well in advance so that the last minute rush can be avoided to know the farm household's expenditure pattern and enable the farmer to exercise a check on farm costs, the farmer in preparing the farm business plans for the ensuing years, the banker for revising the scale of finance, rescheduling loans, etc., and finally, as a tool of financial control to the farmer.

Break even analysis

In any business, there is a point where total costs become equal to total revenues and that point is called as Break Even Point and the corresponding output is known as Break Even Output (BEO).

This means that at this point, the business is making no profit/no loss. Break even point is the minimum point of average total cost. A farmer must produce atleast this amount of product to cover the total cost of production. Whatever is produced above this point will be the profit for the farmer. The point where the farmer recoups his investment is the Break Even Point. There are two approaches to measure the Break Even Point:

Linear approach

Here the sale price of output remains constant for all the output sales. Here the total cost curve and the total revenue curve are linear that is these two curves are straight lines, where the total revenue curve cuts the total cost curve in the Break even point and the corresponding output is known as Break even output.

Break Even Point = Total Fixed Cost/(Selling Price per Unit of Output – Variable Cost per Unit of Output)

Margin of safety

The margin of safety of a farmer is the difference between its normal capacity and break even output. Margin of safety indicates the shock absorbing capacity of the farmer in times of risk and uncertainty. In other words, it reflects the financial strength of the enterprise.

Margin of safety = Normal capacity – Break even output

Margin of safety in monetary terms = Revenue of the total output – Revenues from Break even output.

Curvilinear approach

Here the total revenue changes over the period of time, since the price changes, one output sales to the other. Generally, the curvilinear approach is used for perennial crops and also in business where the gestation period is very long.

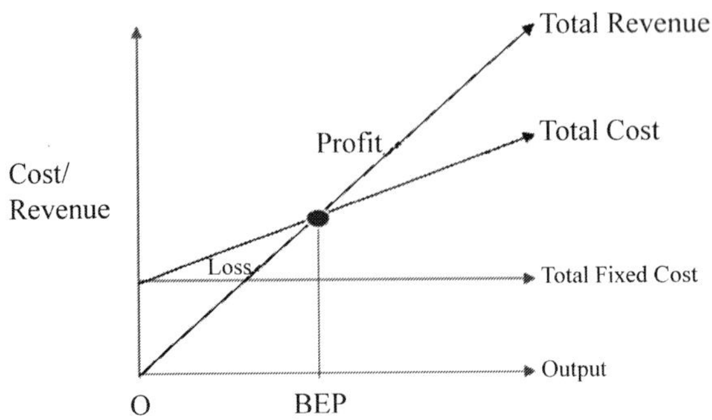

Shut down point

Shut down point is the minimum point of average variable cost. A farmer must produce atleast this amount so that he will be able to cover the variable cost of production. If the total revenue curve goes below this point, it is better to close the business instead of incurring losses.

So this point is called as Shut down point.

25

Bank Support and Insurance for Livestock Enterprises

Scheme

The needy livestock farmer visits the banks in the local area and enquire with the bank manager about the livestock projects and after having discussion with him, he visits the technical expert. A scheme can be prepared by a beneficiary after consulting local technical persons of State animal husbandry department, DRDA, SLPP, etc. livestock co-operative society/union/federation/commercial livestock farmers. If possible, the beneficiaries should also visit progressive livestock farmers and government/military/agricultural university livestock farm in the vicinity and discuss the profitability of livestock farming. A good practical training and experience in livestock farming will be highly desirable. The livestock co-operative societies established in the villages as a result of efforts by the Livestock Development Department of State Government and National Livestock Development Board would provide all supporting facilities particularly marketing of fluid milk. Nearness of livestock farm to such a society, veterinary aid centre, artificial insemination centre should be ensured. There is a good demand for milk, if the livestock farm is located near urban centre. The scheme should include information on land, livestock markets, availability of water, feeds, fodders, veterinary aid, breeding facilities, marketing aspects, training facilities, experience of the farmer and the type of assistance available from State Government, livestock society/union/federation.

The scheme should also include information on the number of and types of animals to be purchased, their breeds, production performance, cost and other relevant input and output costs with their description. Based on this, the total cost of the project, margin money to be provided by the beneficiary, requirement of bank loan, estimated annual expenditure, income, profit and loss statement, repayment period, etc. can be worked out and shown in the Project report.

Scrutiny of Schemes by Banks

The scheme so formulated should be submitted to the nearest branch of a bank. The bank's officers would assist in preparation of the scheme for filling in the prescribed application form. The bank will then examine the scheme for its technical feasibility and economic viability.

Technical Feasibility

Nearness of the selected area to veterinary/breeding/milk collection centre and the financing bank's branch.

Availability of good quality animals in nearby livestock market.

Availability of training facilities.

Availability of good grazing ground/lands.

Green/dry fodder, concentrate feed, medicines, etc.

Availability of veterinary aid/breeding centres and marketing facilities near the scheme area.

Capability of the owner and employees such as technical knowledge and skill.

Economic Viability

Unit cost of livestock .

Input cost for feeds and fodders, veterinary aid, breeding of animals, insurance, labour and other overheads.

Output costs, i.e. sale price of livestock products, manure, gunny bags, young ones, other miscellaneous items etc.

Income-expenditure statement and annual gross surplus.

Cash flow analysis

Repayment schedule (i.e. repayment of principal loan amount and interest).

Other documents such as loan application forms, security aspects, margin money requirements, etc. are also examined.

A field visit to the scheme area is undertaken for conducting a techno-economic feasibility study for appraisal of the scheme.

Break Even Point, Investment Analysis (particularly, IRR), Payback period, Marketing process.

Sanction of bank loan and its disbursement

After ensuring technical feasibility and economic viability, the scheme is sanctioned by the bank.

The loan is disbursed in kind in 2 to 3 stages against creation of specific assets such as construction of sheds, purchase of equipments and machinery, purchase of animals and recurring cost on purchase of feeds/fodders for the initial period of one/two months.

The end use of the fund is verified and constant follow-up is done by the bank.

Lending terms

Each Regional Office (RO) of NABARD (www.nabard.org) has constituted a State Level Unit Cost Committee under the Chairmanship of RO-in-charges and with the members from developmental agencies, commercial banks and cooperative banks to review the unit cost of various investments once in six months. The same is circulated among the banks for their guidance.

These costs are only indicative in nature and banks are free to finance any amount depending upon the availability of assets.

Margin money

NABARD had defined farmers into three different categories and where subsidy is not available the minimum down payment as shown below is collected from the beneficiaries.

Insurance in livestock sector

Livestock insurance in India is a multi-agency programme. General Insurance Corporation (GIC) along with its subsidiaries – United India Insurance Company Ltd., New India Assurance Company Ltd., Oriental Insurance Company Ltd., and National Insurance Company Ltd., is carrying out livestock insurance. The insurance market was liberalized only in the year 2000. After this, understanding the volume of business, private sector (BASIX-Royal Sundaram) have also entered into the market. The type of insurance, procedure, claim details, etc. are listed below.

Cattle insurance

Under this insurance, animals are covered against death due to diseases or accident (including fire/lightning/famine/flood cyclone) surgical operation, strike, riot, civil commotions risk.Generally there are three types in it:Cattle insurance,Foetus (Unborn Calf Insurance) andCalf heifer rearing insurance.

Sheep and Goat insurance

This scheme is also governed under Market Agreement.

Policy provides indemnity to indigenous cross-bred and exotic sheep and goat against death due to accident (including fire, lightening, flood, cyclone, famine, strike, riot and civil commotion) and disease. Earthquake and landslide covers are also provided. Standard and common exclusions apply as per Cattle Policy. Animals are identified by means of small brass buttons ear tags. Animals under scheme category enjoy certain benefits in premium rate and claim procedure.

Pig, Horse, Donkey, Yak, Mule insurance etc., are also available.

Poultry/Duck Insurance

The cover is available to the poultry/duck farm owned by the farmers.

Insurance covers all types of exotic and cross breed poultry birds and ducks against death due to accident (including fire, lightning, famine, riot and strike and civil commotion) or diseases as per Poultry Insurance Policy.

Animal driven cart insurance

This insurance covers carts, tongas and coaches drawn by buffaloes, bulls, bullocks, horse, mule, donkeys and camels and also the animals pulling it. T.P. liability and death, disablement of the driver as per Animal driven cart Insurance policy.

Cattle insurance

The scheme covers the following animals, whether indigenous, exotic or cross-bred.

Milch Cows and Buffaloes

Calves / Heifers

Stud Bulls

Bullocks (Castrated Bulls) and Castrated Male Buffaloes

Animals within a specified age group are accepted under the Standard Insurance Scheme. Sum insured under the policy will be the market value of the animal. Indemnity under the policy will be the sum insured or market value prior to illness whichever is less. The indemnity is limited to 75% of sum insured in case of a PTD claim. The basic premium rate per annum is 4% of the sum insured. Long term policies are also issued with long term discounts. The premium rates under the policy are concessional for covering animals under government subsidized schemes. Group discounts are also available.

Insurance coverage

The policy shall give indemnity for death due to.

- Accident (due to fire, lightning, flood, inundation, storm, hurricane, earthquake, cyclone, tornado, tempest and famine).
- Diseases contracted or occurring during the period of the policy.
- Surgical Operations.
- Riot and Strike.

The policy can also be extended to cover PTD on payment of extra premium;

- Permanent total disability which, in the case of milch cattle result in permanent and total incapacity to conceive or yield milk.
- PTD which in the case of stud bulls results in permanent and total incapacity for breeding purpose.
- In case of bullocks, calves / heifers and castrated male buffaloes results in permanent and total incapacity for the purpose of use mentioned in the proposal form.

Documents to effect insurance coverage

- Proposal form
- Veterinary health certificate from a qualified veterinarian giving the age, identification marks, health, and market value of the animal in the prescribed format.

Identification of animal

All insured animals should be suitably identified by natural identification marks and color should be clearly noted in the proposal form and Veterinarian's Report.

Ear tags made of suitable material are applied to the ear of the animals and the code number is entered into the Veterinary Health Certificate.

Photographs of animals may be insisted in case of high value animal.

Claim procedure

In the event of death of an animal, immediate intimation should be sent to the insurers and the following requirements should be furnished:

- Duly completed claim form.
- Death certificate obtained from qualified Veterinarian on Company's form.
- Postmortem examination report if required by the Company.
- Ear tag applied to the animal should be surrendered. The condition of 'No Tag- No claim' will be applied if the tag is not surrendered.

Claim procedure for PTD claim

- A certificate from the qualified veterinarian to be obtained.
- The animal will be inspected by the company's Veterinary Officer also.
- Complete chart of treatment, medicines used, receipts, etc. should be submitted.
- Admissibility of claim will be considered after two months of Veterinary Doctor / Company Doctor's report.
- The indemnity is limited to 75% of sum insured.

Sheep and Goat insurance

Highlights

- All indigenous, crossbred and exotic sheep and goat will be covered under the Scheme.

Scope

- The policy provides indemnity against death of sheep and goats due to accident including fire, lightning, flood, cyclone, famine, earthquake, landslide, strike, riot or diseases contracted or occurring during the period of insurance.

Sum insured

- The market value of sheep and goats varies from breed to breed, from area to area and from time to time.
- The examining veterinarian's recommendations is considered as the proper guide for acceptance of insurance as well as for settlement of claims.
- Sum insured will not exceed 100% of market value.

Claim procedure

- In the event of death, immediate intimation should be given to the Company and the Insured should furnish the following documents and required information.
- Duly completed claim form.
- Death certificate from a veterinarian on Company's form
- Post-mortem examination report, if required by the Company.
- Ear tag wherever applicable.

Poultry insurance

Highlights

- This is a comprehensive insurance scheme applicable to poultry farms consisting of layer birds, broiler birds and parent stock (Hatchery) which are exotic and crossbred.
- All birds in a farm should be covered. After issuing policy, if additional birds are introduced in the farm, immediate notice to be given to insurer otherwise claim will be repudiated.
- The scheme is applicable to poultry farms consisting of minimum number of birds as specified.

The scheme is available for insuring birds in the following age groups

Broilers	• 1 day to 8 weeks • 1 day to 6 weeks
Layers	• 1 day to 20 weeks • 21 weeks to 72 weeks • 1 day to 72 weeks
Hatchery Birds (Parent Stock)	• 1 day to 72 weeks

The premium rates are applicable on per cent basis which are applicable to the peak value of birds in the applicable categories.

- The sum insured is the peak value and for broilers it is Rs 45 and for layers Rs 75. There is a week wise valuation table in-built in the policy which is applied for calculating indemnity. In case of parent, stock the same is negotiable.
- The policy is charactersied by excess and final indemnity is restricted to 80% (60% in case of Gumboro).

- The scheme is characterized by No claim discounts as well as good feature discount.

Insurance Coverage

- The policy shall provide indemnity against death of birds due to accident (including fire, lightning, flood, cyclone, storm, tempest, earthquake, strike, riot, act of terrorism) or diseases contracted or occurring during the period of insurance subject to the exclusions.

How to Effect Insurance

- Proposal form.
- Veterinary Health Certificate from a qualified veterinarian.
- All birds in the farm should be covered. Farm should follow standard package of practices, vaccination schedule, deworming and debeaking.
- Farm should maintain essential records as per insurers specifications.

Claim Procedure

- In the event of death of birds, immediate intimation should be given to the Company and the Insurer should be supplied with the following documents and required information:
    - Duly filled in claim form.
    - Vet. P.M. Report for sample birds.
    - Daily records of mortality, feeding, etc.
    - Purchase invoices for the birds.
    - Any other point to substantiate the loss like photographs, medical bills, etc. as and when required.
- In case of alarming death/outbreak of epidemic nature, immediate notice within 12 hours should be given to the Company and all birds should be segregated and produced to the representative of the Company or to any person authorised by the Company for inspection.
- Daily mortality details should be sent to the Company on weekly basis failing which report will be treated as nil for that particular week.
- Delay in reporting of the claim should be avoided and if there is delay for more than three days the claim would be treated as non-standard.
- In case of doubtful claims/ farms for which claim ratio is adverse, Technical Report from an expert may be insisted for settlement of claim.

26

Approaches to Preparation of Entrepreneurial Projects on Livestock

- A project is a specific plan or design presented for consideration.
- It is a location specific activity with specific objectives, time and cost limitations and of non-repetitive nature.
- In banking, projects refers to an activity in which financial resources are expended to create capital assets that produce benefits over an extended period of time and which logically lends itself to planning, financing and implementing as a unit. Whereas, UNIDO defines a project as a proposal for an investment to create and or develop certain facilities in order to increase the production of goods/services in a community over a certain period of time.
- Projects are common term used by many to denote specific action plans.
- Project can be long term or short term, limited or comprehensive, single sector concentrated or multi sector concentrated.
- Project Evaluation is a step-by-step process of collecting, recording and organizing information about project results, including short-term outputs (immediate results of activities, or project deliverables), and immediate and longer-term project outcomes (changes in behaviour, practice or policy resulting from the project).
- Common rationales for conducting an evaluation are:
    - response to demands for accountability;
    - demonstration of effective, efficient and equitable use of financial and other resources;
    - recognition of actual changes and progress made;
    - identification of success factors, need for improvement ;
    - validation for project staff and partners that desired outcomes are being achieved.

Importance

- Evaluating project results is helpful in finding answers to key questions like
  - What progress has been made?
  - Whether the desired outcomes were achieved, if not why?
  - Are there ways that project activities can be refined to achieve better outcomes?
  - Do the project results justify the project inputs?

Project: can be defined thus as

- A scientifically evolved work plan
- Devised to achieve a specific objectives
- Within specified time limit
- Consuming planned resources

Identifying the Project

- The first phase of project management is concerned with identifying the project to achieve the desired objectives.
- The initial task coming under project identification is to find out the sources of the project.
- Agencies like government organisations, international institutions like WHO, World Bank, UNDP, Non GovernmentalOrganisations can serve as the better source of projects.
- Progressive farmers, successful entrepreneurs, technical experts, Bankers, Media, National priorities and Thrust areas of Development also serve sources for Identification of Projects.

Project need analysis

- The aspects included under project need analysis are the beneficiaries (target group), problem, solutions, and decisions.
- The problem should exhibit the necessity of immediate intervention.
- The focus should be to identify the beneficiaries (target group).
- The solutions should solve the original problem.

- The decision to take up the project lies on how these three aspects problem, solutions and beneficiaries are important to project intervention.

Problem formulation and statement of the problem

- The crux of the project lies in the problem formulation process.
- The project team should have detailed understanding of the problem, scope, intervention areas and the out come of the project to be hypothesized.
- Based on a multi phased understanding and analysis, describe the problem to be addressed and resolved.

Project planning

- Project planningcan be defined as a scientific and systematic process, in which logical linkages are clearly established among various element of projects. Successful implementation of the project lies on effective project plan.
- Based on the anticipated goals and objectives the project planning shall be made.
- The project plan is the blue print of the project.
- Effective planning gives proper direction in the implementation of the project and it further helps in adequate monitoring and evaluation.
- For the implementation of plan, an activity chart has to be prepared.
- The activity chart consists of all the proposed activities in the implementation process, including the start date, calendar for the entire project, dates of monitoring and evaluation periods, finishing stages, series of out puts, slack time and responsible person who is going to coordinate the activities etc.

Project budget

- The project budgeting phase is in the project formulation phase.
- Two types of budgets are to be made.
- One is the cost category budget (materials, administration, capital; expenditures etc) and the second is the activity budget.
- This project budget is to calculate the cost of each project inputs.
- The estimation of the project cost should be made on fairly realistic sense of financial values.

- In the multi year projects the inflation rate also has to be anticipated in advance.

Approaches in preparation of livestock entrepreneurial project

- Different approaches are followed while preparing Entrepreneurial project on livestock.
- Based on the technical knowledge, past experience and guidance from the subject matter specialist, the entrepreneur himself can choose the activity, budget, location etc., taking into account the resources available with him and the market demand for the products.
- After choosing the activity, he can assess it's profitability by preparing the Entrepreneurial project.
- While preparing the livestock project , the following aspects have to be adhered.

Institutional - Organizational - Managerial Aspects

- A whole range of issues in project preparation revolves around the overlapping institutional, organizational and managerial aspects of projects, which clearly have an important affect on project implementation. The socio-cultural patterns and institutions of those, the project will serve must be considered.
- The organizational proposals should be examined to see that the project is manageable. The analyst must examine the ability of the available staff to judge whether they can administer such large-scale activities such as Dairy processing unit, Integrated poultry complex(feed mill, hatchery, layers unit and processing) etc.,. When managerial skills are limited, provision may have to be made for training.

Social aspects

- There is a greater need for analysts to consider the social patterns and practices of the clientele a project will serve. More and more frequently, project analysts are also expected to examine carefully the broader social implications of the proposed investments.The project should not affect the local sentiments of the region. Cattle rearing for beef marketing, pork production and sales tanneries etc., are some of the examples. If the social aspect is not taken care of, the project may face severe opposition from the local people, which could ruin the profitability of the project. Though the project may be technically and economically feasible, it could not be processed, if it affects the local people sentiments or their livelihood.

Commercial aspects

- On the output side, careful analysis of the expected market for the project's production is essential to ensure that there will be an effective demand at a remunerative price. Where will the products be sold? Is the market large enough to absorb the new production without affecting the price? If the price is likely to be affected, by how much? Is the product meant for domestic consumption or for export? Does the proposed project produce the grade or quality that the market demands? Since the product must be sold at market prices, a judgment about future government price supports or subsidies may also be considered.Ifthe demand is not estimated or forecasted accurately, it may end in over production or missed sale opportunities.

Financial aspects

- The financial aspects of project preparation and analysis encompass the financial effects of a proposed project on each of its various participants. In livestock projects the participants include farmers, private sector firms, public corporations, project agencies, and perhaps the national treasury.
- The farm budget becomes the basis for shaping the credit terms to be made available. The analyst must judge whether farmers will need loans to finance on-farm investment (and if so, what is the margin money the farmers should invest from their own resources) or to meet some production costs, and whether seasonal short-term credit should be provided for working capital to finance inputs and pay for hired labor. In long term projects , the analyst should judge, whether the farmers have adequate capacity to lead their life till the returns are expected or any special financial arrangements need to be created. The analysis of farm income will also be helpful in assessing the incentives for farmers to participate in the project. What will be the probable level of change in farm income? When it is expected? How likely are price changes or fluctuations could affect farm income? What will be the effect of subsidy arrangements on farm income, and what changes in government policy might affect the income earned by farmers?

Economic aspects

- The economic aspects of project preparation and analysis require a determination of the likelihood that a proposed project will contribute significantly to the development of the farm economy and total economy and whether it justifies using the scarce resources it reuired. The point of view taken in the economic analysis is that of the society as a whole. The financial and economic analyses are thus complementary-the financial analysis takes the viewpoint of the individual participants and the economic analysis that of the society.

27

Procurement Management, Quality Issues, Standardization, Grading and Packaging

Procurement is acquisition of goods and services.

Procurement includes:

- Planning the acquisition
- Planning the contracting
- Requesting proposals
- Selecting a vendor
- Administering the contract
- Closing the contract

Planning the acquisition

It is based on goals of an enterprise acquisition varies – depends on what, when and where to produce. Based on these factors acquisition requirements are arrived.

Planning the contract

Request vendor costs and support for technical requirements from only those vendors that support user requirements. Reduce the time to procure a system by limiting initial vendor proposals to scripted demonstration of user requirements. Maintain consensus by working with key users as they prepare requirements, conduct vendor demonstrations and select the best option.

Requesting the proposals

Identify vendors that support user needs, provide similar products to competitors and/or have existing relationships with your organization. Prepare a vendor short-list and solicit proposals. Prepare solicitation document and administer vendor solicitation process.

Select the vendor

Evaluate vendors during demonstrations and request finalists' costs and support for technical requirements. Check references and conduct site visits and select vendor supporting most user requirements at lowest cost.

Negotiate a contract

Prepare an agreement. Assemble your negotiating team, including project manager and an attorney with system procurement experience. Identify, prioritize and share negotiation issues with vendor. Obtain and evaluate vendor response. Prepare fallback response and share with vendor and narrow issues to short-list and conduct face-to-face negotiations

Administer the contract

Use contract scope of services, project schedule and budget as standards. Monitor vendor compliance. Identify deviations and define agreed upon corrective actions. Prepare change orders/contract amendments where required by corrective actions. Monitor and document successful completion of corrective actions.

Close the agreement

Compare deliverable results to deliverable acceptance criteria included in contract scope of services. Identify corrective actions if the vendor does not adhere to the acceptance criteria. Review updated deliverable to confirm compliance. Accept and pay vendor for deliverable when it complies with acceptance criteria.

Standardisation and grading

Standardization is the process of fixing certain norms for the product. These norms are established by customs or tradition or by certain authority.

Standardization is a application of standard to goods meant for marketing with a view to further sub dividing them into several grades or classes. Standardization means setting standard of quality.

The following are some of the factors on the basis of which standards are set:

- Quality
- Quantity
- Measurement and
- Size

The prevention of Food Adulteration Act, Agmark and Indian standard Institute (ISI) prescribed some minimum standards for fat and solids non-fat contents in respect of milk sold in different forms including raw pasteurized, flavoured etc. Standards of milk products for milk fat, total solids, moisture content, and other constituents-PFA. Chemical standards and moisture contents in ghee have been prescribed under the Agmark, Indian standards Institution (ISI), laid down standard for the fermented milk products.

Advantages of standardization

- Uniformity in quality
- Differential pricing
- Increased in demand
- Elimination of risk
- Expanding the market
- Helps to reduce inventory items

Grading

Grading means separating the products according to established standards. Grading is an important function of standardization. Grading is categorizing the produce into different lots, each containing similar characteristics. The characteristics could be one or more of the following type:

Size – Big, medium, small, long, short, roundish, oblong etc.

Flavour – which in turn speaks of taste or class

Content – Ingredients

Location oriented – for some products - Assam tea, Mysore silk.

Having specific tastes, shape, colour etc.

Examples

- Butter: AA, A, B C
- Eggs: AA, A, B
- Beef: USDA Prime, USDA Choice, USDA Select, USDA Standard

Milk grades and their standards:

Milk	Fat %	SNF %
Buffalo milk	6	9
Cow milk	3.5	8.5
Goat/Sheep milk	3.5	9
Standardized milk	4.5	8.5
Recombined milk	3.0	8.5
Toned milk	3.0	8.5
Double toned	1.5	9.0
Skim milk	0.5	8.7

Other grades of milk

- Grade I- Fresh milk completely free from off-flavours, abnormal colours and visible foreign materials, such milk when tested Methyl Blue Reduction (MBR) should give more than five and half hrs time.
- Grade II - Milk having off-flavours such as cowy/barny, flat, foreign, metallic, or rancid to a moderate degree and MBR time between two and half hours to five and half hours. Presence of small amounts of foreign material placed under this category.
- Grade III - Milk having off-flavours such as acidic, bitter, weedy, oxidized, metallic and extraneous material distinctly visible in great amount is classified as grade III milk. This milk has less than two and half hours MBR time.

Grading of eggs

Classification of eggs according to characteristics that have an economic value – weight

According to BIS - egg grades

Grade	Weight (g/egg)
A Extra large	≥ 60
A Large	53-59
A Medium	45-52
A Small	38-44

Grading of wool

- American or Blood system –it is based on purity of the breed
- British or Spinning count system – it is based on spinning count – No. of hanks per yarn of 512m in 450g of wool.

- Indian System -Grading centres in Jaipur, Bikaner, Jodhpur, Panipat, Ludhiana and Amritsar.

Letter System

Letter	Quality
Super A	Superfine wool
A	Fine wool
B	Medium wool
C	Strong wool
D	Coarse wool

- Number system – (30's-80's) fineness
- Color system - White color, light yellow, medium, heavy yellow, black/ brown (rejected)
- Vegetable matter content

  Light burr – 3% burr

  Medium burr – 3-6%

  Heavy burr - >6%

Advantages and importance of grading

- Production of Large Scale
- Increase in Sales
- Quality Certainty
- Easier to understand quality available for each grade
- Price comparison by consumers is easy to due to grade identity
- Create competition in the market

Problems in standardisation and grading

- Lack of Standards & Grades
- Misuse of Standards & Grades
- Lack of Public Consciousness
- Lack of Testing Facilities
- Lack of consumer awareness of grades.
- Perishabililty and its impact on grades

Trade and quality of products

AGMARK is the acronym for agricultural marketing. It is a quality certification mark under central agricultural produced (Grading & Marketing) ACT, 1937. AGMARK is done for commodities of internal consumption like ghee, vegetable oil butter, etc. The AGMARK label indicates the products meet certain standards of purity and quality. Labels of different colors are used to indicate the grade of the products.

ISI ACT was passed in1952. This ACT gave power to the institute to the test the quality and characteristics of agriculture product and mark them with "AGMARK". It also gave power to the producers of quality product to use mark '959'.

Excellence in food quality and safety has taken a tangible form with the advent of ISO 9000 Quality Management System and Hazard Analysis Critical Control Points (HACCP) standards.

ISO 9000 encompasses all the activities of a company to ensure that it meets its quality objectives, while HACC is directed towards ensuring food safety. The ISO 9000 standards were brought by the International Organization for Standardization (ISO) and the HACCP standards by the Code Alimentarius Commission (C AC).

These standards have assumed importance worldwide both as an essential requirement to tap the market potential and as a marketable feature of the company. Since the global market has become more demanding in terms of quality, safety and timely delivery, installation of the ISO 9000 Quality Management System and HACCP by the food industry is essential for getting a competitive international edge.

Packaging of livestock products – necessities and uses

- Containment – hold the content and keep it till used
- Protection & preservation – mechanical deterioration, light, oxygen, heat, gases, microorganisms, insects
- Information – use, shelf life, storage conditions, ingredients, nutritional values, health claims, description of the product
- Suitability for the process – performance on production line for high speed production with least stoppage
- Convenient – production, storage, use (size & shape, weight, "cook inside" "ready to eat"' easy opening).

- Availability – seasons, location
- Appearance – graphics, attractive

Films used for food packaging are

Typical application	Type of laminate
Crisps, snacks, confectionery, ice cream, biscuit	PVDC/PP/PVDC/PP
Bakery products, cheese, confectionery, dried fruits, frozen vegetables	PVDC/PP/PE
Coffee, dried milk, bag-in-box, potato flakes, frozen foods, MA packaged foods	Met-PET/PE
Retort pouches (cook-inside package)	High barrier PET/PP Or PET/ Aluminum/PP
Vacuum packs for bulk fresh meat, cheese	PE/Aluminum/PP
Dried soup, dried vegetables, chocolate, buttor	PE/Aluminum/Paper
Bag-in/box packaging	PE/mulAinium/PE/PVDC/PA

Where: PP – polypropylene, PVDC – Polyvinylidene chloride, PVC – polyvinyl chloride,

PS – polystyrene, PET – polyethylene terephthalate

28

Retail Marketing, Sales Operations and Management, Advertising, Marketing of Services

Retailing

Retailingincludes all activities involved in selling and providing goods and services to ultimate consumers for personal or household use.

Classification of retail establishments

Based on ownership

- Independent retailer- one store ownership
- Chain retailer- many stores but owner is one
- Franchise – many owners of many stores

Basic forms of franchises are

Dealer agrees to sell certain products provided by a manufacturer, but can use any sales tactics he chooses.

Ex-Michelin Tires, Avon

Dealer must sell the franchiser's product in the exact way the franchiser prescribes.

Ex – McDonalds, Wendy's

Business Format Franchising

Classification based on level of services

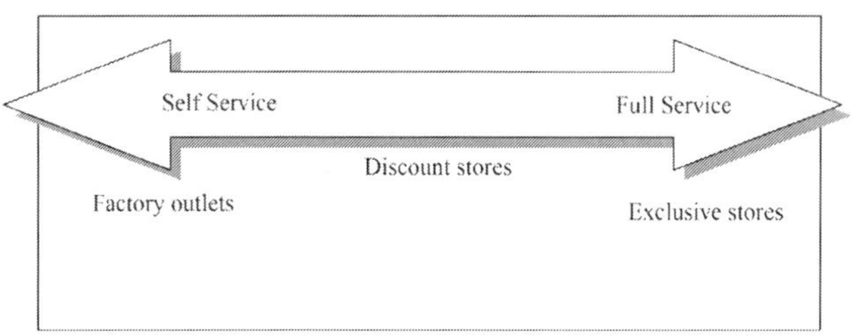

In self service type producer himself sell the produce through their own factory outlets. Discount stores procure from producers in bulk at a lower price. In exclusive stores separate categories of products are sold like- electronic store, cloth store etc.

Classification based on product offering

The mix of products offered to the consumer by the retailer, which is also called as product assortment.

Deep & narrow products Or Shallow & broad like Big Bazaar

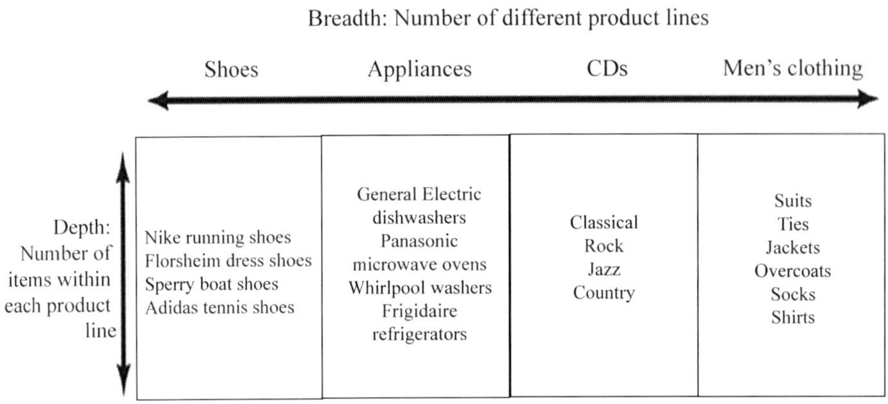

Depth of production line

1. Speciality outlet- only single product at different version- all high end mobile phones
2. Category killers

Breadth of product line

1. General Merchandise stores – footwear store
2. Scrambled Merchandising- involves offering several unrelated product lines in a single store.

Types

Departmental stores- Very large stores offering a huge assortment of "soft" and "hard goods; often bear a resemblance to a collection of specialty stores. A retailer of such store carries variety of categories and has broad assortment at average price. They offer considerable customer service.

Speciality stores- A typical speciality store gives attention to a particular category and provides high level of service to the customers. A pet store that specializes in selling dog food would be regarded as a specialty store. However, branded stores also come under this format.

Supermarket- It is a self-service store consisting mainly of grocery and limited products on non food items.

Convenience store- It is essentially found in residential areas. They provide limited amount of merchandise at more than average prices with a speedy checkout. This store is ideal for emergency and immediate purchases as it often works with extended hours, stocking everyday.

Discount stores- These tend to offer a wide array of products and services, but they compete mainly on price offers extensive assortment of merchandise at affordable and cut-rate prices. Normally retailers sell less fashion-oriented brands.

Non store marketing

1. Automatic vending- employ machines
2. Direct Marketing

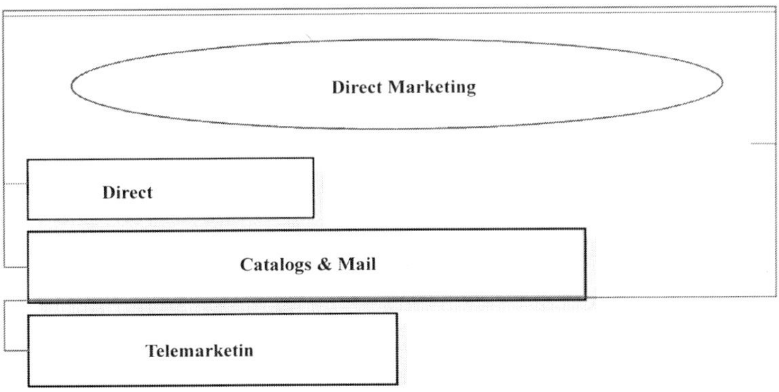

3. Electronic retailing

Retailing Mix

The **retailing mix** includes the activities related to managing the store and the merchandise in the store, which includes retail pricing, store location, retail communication, and merchandise.

Choosing the retailing mix depends on

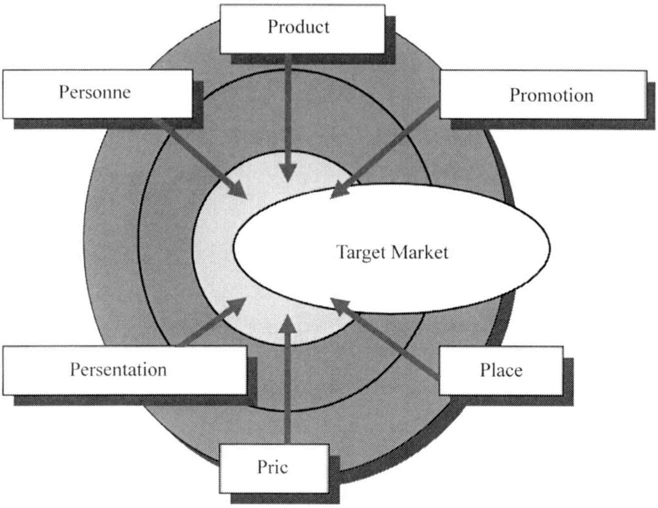

Retailing strategy- **pricing** depends on

- **How much mark-up?**
  - **Allow for Shrinkage and discounting** (**Shrinkage** is the breakage and theft of merchandise by customers and employees.)

Retailing strategy – Location

- **Central Business District- Parasites**(Parasite stores do not create their own traffic. They make money based on their proximity to things that will draw foot traffic. (bigger stores, train stations, airports, office buildings, etc.)
- **Regional Shopping Centers - Anchor Stores** (A large store, such as a department store or supermarket, that is prominently located in a shopping mall to attract customers who are then expected to patronize the other shops in the mall.)
- **Strip Location - Destination stores, Power centers** (Stores that generate customers from larger trading areas than their neighbors or competitors and power centers are huge shopping strips with multiple anchors and often a supermarket)
- **Multichannel Retailers** – (Multichannel retailers utilize and integrate a combination of traditional store formats and non-store formats such as catalogs, television, and online retailing)

Presentation of retail shops

Factors in Creating Store's Atmosphere

- Employee type and density
- Merchandise type and density
- Fixture type and density
- Sound
- Odour
- Visual factors

Factors in personnel decisions

- How many
- How knowledgeable
- How hopeful/ invasive
- Fit the image of the product
- Good personal sellers

Advertising

Advertise is a message designed to promote a product, a service, or an idea. The purpose of advertising is to sell products or services.

Objectives of advertising

- To introduce a new product by creating interest for it among the prospective customers.
- To support personal selling programme. Advertising maybe used to open customers' doors for salesman.
- To reach people inaccessible to salesman
- To enter a new market or attract a new group of customers.
- To light competition in the market and to increase the sales
- To enhance the goodwill of the enterprise by promising better quality products and services.
- To improve dealer relations. Advertising supports the dealers in selling the product. Dealers are attracted towards a product which is advertised effectively.

- To warn the public against imitation of an enterprise's products.

Advertising techniques

1. **Basic appeals**
   - Biological
     - Focus on consumer's basic needs for health and security
   - Emotional
     - Focus on the consumers' feelings (love, romance, pride)
   - Rational
     - Focus on the consumer's reasoning abilities (cost, safety, convenience)
   - Social
     - Focus on the way that social pressures influence consumer behaviour (odour, weight, acne, fashion)
2. **Attention-getting headlines**
   - A successful headline leads a person into reading the rest of the ad.
   - Some headlines attract attention by promising the reader a personal benefit, such as savings or improvement in physical appearance.
3. **Slogans**
   - Short phrases that a company uses over and over in its ads.
   - Good slogans are easy to remember and stick in people's minds.
4. **Testimonials**
   - Aadvertisements in which a person endorses a product.
   - The person may be someone who looks like the average user of the product or it may be a movie or TV star, athlete or other celebrity.
5. **Product characters**
   - Fictional people and cartoon animals or characters used in advertisements over a long period of time (McDonald, KFC)
6. **Comparison of products**
   - Used most frequently to sell products that compete heavily with other brands.

- Advertisers compare their product with similar brands and point out the advantages of using their brand.

7. **Repetition**

- One of the most basic techniques advertisers use to get their message across, whether it is a commercial broadcast several times a day or an ad published frequently.
- Repetition can help build or reinforce a company's reputation. Advertisers also believe that the more people see or hear an advertisement, the more likely they are to accept the message and want the product.

Types of ads

- **Promotional advertising**

Promotional advertising is advertising that is designed to increase sales by

- creating an interest in products
- introducing new products and businesses
- explaining a product
- supporting personal selling efforts
- creating new markets

- **Institutional advertising**

Institutional advertising attempts to create a favorable impression (image) and goodwill for a business or an organization. Purpose is to develop a positive image by presenting information about a company's role in the community, important public issues and topics of general interest.

Advertising media

Media are the agencies, means or instruments used to convey messages. Advertising reaches people through various forms of mass communication. These *media* include newspapers, magazines, television, radio, the Internet, direct mail, outdoor signs, transit signs, window displays, point-of-purchase displays, telephone directories, novelties.

Three Categories of Advertising Media:

- Print media
- Broadcast media
- Specialty media

Print media can include any of the following:

- Newspapers
- Direct Mail
- Magazine
- Outdoor Advertising
- Directory Advertising
- Transit Advertising

Newspapers

Approximately 55% of adults read the newspaper every day.

Shopper- A community newspaper which contains no editorial content and is delivered free to persons who live in certain areas (full of ads)

Advantages & disadvantages of newspaper advertising

- Large readership
- Known circulation (easy to target)
- Low cost
- Timely and flexible
    - Wasted circulation
    - Disposable (short lifespan)
    - Poor quality advertising

Magazine Classifications: Local, Regional, National weeklies, Monthlies and Quarterlies

Advantages & disadvantages of magazine advertising

- Easy to target your market
- Read slowly and thoroughly
- Good print quality
- Longer life span because they are kept of an extended period of time
    - Less mass appeal within a geographic area
    - More expensive than newspapers
    - Not timely or flexible (long lead times)

Direct mail advertising (Junk Mail)

- Advertising that is sent directly to prospective customers through the mail
- (More than $80 billion in goods and services sold annually through direct mail)
- Have you ever bought anything through direct mail advertising?
- What do you do with it when you get it?

Advantages & disadvantages of direct mail advertising

- Advertiser can be highly selective
- Flexible and secretive
- Wide choice of formats
- Can use coupons or other incentives
- Can directly make the sale
    - Low level of response (-1%)
    - High costs
    - Poor image (junk mail) often not read

Outdoor advertising

- Non-standardized outdoor signs are used by local firms at their place of business or in other locations throughout the community.
- Standardized outdoor signs are available to local, regional or national advertisers.

Three types of standardized outdoor signs

- **Posters** - Preprinted sheets put up like wallpaper on outdoor billboards (McDonalds)
- **Painted bulletins** - Painted billboards that are changed every 6 months to a year
- **Spectaculars** - outdoor signs using lights, moving parts and are situated in high traffic areas or cities

Advantages and disadvantages of outdoor advertising

- Highly visible
- Relatively inexpensive
- Permits easy repetition of message
- Can be geographically tailored for target market
    - Short message due to limited viewing time
    - Unknown audience
    - Government regulations

Directory advertising

- Alphabetical listing of businesses
    - Relatively inexpensive
    - Found in 98% of households - all demographics
    - Kept for at least a year - not thrown away
    - Very inflexible due to being printed yearly
    - Wasted advertising (to non-target market)

Transit advertising

- Using public facilities to advertise - such as subways, on buses and taxis, in stations
- Reaches a wide and captive audience
- Economical
- Defined market (usually urban)
    - Unavailable in smaller towns
    - Subject to defacement
    - Restricted to certain travel destinations

Broadcast media- radio, television

Radio advertising

- Prime time is morning and afternoon drive times - advertisers guaranteed concentrated audience

- Ads are available in 15, 30 or 60 second time slots

Advantages and Disadvantages of Radio Advertising

- Select and audience - target their market
- Flexible - can change quickly and easily
- Mobile (can be taken anywhere - shopping, jogging, hiking or driving
    - Short life span
    - Sometimes many stations - have to decide which to use or use them all (more expensive) Distractions - no visual involvement

Television advertising

- The *ultimate* advertising medium because it can communicate with sound, action and color
- Prime time is 7 p.m. - 11 p.m.
- Infomercials - 30 minute commercials

Advantages & disadvantages of television advertising

- All elements for creative message
- Believability
- More personal & effective
- Can reach the masses or target specific interests
- Adaptable to special needs
    - Expensive - the highest production costs - too high for small businesses
    - Audience size is not assured
    - Nuisance - channel surfing - leave during commercials

Specialty media

- Inexpensive, useful items with an advertiser's name printed on them - usually given away

Other Types of Advertising Media

- Sports Arena Billboards
- Movie theater commercials

- Hot air balloons, blimps, skywriting, banners
- shelf ads, shopping cart ads, coupon machines, receipt ads

Marketing of services

A service is defined as any activity or benefit that one party can offer to another which is essentially intangible and does not result in the ownership of anything.Most company offerings to customers contain an element of service and this is illustrated by the service continuum.

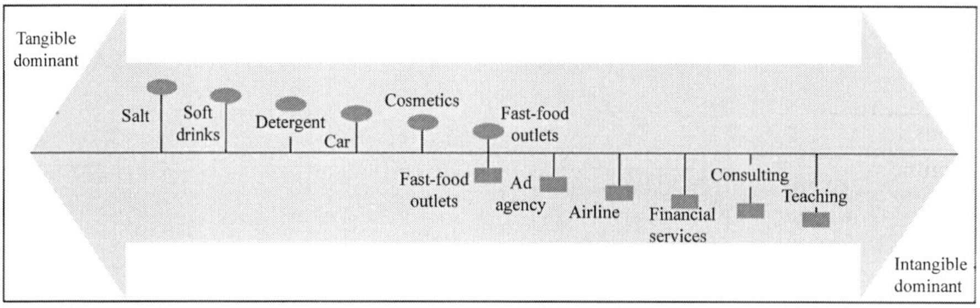

Categorising offerings along the service continuum

- ***Pure tangible goods***
  - toothpaste
- ***Tangible goods accompanied by one or more service***
  - computer and warranty
- ***Hybrid offer consists of equal parts of goods and services***
  - restaurants
- ***Service with accompanying minor goods***
  - air travel
- ***Pure service***
  - haircut

Service characteristics

i. Intangibility- Cannot be seen, tasted, felt, heard or smelt before they are bought. Service providers need to manage the evidence by providing evidence of the benefits.

ii. Inseparability- Services produced and consumed simultaneously. Cannot be separated from providers, whether people or machines. Customers are always involved

iii. Variability - Quality may vary greatly depending on who provides the service, when and how. Staff need to know how to do something well. Staff must be well motivated to maintain high standards of service.

iv. Perishability - Services cannot be stored for later sale or use

v. Lack of ownership- No physical product is exchanged and therefore nothing owned.

Difference between services and goods

Goods	Services	Implications
Tangible	Intangible	Services cannot be inventoried, displayed and communicated
Standardized	Heterogeneous	Each time experience differs. Services quality depends on many uncontrolled factors
Production separate from consumption	Simultaneous production and consumption	Costumer participation in and affect the transaction. Mass production is difficult
Non perishable	Perishable	Services cannot be returned, resold or stored, cannot be owned.
Right of ownership	No ownership	

Marketing strategies for service firms

The service component and support processes of product offerings are rapidly becoming the competitive advantage in winning customer loyalty.

In services, the last experience
remains uppermost in your mind.
Therefore,
it is not enough to be good,
you have to be consistently good
Services marketing triangle

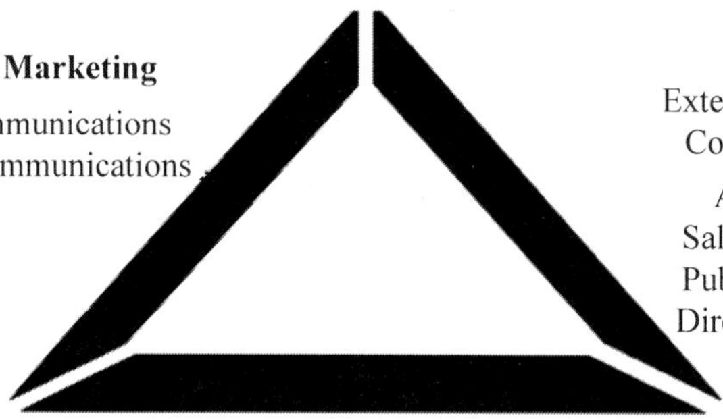

Internal marketing

- It enables service marketers to deliver promises to customers.
- It shows- constituent individual and dept.s who are considered to be each other's customers.
- Marketing conducted by a service firm to train and effectively motivate its customer contact employees and all the supporting service people to work as a team to provide customer satisfaction.

External marketing

- The link between an organisation and its customs is the external marketing process. It represents the promises which organisation make to their customers with reference to products or services they offer.
- Key role in formation of custom's expectations, because their expectations are affected by the services provider's direct and indirect marketing massages.

Interactive marketing

- It is about the keeping the promises made by the organisation to the customers along with delivering a quality services to the customers
- It is actual contact between the service employees and the customers and is called the "moment of the truth" or the service encounter.
- Marketing that recognises that the perceived service quality depends heavily on the buyer-seller interaction.
- Emphasis on relationship marketing.

Services marketing mix

- Service offering (product)
- Price
- Distribution
- Promotion
- People
- Processes
- Physical evidence (Environment)

Service offering (product)

Two types

- Core services offering- intangible
- Secondary services offered- tangibles + augmented with elements of the services

Price -It influences customers' expectations, purchase decisions and evaluation of service quality.

Distribution (Place) - Refers to the availability and accessibility of service offerings to customers. Involves decisions regarding physical location and which intermediaries use to provide the services.

Promotion

Service promotional objectives

- To develop an awareness or interest in the organisation and its services
- To communicate the benefits of purchasing a service

- To build a positive image of the organisation
- To differentiate the organisation from its competitors
- To remind customers of the existing of the services and the service organisation

People- People as an element in service mix include all the human actors – the employees (internal customers) the buyers (external customers) and other customers – who play a part in service delivery. Influence the buyer's perception of choice in the service environment.

Service quality is directly proportional to employee Satisfaction

Processes - Processes are the actual procedures, mechanisms and flow of activities by which services are delivered.

Importance

- The customers are participants in the service processes
- Service processes are difficult to structure
- Outcome is depend on both internal and external factors
- Service processes play an internal part in customers satisfaction

Physical evidence (Environment)- Where the service provider delivers the service and where customers and organisation interact, facilitate communication.

- Help develop an image in the mind current and prospective customers.
- Brochures, letterheads, business cards, report formats, equipments and physical facilities

29

Expectations From A Veterinary Professional

Veterinary practice has gone through different phases with different components

- Phase I - Patient and Veterinarian: objective was only to treat illness of the patient by veterinarian.
- Phase II – Patient - Veterinarian – Owner: Veterinarian was to take recognition of owner and his/her needs.
- Phase III - Patient - Veterinarian – Owner – Law: Additional responsibility on veterinarians to work as per the law (e.g. Registration at VCI, Veterinary jurisprudence, Giving evidence at court of law, Health certificates, Death certificate, Cruelty to animals, export and import law, euthanasia rules, etc.)
- Phase IV - Patient - Veterinarian – Owner – Law – Environment: Further added responsibility to protect environment. E.g. Biomedical waste management.

1. Basic B.V.Sc and A.H degree is no more acceptable specialization and additional qualification, computer knowledge and communication skills is expected by the professionals.
2. Upgradation of knowledge: Refresher courses, on hand training, wet lab practice are need of the hour.
3. Upgrading diagnostic knowledge by way of learning newer diagnostic tests, procedures cannot diagnose a case based on only clinical observation.
4. In certain fields like poultry industry veterinarian has to develop integrated approach, he/she needs to be a pathologist, nutritionist, management specialist and clinician – "All in one" vet is needed.

5. Industry definitely looks into financial return from the veterinarian, industry is finance driven. Just handling single case on day to day basis is gone. all efforts and inputs are decide on the production improvement and financial benefit. Veterinarian has to spell out what is the extra benefit expected by a newer procedure, alterations and facilities.
6. Industry looks for a "team player" who has good interpersonal skills, leadership qualities and human resource developer rather than a veterinarian who has a good academic performance.
7. Communication skill is deciding factor many times in recruitment, assigning new responsibilities etc.
8. Strict office hours do not apply anymore. Your office time is decided by who efficiently discharge your duties/ responsibilities. Slower you are longer is your office hours.
9. Payment in terms of monthly salary will disappear in next couple of years. It is responsibility driven assignment on contract basis.
10. Research and field trials become part of every veterinarian working in any aspect of veterinary profession.
11. Marketing of goods, services etc. become a part of veterinarian responsibility. Industry looks for a Techno-commercial veterinarian rather than just technical officer.
12. Client education is gaining importance and effective client education becoming integral part of the veterinarian's life.
13. Integrity, transparency, tolerance are traits demanded by a veterinarian – industry do not tolerate any shortfalls in this area.
14. Slowly the gap between boss and worker is reducing and veterinarian has to adjust to this changing scenario.
15. Small is not beautiful: not anymore. Mass production, integrated business approach, wider networking and bigger area of operation is the key word in the corporate houses. So veterinarian is expected to adapt to this new approach in the business.
16. Ethics – all are important, veterinarian is expected to uphold the dignity of the veterinary profession.

Concept of wellness Veterinarians

Wellness veterinarian focus on building their loyal client base by making them happy and make them come back as need. Weakness of Veterinary practitioner to be avoided like too dominant attitude in profession, talks too much, listen too little, does not follow structured protocols, little knowledge in some fields, does not provide clear instructions, not willing to invest in discussion.

- In the face of unprecedented competition, the veterinarian and his/her team must provide their patients & clients the best scope of medical and surgical care but also a variety of services and products .For some veterinarians these services & products are not considered to be "ethical" or part of their responsibility. However in the eyes of the owners, the veterinarian is **the expert**, so it is quite normal and "expected" that he or she would fulfill these needs. The "animal doctor" is expected to propose such services or products. However, it is well known that there is a potential cultural conflict. Most veterinarians will mention that they have not studied medicine and surgery to "sell dog food, or shampoos". In such case the barrier is the veterinarian, not the owner.

Expectations & needs

- There are several kinds of expectations. Those who are expressed or so-called 'explicit' and those who are not expressed by the customers or so-called 'implicit' expectations. It is quite important to know what are the client's implicit expectations since by definition these will not be mentioned by people. A perfect example is the fact that people expect the personnel and staff in a veterinary clinic to have a ' professional medical look' (white or medical types of clothes...), if it is not the case, people may be surprised or even upset...but they will not mention it... it is implicit for them. Veterinarians specifically need to have a good understanding of that category of expectations. Some classical implicit expectations of the consumers include:
    - Availability (no wait, flexible hours, easy access & parking, sufficient stock, etc.)
    - Patience (Clients expect their Doctor to be patient with them, allow sufficient time for them)
    - Explanatory (Answering the questions calmly, not avoiding them, clarify their doubts and explains even the minute details)
    - Transparency (prices should be clearly marked, invoices should be itemized, etc.)
    - Choice (various products & services, 'freedom of choice', etc.)
    - Environment (comfortable, neat, clean, odorless, friendly, modern, etc.)

  - Clarity of the offer (prices listed, estimations, badges, etc)
  - Services (various services adapted to their needs as pet owners)
- Various surveys have shown that what clients were looking for in a veterinarian was by order of importance his or her:
  - kindness
  - affordability
  - availability
  - capacity to listen, and only after:
  - his or her competency!
  - approach
- Measuring client satisfaction in a practice can help maintain a more stable, satisfied client base. Satisfaction will often be a measure of client perception of quality. The highly satisfied client will feel they have received a high quality service, whereas the dissatisfied client will be disappointed by the quality of service.
- Client service is the ability to meet client requirements. Services are experienced, and veterinarians, as service providers, are as much in managing the client's experience as in providing technical expertise.
- "Any business that wants to succeed must be aware of its customer's requirements...failure to do so is a missed opportunity to satisfy client needs and to maximize profits." Many practitioners are focused on the medical & technical issues. They do not realize that their services do not match necessarily what their clients expect and do not **listen** to them.

30

Eco Jobs and Sustainable Development Through Livestock Production

A Eco/green job, also called a green-collar job is, according to the United Nations Environment Program "work in agricultural, manufacturing, research and development (R&D), administrative, and service activities that contribute(s) substantially to preserving or restoring environmental quality. Specifically, but not exclusively, this includes jobs that help to protect ecosystems and biodiversity; reduce energy, materials, and water consumption through high efficiency strategies; de-carbonize the economy; and minimize or altogether avoid generation of all forms of waste and pollution.

- Livestock play a vital role in rural economy. The combination of livestock and crop farming enables complementarity through productive utilisation of farm by-products and conservation of soil fertility, thus increasing rural farm income. Apart from providing food products like milk, egg and meat, livestock sector generates productive employment and valuable supplementary income to the vast majority of rural households, majority of whom are small and marginal farmers and landless labourers. Growing human population, increasing urbanisation, rising domestic incomes and changing lifestyles in the country have led to increasing demand for livestock products. Livestock like cattle (bulls and cows), buffaloes, sheep and goat are an integral part of India's socio-economic life. Animal husbandry is a part of agricultural economy. It directly supports about five per cent (20 million) of our population. India has two per cent of the geographical area and accounts for 15 per cent of livestock population (400 million). Cows and buffaloes comprise 56.5 per cent of world population.India ranks first, second, third and fifth in buffalo, cattle and goat, sheep and poultry population in the world, respectively. (Economic Survey, 2008-09). The total livestock population of Tamil Nadu stood at 249.42 lakhs which comprises 4.94, 1.69, 9.10, 6.58 and17.7 per cent of the cattle, buffalos, sheep, goat and poultry population of the country (17th livestock census All India Summary Report, 2004).

Sustainable livestock production strategies

- Proper management and nutrition are essential to the health and well being of domestic animals; particularly livestock species that are expected to maintain a high level of production while relying on livestock owners to meet all their physiological and behavioral needs. As livestock production becomes more intensified, the need to ensure that management and nutrition do not limit only to animal health or productivity increases. Best management practices have to be followed in biosecurity management of livestock and also in handling livestock manure.

- Management and nutrition are also central to the prevention and control of many infectious and noninfectious diseases besides high-level production performances. Although infectious diseases require the presence of a specific infectious organism(s), the mere presence of the causal microbe is not usually sufficient to assure that disease will develop. Other environmental and host factors influence whether the infected animal develops clinical disease or has reduced productivity as a result of the infection.

- The most effective method of preventing infectious disease is to eradicate and exclude the organism(s) causing the disease. Often, this is impossible or impractical. It becomes necessary to control the infectious disease by minimizing circumstances that favor the spread of the infectious agent, mitigating the environmental circumstances that contribute to development of the disease in the presence of the infectious agent, and minimizing circumstances that increase the host's susceptibility.

- Proper nutritional management is essential to animal health and productivity and thereby reduce the uses of scarce resources which are essential for sustainability. Nutrition plays a significant role in influencing the animal's susceptibility to disease as well as in managing certain diseases . Rations/diets must be formulated to provide for the basic physiologic needs (eg, energy, protein, fats, carbohydrates, vitamins, minerals) of the animal and to ensure optimal growth and productivity.

- Loss of biodiversity is another continuing danger to soil.

- Watershed management can partly take care of such ill-effects, which consists of conservation of soil, biomass and water resources, development of reclaimable areas, introduction of improved crop production practices, etc.

Sustainable production measures

- Many different management practices can improve a livestock operation's production efficiency and reduce greenhouse gas emissions. Improved livestock management reduces atmospheric concentrations of carbon dioxide through the mechanism of soil carbon sequestration on grazing lands.
- As plants grow, they remove carbon dioxide from the atmosphere. Even though grazing cattle harvest a large portion of the plant material, through good management residues accumulate and increase the amount of organic matter in the soil. Some of this organic matter will remain in the soil or plant root system for long periods of time instead of being released back into the atmosphere as carbon dioxide. Some of the most effective practices include

Improving grazing management

- Soil testing, followed by the addition of proper amendments and fertilizers
- Supplementing cattle diets with needed nutrients
- Developing a preventive herd health program
- Providing appropriate water sources and protecting water quality
- Improving genetics and reproductive efficiency

Livestock waste management

- Livestock waste contains many microorganisms such as bacteria, viruses, and protozoa. Some of these microorganisms do not cause sickness in animals or humans. However, some others are pathogens, meaning they are capable of causing disease in animals and/or humans. Irrespective of the size of their farms, all livestock producers have an important role in limiting pathogen movement from their operation to the environment. Waste management provide livestock producers to control pathogens in their production system. The Best Management Practices (BMPs) are pertaining to animal management and housing, dietary modifications, production management, land application of manure, and the chemical and biological treatment of stored manure.

Animal husbandry and greenhouse gases

- The two major greenhouse gases produced by animal husbandry are methane and nitrous oxide. Their concentrations have increased considerably over the past 120 years. In this period the atmospheric CH4 concentration has more than doubled and the N20 concentration has risen by more than 30 per cent. One source of CH4 in animal husbandry is the fermentation of feed in the stomach of ruminants and non-ruminants. Due to their ability to digest cellulose, ruminants account for the greater share in the production of CH4. Another source of CH4 associated with animal husbandry is the decomposition of animal wastes. These mainly consist of organic material, which produces CH4 when decomposed under anaerobic conditions. The source of nitrous oxide due to animal husbandry is the decomposition of animal wastes. Any further intensification of animal husbandry will increase the amount of animal waste, making a further increase in N20 emissions likely.

Interventions for sustainable livestock production

- Policy instruments fall into three main groups: (a) price policies, (b) institutional policies, and(c) policies promoting technological change. Price policies are the responsibility of national governments, although they may be influenced by international agencies, such as customs unions, the World Bank or the WTO. However, national and local governments, private individuals orassociations, development agencies and Non-Government Organizations introduce institutional and technological changes.

- Price policies can be categorized into (i) trade policy, (ii) exchange rate policy, (iii) tax and subsidy policy, and (iv) direct interventions such as floor and fixed prices. Trade policy, from a developing country's perspective, should include continued pressure, through international fore such as the WTO, on developed countries to reduce tariffs and other barriers aimed at supporting their own producers. However, greater benefits might be achieved by reducing levels of protection for industrial s ectors within the developing countries, as such protection raises input costs and effectively taxes agricultural producers. Taxes, subsidies and governments' direct market interventions have usually failed to bring lasting benefits. There remains a case for limited use of subsidies for disaster relief and to promote the use of new inputs, such as vaccines or drugs. Alternatively moderate taxes on livestock producers might be used to recover costs of providing public goods such as disease control or eradication programmes.

- Policies for the promotion of appropriate institutions have a major impact on livestock development. The authors of a review of about 800 livestock development projects found that most had failed to bring about significant sustainable improvements in livelihoods of the poor.

- Institutional development is also needed for the provision of credit, animal health services and genetic material. The introduction of new technology must be accompanied by the strengthening of the institutional framework required for its implementation. The other key area, where institutional change is essential for the success of livestock development, is that of marketing, including transport, processing and selling. As marketing activities exhibit economies of scale, large commercial operations are most likely to be cost-effective. Unfortunately, in negotiating contracts with such companies, small-scale producers are in a weak position, lacking market power and information on patterns of supply, demand and prices. Thus in promoting institutional development, there is a need for dissemination of market information, and encouragement of co-operative group action and participation by small-scale producers to strengthen their bargaining position.
- Technological change may be promoted by supporting research and development and the dissemination of information to farmers. Public funding for agricultural research, and particularly for livestock research, has declined over recent decades. Since much research output provides public goods it is unlikely to receive adequate funding from the private sector. The decline in public sector funding should therefore be reversed.
- An appropriate institutional framework must be developed to integrate a farmer participatory systems approach with science-based adaptive and applied research, depending on collaboration between producers, and natural and social scientists. The national research organizations must take responsibility for research prioritization, ensuring that it is appropriate for relative resource availability, taking into account the needs of the poor, and coordinating donor assistance. To improve food security in a sustainable manner, developing countries will often require an investment in their agricultural research system at a level of 1 percent of the value of agricultural output over the short term and 2 percent in the long term.
- Areas of research deserving attention include animal and veterinary public health measures, improvements in forage crops and utilization of crop by-products, and improvements in husbandry and management of production systems. Local breed improvement is a slow process and crossbreeding with, or adopting, exotic breeds generally more easily achieve increases in production. Technical research has to be complemented by socio-economic research into the institutional framework for the allocation of natural resources, credit, and labor hire,

the delivery of inputs and the processing and marketing of livestock products. Research is needed to describe and analyze the strengths and weaknesses of existing institutions and to propose and test alternatives for improvement. In addition, socio-economists are needed to contribute to the research prioritization process, by assessing likely costs and benefits of proposed research projects.

Part E
Livestock Business Management

31

Management

Popularly the term management is used to refer to the group of managerial personnel of an enterprise. But the use of the term management in this sense is not correct, because the managerial personnel of an enterprise are usually designated as 'managers', 'executives' or administrators. Strictly speaking the term management refers to functional concept of management. Management refers to the sum total of all those functions or activities, which relate to the laying down of policies, plans and purposes, securing men, money, machinery needed for the achievement of the organisational objectives, putting all of them into operation and supervising and checking their performances in order to ensure the productive use of human and material resources for the maximum benefit or profit of the organisation, its employees and society in general.

Management is the sum total of five principal functions namely planning, organising, staffing, directing and controlling. The functional areas of management include: a) Financial management, b) Personnel management, c) material management, d) Production management, e) marketing management and f) Office management.

Relationship between Administration and Management

It is very difficult to make a clear demarcation between administrative functions and managerial functions. Therefore in practice, no distinction is made between the terms, administration and management. There will be no two separate sets of management personnel required to perform administrative functions and managerial functions. Therefore, to club the meaning of administration and management, the term management itself is classified into two categories namely, a) Administrative Management and b) Operative management.

a) Administrative management is primarily concerned with the determination of the goals and policies of an enterprise while the b) operative management is concerned with the implementation of policies laid down by the administrative management in the achievement of the goals of the enterprise.

Management is often divided into Top management, Middle management and Lower management. The top and middle management is more concerned with administrative management, policy making and goal setting, while the lower management is concerned with the operational management that is implementation of policies laid down by the administrative management.

Relationship between Management and Organisation

The term organization is use in different senses. It refers to: a) work or activity of bringing together various factors of production such as land, labour and capital in order to achieve the desired objectives of an enterprise. This is the economic concept. b) It refers to the name of a company or a firm or Concern such as BEL, HMT etc. Here the term organization is used as a noun form. c) However, when the term Organisation is used as a management concept, it refers to the organizational structure or skeleton (of an enterprise) which provides for 1) the identification of various activities required to be performed for the accomplishment of the objectives of the enterprise, 2) division of objectives into logical and convenient groups, 3) allocation of activities into different departments and each department being provided with properly qualified personnel and facilities, 4) fixing responsibilities on the departments and on the individuals, 5) delegation of sufficient authority to subordinates for effective operation and 6) co-ordination of the activities of the different departments and individuals to ensure co-operation and unity for the accomplishment of the desired objectives.

However, the main difference between management and organisation is that, management is an executive function in that and it is mainly concerned with execution of things, while organisation performs the organic function in that and, it is concerned with putting together, the different parts or divisions of the enterprise into efficient working order.

Functions of Management

Management has been described as a social process involving responsibility for economical and effective planning & regulation of operation of an enterprise in the fulfillment of given purposes. It is a dynamic process consisting of various elements and activities. These activities are different from operative functions like marketing, finance, purchase etc. Rather these activities are common to each and every manger irrespective of his level or status.

Different experts have classified functions of management. According to *George & Jerry*, "There are four fundamental functions of management i.e. planning, organizing, actuating and controlling".

According to Henry Fayol, "To manage is to forecast and plan, to organize, to command, & to control". Whereas Luther Gullick has given a keyword '**POSDCORB**' where P stands for Planning, O for Organizing, S for Staffing, D for Directing, Co for Co-ordination, R for reporting & B for Budgeting. But the most widely accepted are functions of management given by KOONTZ and O'DONNEL i.e. **Planning**, **Organizing**, **Staffing**, **Directing** and **Controlling**.

For theoretical purposes, it may be convenient to separate the function of management but practically these functions are overlapping in nature i.e. they are highly inseparable. Each function blends into the other & each affects the performance of others.

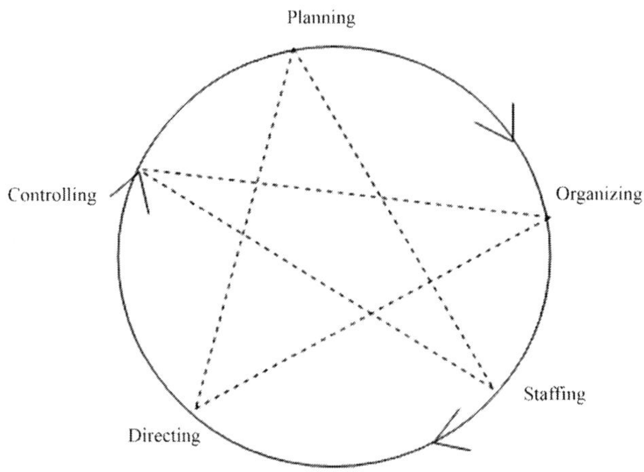

1. Planning

It is the basic function of management. It deals with chalking out a future course of action & deciding in advance the most appropriate course of actions for achievement of pre-determined goals. According to KOONTZ, "Planning is deciding in advance - what to do, when to do & how to do. It bridges the gap from where we are & where we want to be". A plan is a future course of actions. It is an exercise in problem solving & decision making. Planning is determination of courses of action to achieve desired goals. Thus, planning is a systematic thinking about ways & means for accomplishment of pre-determined goals. Planning is necessary to ensure proper utilization of human & non-human resources. It is all pervasive, it is an intellectual activity and it also helps in avoiding confusion, uncertainties, risks, wastages etc.

2. Organizing

It is the process of bringing together physical, financial and human resources and developing productive relationship amongst them for achievement of organizational goals. According to Henry Fayol, "To organize a business is to provide it with everything useful or its functioning i.e. raw material, tools, capital and personnel's". To organize a business involves determining & providing human and non-human resources to the organizational structure. Organizing as a process involves:

- Identification of activities.
- Classification of grouping of activities.
- Assignment of duties.
- Delegation of authority and creation of responsibility.
- Coordinating authority and responsibility relationships.

3. Staffing

It is the function of manning the organization structure and keeping it manned. Staffing has assumed greater importance in the recent years due to advancement of technology, increase in size of business, complexity of human behavior etc. The main purpose of staffing is to put right man on right job i.e. square pegs in square holes and round pegs in round holes. According to Kootz & O'Donell, "Managerial function of staffing involves manning the organization structure through proper and effective selection, appraisal & development of personnel to fill the roles designed un the structure". Staffing involves:

- Manpower Planning (estimating man power in terms of searching, choose the person and giving the right place).
- Recruitment, Selection & Placement.
- Training & Development.
- Remuneration.
- Performance Appraisal.
- Promotions & Transfer.

4. Directing

It is that part of managerial function which actuates the organizational methods to work efficiently for achievement of organizational purposes. It is considered life-spark of the enterprise which sets it in motion the action of people because planning, organizing and staffing are the mere preparations for doing the work. Direction is that inert-personnel aspect of management which deals directly with influencing, guiding, supervising, motivating sub-ordinate for the achievement of organizational goals. Direction has following elements:

- Supervision
- Motivation
- Leadership
- Communication

Supervision- implies overseeing the work of subordinates by their superiors. It is the act of watching & directing work & workers.

Motivation- means inspiring, stimulating or encouraging the sub-ordinates with zeal to work. Positive, negative, monetary, non-monetary incentives may be used for this purpose.

Leadership- may be defined as a process by which manager guides and influences the work of subordinates in desired direction.

Communications- is the process of passing information, experience, opinion etc from one person to another. It is a bridge of understanding.

5. Controlling

It implies measurement of accomplishment against the standards and correction of deviation if any to ensure achievement of organizational goals. The purpose of controlling is to ensure that everything occurs in conformities with the standards. An efficient system of control helps to predict deviations before they actually occur. According to *Theo Haimann*, "Controlling is the process of checking whether or not proper progress is being made towards the objectives and goals and acting if necessary, to correct any deviation". According to Koontz & O'Donell "Controlling is the measurement & correction of performance activities of subordinates in order to make sure that the enterprise objectives and plans desired to obtain them as being accomplished". Therefore controlling has following steps:

a. Establishment of standard performance.

b. Measurement of actual performance.

b. Comparison of actual performance with the standards and finding out deviation if any.

c. Corrective action.

Henri Fayols 14 Principles of Management

A principle refers to a fundamental truth. It establishes cause and effect relationship between two or more variables under given situation. They serve as a guide to thought & actions. Therefore, management principles are the statements of fundamental truth based on logic which provides guidelines for managerial decision making and actions. These principles are derived: -

a. On the basis of observation and analysis i.e. practical experience of managers.

b. By conducting experimental studies.

There are 14 Principles of Management described by Henri Fayol.

1. Division of Labor

a. Henri Fayol has stressed on the specialization of jobs.

b. He recommended that work of all kinds must be divided & subdivided and allotted to various persons according to their expertise in a particular area.

c. Subdivision of work makes it simpler and results in efficiency.

d. It also helps the individual in acquiring speed, accuracy in his performance.

e. Specialization leads to efficiency & economy in spheres of business.

2. Party of Authority & Responsibility

a. Authority & responsibility are co-existing.

b. If authority is given to a person, he should also be made responsible.

c. In a same way, if anyone is made responsible for any job, he should also have concerned authority.

d. Authority refers to the right of superiors to get exactness from their subordinates whereas responsibility means obligation for the performance of the job assigned.

e. There should be a balance between the two i.e. they must go hand in hand.

f. Authority without responsibility leads to irresponsible behavior whereas responsibility without authority makes the person ineffective.

3. Principle of One Boss

a. A sub-ordinate should receive orders and be accountable to one and only one boss at a time.

b. In other words, a sub-ordinate should not receive instructions from more than one person because -

   It undermines authority

   - Weakens discipline
   - Divides loyalty
   - Creates confusion
   - Delays and chaos
   - Escaping responsibilities
   - Duplication of work
   - Overlapping of efforts

c. Therefore, dual sub-ordination should be avoided unless and until it is absolutely essential.

d. Unity of command provides the enterprise a disciplined, stable & orderly existence.

e. It creates harmonious relationship between superiors and sub-ordinates.

4. Unity of Direction

a. Fayol advocates one head one plan which means that there should be one plan for a group of activities having similar objectives.

b. Related activities should be grouped together. There should be one plan of action for them and they should be under the charge of a particular manager.

c. According to this principle, efforts of all the members of the organization should be directed towards common goal.

d. Without unity of direction, unity of action cannot be achieved.

e. In fact, unity of command is not possible without unity of direction.

Basis	Unity of command	Unity of direction
Meaning	It implies that a sub-ordinate should receive orders & instructions from only one boss.	It means one head, one plan for a group of activities having similar objectives.
Nature	It is related to the functioning of personnel's.	It is related to the functioning of departments, or organization as a whole.
Necessity	It is necessary for fixing responsibility of each subordinates.	It is necessary for sound organization.
Advantage	It avoids conflicts, confusion & chaos.	It avoids duplication of efforts and wastage of resources.
Result	It leads to better superior sub-ordinate relationship.	It leads to smooth running of the enterprise.

Therefore it is obvious that they are different from each other but they are dependent on each other i.e. unity of direction is a pre-requisite for unity of command. But it does not automatically comes from the unity of direction.

5. Equity

a. Equity means combination of fairness, kindness & justice.

b. The employees should be treated with kindness & equity if devotion is expected of them.

c. It implies that managers should be fair and impartial while dealing with the subordinates.

d. They should give similar treatment to people of similar position.

e. They should not discriminate with respect to age, caste, sex, religion, relation etc.

f. Equity is essential to create and maintain cordial relations between the managers and sub-ordinate.

g. But equity does not mean total absence of harshness.

h. Fayol was of opinion that, "at times force and harshness might become necessary for the sake of equity".

6. Order

a. This principle is concerned with proper & systematic arrangement of things and people.

b. Arrangement of things is called material order and placement of people is called social order.

c. Material order- There should be safe, appropriate and specific place for every article and every place to be effectively used for specific activity and commodity.

d. Social order- Selection and appointment of most suitable person on the suitable job. There should be a specific place for every one and everyone should have a specific place so that they can easily be contacted whenever need arises.

7. Discipline

a. According to Fayol, "Discipline means sincerity, obedience, respect of authority & observance of rules and regulations of the enterprise".

b. This principle applies that subordinate should respect their superiors and obey their order.

c. It is an important requisite for smooth running of the enterprise.

d. Discipline is not only required on path of subordinates but also on the part of management.

e. Discipline can be enforced if -

- There are good superiors at all levels.
- There are clear & fair agreements with workers.
- Sanctions (punishments) are judiciously applied.

8. Initiative

a. Workers should be encouraged to take initiative in the work assigned to them.

b. It means eagerness to initiate actions without being asked to do so.

c. Fayol advised that management should provide opportunity to its employees to suggest ideas, experiences& new method of work.

d. It helps in developing an atmosphere of trust and understanding.

e. People then enjoy working in the organization because it adds to their zeal and energy.

f. To suggest improvement in formulation & implementation of place.

g. They can be encouraged with the help of monetary & non-monetary incentives.

9. Fair Remuneration

a. The quantum and method of remuneration to be paid to the workers should be fair, reasonable, satisfactory & rewarding of the efforts.

b. As far as possible it should accord satisfaction to both employer and the employees.

c. Wages should be determined on the basis of cost of living, work assigned, financial position of the business, wage rate prevailing etc.

d. Logical & appropriate wage rates and methods of their payment reduce tension & differences between workers & management creates harmonious relationship and pleasing atmosphere of work.

e. Fayol also recommended provision of other benefits such as free education, medical & residential facilities to workers.

10. Stability of Tenure

a. Fayol emphasized that employees should not be moved frequently from one job position to another i.e. the period of service in a job should be fixed.

b. Therefore employees should be appointed after keeping in view principles of recruitment & selection but once they are appointed their services should be served.

c. According to Fayol. "Time is required for an employee to get used to a new work & succeed to doing it well but if he is removed before that he will not be able to render worthwhile services".

d. As a result, the time, effort and money spent on training the worker will go waste.

e. Stability of job creates team spirit and a sense of belongingness among workers which ultimately increase the quality as well as quantity of work.

11. Scalar Chain

a. Fayol defines scalar chain as 'The chain of superiors ranging from the ultimate authority to the lowest".

b. Every orders, instructions, messages, requests, explanation etc. has to pass through Scalar chain.

c. But, for the sake of convenience & urgency, this path can be cut shirt and this short cut is known as Gang Plank.

d. A **Gang Plank** is a temporary arrangement between two different points to facilitate quick & easy communication as explained below:

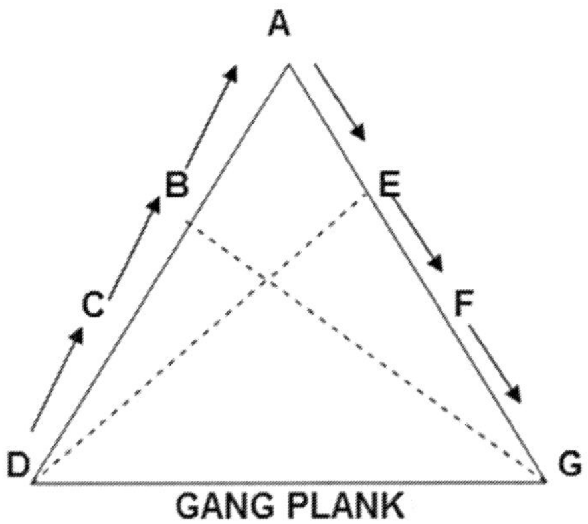

In the figure given, if D has to communicate with G he will first send the communication upwards with the help of C, B to A and then downwards with the help of E and F to G which will take quite some time and by that time, it may not be worth therefore a gang plank has been developed between the two.

e. **Gang Plank** clarifies that management principles are not rigid rather they are very flexible. They can be moulded and modified as per the requirements of situations

12. Sub-Ordination of Individual Interest to General Interest

a. An organization is much bigger than the individual it constitutes therefore interest of the undertaking should prevail in all circumstances.

b. As far as possible, reconciliation should be achieved between individual and group interests.

c. But in case of conflict, individual must sacrifice for bigger interests.

d. In order to achieve this attitude, it is essential that -

- Employees should be honest & sincere.
- Proper & regular supervision of work.
- Reconciliation of mutual differences and clashes by mutual agreement. For example, for change of location of plant, for change of profit sharing ratio, etc.

13. Espirit De' Corps (can be achieved through unity of command)

a. It refers to team spirit i.e. harmony in the work groups and mutual understanding among the members.

b. Spirit De' Corps inspires workers to work harder.

c. Fayol cautioned the managers against dividing the employees into competing groups because it might damage the moral of the workers and interest of the undertaking in the long run.

d. To inculcate Espirit De' Corps following steps should be undertaken -

- There should be proper co-ordination of work at all levels
- Subordinates should be encouraged to develop informal relations among themselves.
- Efforts should be made to create enthusiasm and keenness among subordinates so that they can work to the maximum ability.
- Efficient employees should be rewarded and those who are not up to the mark should be given a chance to improve their performance.
- Subordinates should be made conscious of that whatever they are doing is of great importance to the business & society.

e. He also cautioned against the more use of Britain communication to the subordinates i.e. face to face communication should be developed. The managers should infuse team spirit & belongingness. There should be no place for misunderstanding. People then enjoy working in the organization & offer their best towards the organization.

14. Centralization & De-Centralization

a. Centralization means concentration of authority at the top level. In other words, centralization is a situation in which top management retains most of the decision making authority.

b. Decentralization means disposal of decision making authority to all the levels of the organization. In other words, sharing authority downwards is decentralization.

c. According to Fayol, "Degree of centralization or decentralization depends on no. of factors like size of business, experience of superiors, dependability & ability of subordinates etc.

d. Anything which increases the role of subordinate is decentralization & anything which decreases it is centralization.

e. Fayol suggested that absolute centralization or decentralization is not feasible. An organization should strike to achieve a lot between the two.

Farm Management

Applying the definition of management, the term farm management refers to the sum total of all those activities which relate to raising of a crop, or setting up of a livestock or fishery unit on a piece of land, making it productive by providing judicious inputs like labour, capital, materials, machinery etc., and by employing traditional knowledge, wisdom and modern scientific methods that are economical and ecofriendly so as to obtain maximum profit for the benefit of the enterprise and to the society in general not only during the present day but also on a future date.

Organizational aspects of livestock farm

The organisational structure of a large livestock farm can be presented in the following general way. However, depending on the type of livestock farm, certain divisions may be deleted and others added.

The following is the organisational structure of a large livestock farm:

1. General farm management: This is done by General Manager / Managing Director / Manager of the farm. His duties include overall co-ordination of the various departments of the livestock farm.

2. Estate branch: The Estate officer or Engineer in-charge will be responsible for providing housing, landscaping, erecting various structures for cooling, washing, wallowing etc., required for livestock.

3. Geneticist: His job includes determining the breeding policy, maintenance of breeding and production records, assisting or taking appropriate decisions on livestock purchase etc. There can be separate officer in-charge of purchases for various inputs including the livestock.

4. Nutritionist: His job includes formulation proper nutritional rations to different classes and individual livestock, feed mixing, fixing feeding schedule, feeds and fodder production etc. There can be separate officer in-charge of fodder production who is basically an agriculture graduate, specialised in fodder production.

5. Gynecologist or Reproduction specialist: The gynecologist's job includes heat detection, carrying out artificial insemination, pregnancy diagnosis, pre and postpartum care, treatment of repeat breeders, correction of obstetrical cases, maintenance of individual animal's reproduction records etc. There will be no gynecologist in a poultry farm.

6. Veterinary officer: Duties of veterinary officer include the health care of the livestock, taking prophylactic measures like vaccination, de-worming, sanitary measures, diagnosis and treatment of sick animals, etc.
7. Products Manager: He will be in-charge of products management like harvesting of various products, grading, preserving, transportation and marketing them. All decisions pertaining to product optimisation, economising production, maximising products and obtaining high profits will have to be taken by product manager in consultation with the general manager and other staff.
8. Personnel Manager: In very big livestock organisation, there can be personnel division in-charge of recruitment of office and technical staff including skilled labourers. Maintenance of their individual records, assignment of suitable work, supervision of work, assessment of work, giving promotions to them, looking after their security, work place environment, maintenance of provident fund accounts, savings accounts, maintenance of pension funds, payment of pension, gratuity etc., all form the duties of personnel manager.
9. Officer in-charge of marketing: The duties of marketing officer includes various activities connected with marketing of products. Decisions regarding various products to be produced, their packaging, branding, selecting suitable channels of marketing, price fixation etc., are taken by the marketing officer.

Types of Farming

Based on land utilisation and farming practices followed, the types of farming are as follows:

- Diversified Farming - Many enterprises (Livestock, Fruit crop, Poultry, etc.)
- Specialised Farming - Main enterprise (Dairy farming or Sheep farming etc.)
- Mixed Farming (Crop + Livestock enterprise)
- Irrigated or Dry Farming - When rainfall is less than 50 cm.
- Ranching - Land is not tilled.

System of Farming

Based on type of ownership to land and methods of agriculture used in operating the land, the system of farming is given as follows:

1. Peasant Farming
2. Co-operative Farming
3. State Farming
4. Capitalistic Farming and
5. Collective Farming

Farm Records: Farm Records are also useful in making farm management decisions. Enterprise record system which include farm income statement, listing of receipts and expenses by enterprise, listing of account payable and receivable, a depreciation schedule, inventories and a pay roll record is very helpful as a tool in farm management.

A. Farm Records

1. Physical

- Farm map
- Labour record
- Feed record
- Machinery use register, etc.

2. Financial

- Farm inventory record
- Farm financial register
- Purchase register
- Wage register, etc.

3. **Supplementary**

- Rainfall register
- Hire register
- Stationary register, etc.

B. Credit Supply to Farm

Loans from Banks

- Short-term loan
- Medium-term loan
- Long-term loan

Private lending agencies

C. Farm Efficiency Measures

Physical efficiency measures	*Financial efficiency measures*
Aggregate measures	**Aggregate measures**
- Total production,	-Gross income
- Number of Livestock, etc.	-Gross profit
	-Net worth, etc.
Ratio measures	**Ratio measures**
-Land use efficiency	- Cost ratio
-Labour efficiency	- Capital ratio
-Machinery efficiency, etc.	- Income ratio, etc.

Thus the farm management covers all aspects of farming, which have a bearing on the economic efficiency of the farm.

Farm Budgets

Complete Budgeting: It refers to estimation of returns for the entire farm business. For example, if a farm has crops, dairy, poultry and fishery, the statement showing the estimated returns and expenses of all those enterprises together with a complete budget.

Partial Budgeting: If a separate estimate of the returns and expenses for each enterprise in the farm is made, it is called a partial budgeting. For instance the budget for the poultry unit alone or only the dairy or for a particular crop will be a partial budget. Partial budgets are commonly used to estimate the effects or outcomes of possible adjustments in the farm business before such adjustments are actually made.

Approaches to Management – Top 9 Approaches

1. Scientific Management approach.
2. Management Process or Administrative Management approach.

3. Human Relations approach.
4. Behavioural Science approach.
5. Quantitative or Mathematical approach.
6. Systems approach.
7. Contingency approach.
8. Operational approach.
9. Empirical approach.

1. Scientific Management Approach

The establishment of formal organisation structure, formal lines of authority, factory systems and procedures had to be undertaken for coordinated effort. In order to deal with these problems, a management movement known as 'Scientific Management' was born. Frederick Winslow Taylor (1865-1915) was the first to recognise and emphasise the need for adopting a scientific approach to the task of management. The introduction of the concept of standard time, standard output, standard cost, standardisation of production process, change in the attitude of management and workers to bring about the mutuality of interests are the important landmarks of scientific management. This approach was supported and developed by Henry L. Gantt, Frank Gilbreth, Lillian Gilbreth, Harrington Emerson, etc.

2. Management Process or Administrative Management Approach

The advocates of this school perceive management as a process consisting of planning, organising, commanding and controlling. In the words of W.G. Scott, "It aims to analyse the process, to establish a conceptual framework for it, to identify principles underlying it, and to build a theory of management from them". It regards management as a universal process, regardless of the type of the enterprise, or the level in a given enterprise. It looks upon management theory as a way of organising experience so that practice can be improved through research, empirical testing of principles and teaching of fundamentals involved in the management process. The process school is also called the 'traditional' or 'universalist' school as it believes that management principles are applicable to all the group activities, Henry Fayol is regarded as the father of this school. Oliver Shelden, J.D. Mooney and Chester I. Barnard are among the other important contributors to this approach.

3. Human Relations Approach

The human relations approach is concerned with the recognition of the importance of human element in organisations. Elton Mayo and his associates conducted the world famous Hawthorne Experiments and investigated the myriad of informal relationships, social cliques, patterns of communication and patterns of informal leadership. As a result of these experiments, a trend began which can be phrased as 'being nice to people'. This trend was eventually termed as 'the human relations movement'. The human relations approach revealed the importance of social and psychological factors in determining workers' productivity and satisfaction. It was instrumental in creating a new image of man and the workplace. It put stress on interpersonal relations and the informal groups. "It's starting point was in individual psychology rather than the analysis of worker and work. As a result, there was a tendency for human rationalists to degenerate into mere slogans which became an alibi for having no management policy in respect of the human organisation." Nevertheless, this school has done a unique job in recognising the importance of human element in organisations.

4. Behavioural Science Approach

The 'behavioural science' approach utilises methods and techniques of social sciences such as psychology, sociology, social psychology and anthropology for the study of human behaviour. Data is objectively collected and analysed by the social scientists to study various aspects of human behaviour.

5. Quantitative or Mathematical Approach

This approach stands for using all pertinent scientific tools for providing a quantitative basis for managerial decisions. The abiding belief of this approach is that management problems can be expressed in terms of mathematical symbols and relationships. The basic approach is the construction of a model because it is through this device that the problem is expressed in its basic relationships and in terms of selected objectives. The users of such models are known as operations researchers or management scientists. Linear programming, Critical Path Method, Programme Evaluation Review Technique, Breakeven analysis, Games Theory and Queueing Theory have gained popularity for solving managerial problems these days. These techniques help the managers in improving their decisions by analysing the various alternatives in a scientific manner.

6. Systems Approach

A system is composed of elements or subsystems that are related and dependent on each other. The system approach is based on the generalisation that an organisation is a system and its components are inter-related and inter-dependent. This approach lays emphasis on the strategic parts of the system, the nature of their interdependency, goals set by the system and communication network in the system. Another basic feature of the systems approach is that attention is paid towards the overall effectiveness of the system rather than the effectiveness of subsystems. Under system approach, the overall objectives and performance of the organisation are taken into account and not only the objectives and performance of its different departments or subsystems.

7. Contingency Approach

The latest approach to management is known as 'contingency' or 'situational' approach. Underlying idea of this approach is that the internal functioning of organisations must be consistent with the demands of technology and external environment and the needs of its members if the organisation is to be effective. This approach suggests that there is no one best way to handle any management problem. The application of management principles and practices should be contingent upon the existing circumstances. Functional, behavioural, quantitative and systems tools of management should be applied situationally. There are three major parts of the overall conceptual framework for contingency management – (a) environment; (b) management concepts, principles and techniques; and (c) contingent relationship between the two. The environment variables are independent and management variables (process, quantitative, behavioural and systems tools) are dependent. Every manager has to apply the various approaches of management according to the demands of the situation.

8. Operational Approach

Koontz and O'Donnell have advocated operational approach to management. This approach recognises that there is a central core of knowledge about managing which exists in management such as line and staff, patterns of departmentation, span of management, managerial appraisal and various managerial control techniques. It draws from other fields of knowledge and adapts within it those parts of these fields which are specially useful for managers. "The operational approach regards management as a universally applicable body of knowledge that can be brought to bear at all levels of managing and in all types of enterprises. At the same time, this approach recognises that the actual problems managers face and the environments in which they operate may vary between enterprises and levels". The application of science by a perceptive practitioner must take this into account in finding solutions to management problems.

9. Empirical Approach

According to this approach, management is the study of the experiences of managers. The knowledge based on experiences of successful managers can be applied by other managers in solving problems in future and in making decisions. Thus, the empirical school is based on analysis of past experience and uses the case method of study and research. Managers can get an idea of what to do and how by studying management situations of the past. They can develop analytical and problem-solving skills. They can understand and learn to apply effective techniques in comparable situations.

I. Resource Management

Sources and procurement of material: "Goods well bought are half sold" is a proverbial statement in business circles. Careful selection of sources of supply of raw materials required and the actual process of purchase of raw materials and selection steps in making a successful business enterprise. Because of good quality raw materials, steady supply, their economic pricing without sacrificing on the quality of the raw materials are the factors which contribute to make a good product. A good product sells itself because of its quality, thus justifying the statement –'goods well bought are half sold'.

Purchasing department: This department takes the responsibility of procurement of materials required for the business. It decides on what to buy, when to buy, how mach to buy, how to buy, at what price to buy and negotiates the terms and conditions of purchase.

The responsibilities of the purchase department include buying of various materials and equipments required by the business, storing the materials bought, distribution of the materials to the end users of the business organisation, maintenance of records of purchases, suppliers, stocks and issues. It also performs the advisory function, like it tries to remind the end users regarding the economic usage of the raw materials particularly during the high price time and during the off season.

Factors in buying

1. Quality: The materials to be bought must be of very good quality and according to the specifications as sought by the production wing of the enterprise.
2. Quantity: The quantity of the materials bought must be in accordance to the requirement and storage capacity.
3. Delivery of the materials: The purchasing department should select the suppliers who are reliable and who are prompt in delivering the materials

in time as per the schedule so that the production does not stop or get affected.

4. Price: The price of the materials bought must be as economical as possible without sacrificing the quality of the raw materials bought.

Procurement methods or purchasing methods

1. Concentrated purchases or centralised purchasing: In this type of purchasing the quantity of materials required, the various types of materials required, the quality of the materials required etc., for the entire business organisation is done at a centralised level. Usually the stores purchase officer gets the indent from the end users regarding the quantity of various materials and the time by which the materials required etc. After knowing requirements of the organisation, the stores purchase officer places orders for the bulk materials required, receives the materials from the suppliers, stores the materials and distributes the materials to the end users as per the indents. While this type of purchase has its advantages on the buying price as the quantity bought is large thus attracting some concessions from the suppliers. But this type of purchasing has some of the disadvantages also. If the purchases are not done in time and the end user does not get the materials in time, the production process gets affected. This is very important and significant disadvantage particularly if the end user is a manager of a livestock unit and the indented feeds and the fodder or medicines are not received in time by him from the stores purchase officer. Because feeding livestock or administration of medicines to livestock cannot be delayed.

2. Diversification of purchasing or decentralised purchasing: This type of purchasing is exactly opposite to the centralised purchasing. In order to give certain amount of freedom and flexibility to the end user, the diversification of purchasing is done so that depending upon the need and urgency, the end user can purchase materials and ensure smooth and efficient production. This is particularly useful in very big organisations where too many indents cannot be handled by the centralised purchasing section.

3. Reciprocal buying: In this type of purchasing, different enterprises can be mutually benefited by buying materials or products of one enterprise by another and vice versa. This creates an atmosphere of mutual co-operation and discourages the element of exploitation.

4. Current market purchasing: In this type of buying the entrepreneur will purchase at the prevailing the price, the various materials that will suffice for the current season of production.

5. Speculative purchasing: When the entrepreneur expects a spurt in price in the near future, he can go in for purchasing the materials in the market not only for the current needs but also for the future requirement of the enterprise. By this step some savings can be effected because of anticipated escalation in price at a future date. Some of the raw materials bought at a lower price during current season can even be sold at a future date when the real escalation in price happens. However hoarding of any material is against the welfare principle of economics.
6. Purchasing for a future period: While speculative buying is made more to make some savings or profit when the escalation of price is anticipated, purchasing for a future period is done more to ensure uninterrupted supply of raw material to the production process.
7. Contract purchasing: In this type of purchasing, an entrepreneur can enter into rate contract agreement with the supplier of the materials. According to this type of buying it becomes binding on the supplier and purchaser to carry out business transactions as per the terms of sale including price, mode of delivery, payment etc., as per the rate contract agreement entered into by both the parties. Usually rate contract agreement is made for a specific period usually one year and subsequently fresh rate contract agreement is made after the expiry of the current agreement period.
8. Scheduled buying: In this type of purchasing purchases of materials are made as per the schedule of production. This necessitates more number of purchases and some times may lead to non availability of material when the scheduled production is due.

Organisation of purchasing department

Purchase Manager / Stores Purchase Officer

Price clerk	Follow up clerk	Asst. Purchase	General office	Inspector	Receiving Clerk	Chief stores officer
↓	↓	↓	↓	↓	↓	↓
Checks invoices	Checking deliveries through correspondence and phones	Buying decisions	Purchasing 1.Typist/ computer asst. 2.Stenographer 3. File clerk	inspecting & testing of materials	Comparing of incoming materials with the orders and invoices	Receiving materials ↓ storing issuing Record keeping & filing

Purchasing Procedure

The following are the steps that are followed while purchasing materials:

1. Initiating the purchasing requisition: Depending on the balance of materials in stores, list the materials required, their quantity, specifications, quality and date by which the materials are required. Ensure that the indents from all the end users are taken into account while listing.
2. Securing quotations or bids from the various suppliers.
3. Selecting the source of supply: This is done by verifying the prices, stability of the company which is supplying materials, beneficial terms of sale and delivery.
4. Placing the purchase order: After deciding the source of supply orders may be placed for purchasing materials. While placing the order with the supply make sure to mention a) Order No. b) Quantity, c) Specifications of materials, d) Delivery date, e) Delivery instructions / place of delivery / mode of transport etc., f) Billing instruction, g) Price per unit, h) terms of payment etc.
5. Follow up – Receiving – Inspecting: Once the orders are placed with the supplier, make periodic enquiries regarding the probable date of supply, availability of stock etc. Once the materials are received, check the quantity, quality, specifications, price quoted, billing formalities, etc., and the functioning of the materials or equipments before taking the materials to stock.
6. Once the stock is taken, the materials may be issued to end users as per the indents received and records maintained.
7. Unserviceable, broken articles etc., may be periodically auctioned and receipts credited to the accounts.

II. Financial Management

Business enterprise require finance for three purposes. They are:

a) For financing fixed capital,

b) For financing working capital or floating capital,

c) For financing expansion and improvements.

Raising of capital by a company or an enterprise is through:

1. Owned capital, that is by issue of shares,
2. Borrowed capital, that is, 1) by issue of debentures 2) acceptance of deposits from public and 3) by raising loans from financial institutions.

Financial requirements of a company may be classified into a) Long term finance, b) Medium term finance & c) Short term finance.

A) Long term finance: When the financial requirement is considered for more than seven years, it is considered as long term finance. Long term finance is used to provide fixed capital or fixed assets like building, land, machinery etc. Long term finance can be raised by the issue of shares, debentures, loans from financial institutions like NABARD, ICICI, Nationalised banks etc. Even the profits earned during a previous year may be ploughed back to raise capital.

B) Medium term finance: This refers to financial requirement between 2 to 7 years. This money is used for advertisement expenditure, overhauling of machinery, financing of expansions and improvement. Medium term finance is raised through a) preferential shares, b) debentures, c) public deposits, d) loans from commercial banks (term loans), e) loans from IDBI, ICICI, NABAARD.

C) Short term finance: Short term finance is used to meat working capital expenditure and to carryout day to day business. In case of a large dairy unit, the day to day requirement of feeds and fodder expenditure can be met by short term finance. Short term finance can be raised through: a) trade credit, b) bank credit, c) institutional credit, d) advances received from customers, e) overdraft facility from banks etc.

Some common terms used in financial circles

1. Share: A company's owned capital is divided into large number of equal parts called shares. The share capital of the company is not returned to the share holder with in the life time of company.

Kinds of shares: a) Preferential shares: The rate of dividend on these shares is fixed and the dividend must be paid to them in preference to other shares. b) Equity shares: Non preferential shares are called equity shares.

2. Debentures: It is an instrument (a certificate) issued under the common seal of company acknowledging its debt to some person or persons under certain terms and conditions endorsed on the back of the instrument (certificate). The terms usually refer to the rate of interest, the mode of payment and the security offered for ensuring these payments. Like shares, debentures are also offered to the public.

Main difference between equity share holder and preferential share holder is that equity share holder is a proprietor where as preferential share holder is not a proprietor but has very limited access on management. Equity share holder being the owner, has all voting rights in the management's affairs like electing board of directors etc. A debenturer is only a creditor while an equity share holder is a proprietor.

Sources of Agriculture / Livestock finance

Finance for agriculture can be obtained from

- Money lender
- Credit co-operatives
- Commercial banks
- Government
- Regional Rural Banks

3 R's of credit:

To estimate the rationality of a loan, it is essential to know credit analysis. The considerations involved in credit analysis generally fall into three groups: returns, repayment capacity and risk bearing ability. These are popularly known as the three R's of credit.

Returns

This R of credit has great significance for the creditor as well as the borrower. It requires that both the borrower and the financier should be satisfied with the returns from credit. The problem of determining the profitable use of capital is a part of decision making and it involves selection of enterprises, determining the most economical production techniques and determining the size of each enterprise.

Repayment capacity

It is the test of economic feasibility. It determines the amount the farmer will be able to spare for repayment of loan. It is generally acceptable that if an investment is profitable, the loan can be repaid without any difficulty.

Risk bearing ability

Risk bearing ability implies the capacity to cope with an unexpected low income and unpredictable expenses and losses due to the vagaries of nature and other hazards such as insects, pests, diseases and price fluctuations.

3 C's of credit

They are *character, capacity and capital.* Character implies the borrower's moral qualities, such as honesty, integrity and sense of responsibility which all influence the risk bearing ability and repayment. Capacity signifies the borrower to repay the loan, when it is due and depends upon his income. Capital reflects the net worth of the borrower (assets minus liabilities) which also reflects his repayment and risk bearing ability.

Resource scheduling under limited resources and capacity problems:

Any project which has the report of possible expenditure, revenue earnings and expected profits will have to write the schedule of various activities to be performed when the project is at the actual implementation stage. Keeping in mind the various resources namely the material, money, personnel and the time at the disposal of the entrepreneur, he has to allocate these various resources in order to get the maximum returns from the project. This process of allocating various resources namely men, money, material and fixing the time schedule of various activities of the project or enterprise is called resource scheduling.

The following steps may be considered while resource scheduling.

1. List the various activities to be performed.
2. Fix the date on which the actual start of the enterprise is scheduled.
3. Write the time schedule of various activities on day –1.
4. By visualising the various activities to be performed on the following days and weeks, allocate the various resources and fix the time schedule for those days.
5. Calculate the expenditure for these activities and find out whether such allocation of resources is well with in the technical and economic feasibility.
6. If such allocation is found not with in the ceiling or limits of the availability of resources, think of substitutions or reallocation of resources and ultimately decide upon a feasible, economically viable resource and time allocation.
7. Fix up certain basic rules to be followed by every one involved in the enterprise so that there is maximum utilisation of time, money, material and man power in order to make the enterprise more profitable.
8. There should be periodic examination of the schedule with provision for altering the allocation of various resources depending on the price, availability and other aspects of the resources.

Procedure for norm fixation: Before fixing a norm or standard to a particular production activity, it requires a careful study of practically carrying out the activity under reasonable production circumstances. Further weightage must be given to all the possible minor alterations in the production level with in a permissible limit. Only after such an exercise, one can fix a certain norm to any production activity. It may be the time required, quantities of various resources required etc., for that particular production activities. The following are some of the steps to be followed while fixing a norm or a standard:

1. Based on the targeted production activity and fixing the various resources required for such production, a trial run of the production is carried out.
2. Careful study of every step followed sequentially in such production activity.
3. If found reasonably okay, a tentative norm may be arrived.
4. The various steps followed in the production activity may be discussed with all the personnel / labourers in charge of the said production activity.
5. Based on the practical suggestions received from the concerned personnel, suitable modification in the production activity may be brought about.
6. The modified steps may be adopted and another trial run of the production activity is followed.
7. Make sure that the altered / modified procedure is technically and economically viable without affecting the ultimate profits of the enterprise.
8. Any minor problems or practical hitches may be solved, &
9. Finally fix the norm to be adopted as a routine in the overall production process.

III. Product Management

Principles of product optimisation:

1. Proper selection of raw materials with respect to their quality and at very reasonable price.
2. Substitution of the raw material if possible without affecting the quality of the product provided the substitute to chosen is cheaper than the original.

3. Follow the laws of production, ie, the input – output relationship and see that the output is more in proportion to the input as per the law of increasing returns.
4. Take into consideration the seasonal factors of production and consumption patterns. ie. time the production in such a way so that the consumer gets the product when he wants rather than flooding the market with the product when there is no demand.
5. Efficient utilisation of labour.
6. Minimising wastage of raw materials.
7. Proper storage of the product.
8. Keep the fixed costs at minimum ie. expenditure towards fixed assets like land, building, machinery must be minimum without affecting the quality & quantity of production.
9. Keep the variable costs of production also at minimum.
10. Find the break even point and adjust, production level so that there is larger angle of incidence & wider margin of supply.

Break – Even Analysis / Cost – Volume – Profit Analysis (CVP analysis)

The success of any business is measured in terms of profit and profit is dependent on three basic factors viz. a) cost of production, b) selling price and c) volume of sales ie. total sales. The cost of production determines the selling price required to be fixed to realise the desired level of profit, the selling price determines the volume of sales, the volume of sales directly influences the volume of production and the volume of production intern influences the cost of production. Thus costs of production, volume of production, sales, selling price and profits are interrelated. A study of this interrelationship of cost, volume, sale and profit is called cost – volume – profit analysis or CVP analysis. The most widely known form of cost – volume – profit analysis is the break – even analysis.

The term break even analysis is interpreted or defined in two senses. a) in its narrow sense and b) in its broad sense. In its narrow sense, the break even analysis is concerned with the ascertainment of the break – even point. ie. the level of business activity or the volume of sales where the total costs equal to total sales or revenues (TC = TR). This point is called the "point of no profit & no loss", "balancing point", "neutral point", "equilibrium point", "loss ending point", and "profit beginning point". If production is increased beyond this level, profits will accrue and if it is decreased below this level, loss will occur. Thus, break – even point is the specific level of activity or the volume of sales which breaks the total revenues and total costs evenly or equally ie. TR = TC.

b) In the broad sense, the study of cost – volume – profit relationship up to the point where TR = TC is termed break – even – analysis and beyond this point the study is termed CVP analysis.

Margin of safety is defined as the difference between actual sales and sales at break even point. In other words it is the amount by which the actual volume of sales exceeds the sales at break even point.

In other words, Margin of safety = Actual sales – Break even sales.

The margin of safety is an indication of profitability of a business. Since the fixed costs are covered by the break even sales, the margin of safety or the additional sales over break even sales would naturally add to the profits of organisation. The size of margin of safety indicates the amount of profit. A large margin of safety indicates high profits and low margin of safety indicates low profits. When the margin of safety is low, the following steps may be taken. 1) Increase the volume of sales, 2) Increase the selling price, 3) Decrease the fixed costs, 4) Decrease the variable costs 5) Improve the sales mix ie. substitute unprofitable products by profitable ones.

Break even chart and Angle of incidence: When total sales and total costs are graphically represented, the point at which the total sales line (TS or TR) intersects the total costs line, is called the break even point and the angle formed at this point between the two lines to the right side of the break even point is called angle of incidence. Such a chart is called Break Even chart. A large angle of incidence indicates that profits are made at a high rate and a small angle of incidence indicates that the profits are made at a relatively lower rate. A large margin of safety with wide angle of incidence indicates most favourable position of a business and even the existence of monopoly positions.

Use of break – even – analysis

1. Ascertainment of Break – Even point.
2. Determination of costs and revenues at different levels of output.
3. Product planning – ie. add or remove the product.
4. Activity planning – planning expansion or reduction of business.
5. Profit planning.

6. Make or buy decisions.
7. Equipment selection and replacement decisions.
8. Methods of business promotion.
9. Decisions on distribution channels.
10. Price decision.
11. Suspension or permanent closing down.
12. Forecasting.
13. Performance evaluation.
14. Cost – control.

IV. Personnel Management / Labour Management

Personnel management deals with various activities connected to the personnel or staff of a business organisation. The various functions of personnel management include:

a) Recruitment of staff,

b) Giving proper training to the staff,

c) Putting the right man to the right job,

d) Making decisions of wage structure, promotional policy, merit rating of employees, etc.

e) Taking care of health, safety and recreation of employees,

f) Maintenance of records of service,

g) Payment of gratuity, pension, provident fund, encashment of leave, etc. of the employees at the time of retirement.

Identification of work

Identification of work is the process by which information is collected about the quantity and quality of work, different kinds of works or skills required to be performed in an industry or enterprise. It is some kind of listing of different minute works involved in a production enterprise.

Job analysis

Work of Job analysis is the process by which pertinent information about job contents and job duties, qualifications required for each job, etc. are obtained. Job analysis involves job description and job specification.

Job description

It describes the job and duties involved in the job and also indicates the magnitude and specific details of the job. Job specifications on the other hand specifies the qualifications and qualities of the job holder for the successful performance of the job. The difference between Job description and Job specification can be illustrated with the following example:

Considering the example of milking a cow, the job description gives the details regarding the correct method of milking like the full hand milking and not milking by stretching the teat between thumb and index finger or by pressing the teat between the thumb knuckle and index finger. Details regarding the number of animals to be milked, number of times milking in a day, the timings of milking, maximum time allowed for the completion of milking process in each cow, etc. all go into the job description.

Job specification specifies the qualifications of the job holder. That is in the specific example of a milk man, the qualifications include that he should have prior experience in milking, he should have some knowledge of clean milk production, he should be free from communicable diseases like tuberculosis, he should pay attention towards personal hygiene, like cleanliness, clipping of nails, etc.

Distribution of Labour

It is the process of allocation of right job to the right man at right time in right quantity and right place in order to get optimum quantity of production with assured quality and efficiency.

Types of Labour

1. Hired/Casual - Seasonal
   - For special jobs
2. Temporary - Skilled
   - Unskilled
3. Permanent - Skilled (eg. Milkers, Clerks)
   - Unskilled (eg. Workers, Attendants)

Division of Labour

Division of labour means dividing large tasks into smaller packages of work to be distributed among several people. This work specialization allows an employee to master a task in the shortest time with a minimum skill.

Making of an article is split up into several processes and each process is entrusted to a separate set of workers. This is known as division of labour. It is simply a form of specialization of labour. There are 3 types of division of labour. They are,

a) Simple division of labour

A work is done by the combined efforts of a group of workers. It is difficult to say how much work each one did. Ex. Carrying a heavy almirah lead by a number of people.

b) Complex division of labour

The work is split up into different processes and each worker is assigned a definite part of the work. This is the division of labour proper. Ex. Manufacturing of pins, making of bread etc.,

c) Territorial division of labour

This firm refers to certain localities or cities or towns specializing in the production of some commodities.

Division of Labour or Job specialisation

In the modern industrial type of production the production of an article is split up into a number of processes or operations and each process or operation is entrusted to a worker or to a group of workers who are specialised in that work. The splitting up of production of an article into several operations and the entrustment of each operation to a worker or group of workers specialised in that work is called division of labour. It is also known as specialisation, as each worker or group of workers specialise in only one process of the manufacture of an article.

Advantages of division of labour or job specialisation

1) It increases over all productivity of the enterprise.
2) Large scale production is possible.
3) Lowers the cost of production.
4) Improves quality of the products produced.
5) There is better scope for allotting right job to the right person.
6) There is better scope for utilising the ability of each worker to the fullest extent.

7) Improves the skill of the worker.
8) Less strain for the worker.
9) Saves time and energy.
10) Makes learning a skill for the beginner more easy as the production activity is split into smaller portions.
11) Economy of tools is possible.
12) Use of machines is possible.
13) There is possibility of introducing or finding new innovations by the workers in that field of limited activity entrusted to him.
14) Diversification of job is possible.

Disadvantages of job specialisation

1) Monotony of work.
2) Labourer being a specialist in a particular skill cannot move to another job thus restricting his mobility to another job.
3) Worker becomes ignorant of other jobs.
4) The labourer may lose the sense of pride of work as his contribution to the final product is very little.
5) Retards human development.
6) May create unemployment when the production enterprise utilising the particular skill gets closed due to certain reasons.
7) Exploitation of women and children is possible.
8) Evils of factory system like over crowding, growth of slums etc. are likely to occur.
9) Class conflicts between the employer and employee may occur.
10) Over specialisation is likely to kill the creative instinct of the worker when viewed in a wider and broader perspective.

Labour Supervision

Supervision means overseeing the work performance of the subordinates. In any organisational structure there is direct contact of the immediate superior with that of the subordinate and it is the job of the supervisor to oversee or supervise the work performance of the subordinate.

Taking the example of Directorate of Animal Husbandry and Veterinary Services of any state government, the organisational structure broadly is as follows:Director – Additional Director – Joint Director – Deputy Director –

Assistant Director – Veterinary officer – Livestock Inspector

The Director oversees the work performance of the entire department of Animal Husbandry and Veterinary Services of the entire state with the assistance of the officers down the organisational structure. The Joint Director who is stationed at a divisional head quarter will be supervising the work performance of the subordinate staff coming under his division which usually comprises of a cluster of districts. Similarly, the Deputy Director will look after the work performance of the subordinate staff at the district level and Assistant Director at taluk level. Now we can make a distinction between Supervision and Direction. Supervision and direction although appear to be same, they are different in their scope of work. Direction includes supervision and hence the scope of direction is wider than the supervision. While, a supervisor is directly in contact with the immediate subordinate, usually a grass root level worker and he performs the job of overseeing the work performance of the immediate subordinate. On the other hand the Director supervises the supervisors and is responsible for the over all performance of the entire organisation.

Tenets or Principles of Labour Supervision

In any organisation the ultimate success of transmitting the goals and plans of the organisation depends on the work performance of its staff or personnel. The work performance of the staff in turn depends on several factors like the health of the workers, working condition, wage structure, opportunity for promotion, recognition of the merit of the worker, safety of the workers, retirement benefits, medical facilities, recreational facilities, educational facilities provided to children, housing facilities, transport facilities for commuting between the work place and the place of dwelling, etc. In addition to all these privileges enjoyed by workers, it is also equally important that there is proper accountability for their work.

The supervisors who perform the job of supervision should keep in mind the following broad guidelines in order to promote, protect and realistically achieve the objectives of the organisation through extracting optimum work performance from the workers:

1. Keeping in mind the ability of individual worker based on his qualifications, experience, age and physical ability, assign the job and ensure that the individual performs the individual task in the given time frame.

2. While assigning the work give the details of work schedule, work procedure, provide necessary tools, machinery, materials etc. required for the work.
3. Create proper work atmosphere in the work place by providing clean and ventilated premises, creating friendly atmosphere among workers, giving due respect to workers, causing no harassment to workers, particularly the women employees.
4. Provide safety training, safe tools and equipment to workers and make them safety conscious, thus ensuring safety at work place.
5. Depending upon the provisions of the company or enterprise the supervisor should take part in the process of selecting the employees.
6. Newly appointed workers must be given suitable orientation training in the beginning and at later stages periodic in-service training must be given to update the knowledge and skill of the workers.
7. The supervisor ensures discipline among workers by himself being very regular and punctual.
8. Supervisor must have the ability to lead and motivate the workers and also control the work performance of them by suitable guidance and by taking corrective measures wherever necessary.
9. Supervisor serves as an effective link between the subordinates and the superior authorities.
10. The supervisor transmits the problems of the subordinates to the superiors and thus helps in solving the problems of the subordinates by influencing the higher ups to take suitable policy decisions.

Qualities of a good supervisor

1. He should have good knowledge of the organisation's structure for which he is working for and understand its policies, objectives and goals and also rules and regulations of the organisation.
2. He should be sound in the knowledge of the job that he is supervising and must be able to operate most of the equipments etc. working under him.
3. He should have good communication skills, orderly thinking and should be able to judge people.
4. The supervisor should be mentally alert, physically fit, emotionally stable and cool in temperament.

5. The supervisor must be easily approachable by the subordinates and must have the patience to hear the problems of them and take suitable remedial measures.
6. As the supervisor himself cannot perform all the duties, he should have enough trust in the ability of others and entrust works according to the ability of different workers
7. Supervisor must have the ability to take quick and correct decisions particularly at times of crisis, as in the case of power failures, break down of machinery etc.
8. He should be physically fit and possess good vigour and health.
9. He should lead, inspire and motivate the workers.
10. He should be worthy of emulation.

Pricing Strategies

In terms of the marketing mix some would say that pricing is the least attractive element. Marketing companies should really focus on generating as high a margin as possible. The argument is that the marketer should change product, place or promotion in some way before resorting to pricing reductions.

Penetration Pricing

The price charged for products and services is set artificially low in order to gain market share. Once this is achieved, the price is increased. This approach was used by France Telecom and Sky TV. These companies need to land grab large numbers of consumers to make it worth their while, so they offer free telephones or satellite dishes at discounted rates in order to get people to sign up for their services. Once there is a large number of subscribers prices gradually creep up. Taking Sky TV for example, or any cable or satellite company, when there is a premium movie or sporting event prices are at their highest – so they move from a penetration approach to more of a skimming/premium pricing approach.

Economy Pricing

This is a no frills low price. The costs of marketing and promoting a product are kept to a minimum. Supermarkets often have economy brands for soups, spaghetti, etc. Budget airlines are famous for keeping their overheads as low as possible and then giving the consumer a relatively lower price to fill an aircraft. The first few seats are sold at a very cheap price (almost a promotional price) and the middle majority are economy seats, with the highest price being paid for the last few seats on a flight (which would be a premium pricing strategy). During times of recession economy pricing sees more sales. However it is not the same as a value pricing approach which we come to shortly.

Price Skimming

Price skimming sees a company charge a higher price because it has a substantial competitive advantage. However, the advantage tends not to be sustainable. The high price attracts new competitors into the market, and the price inevitably falls due to increased supply. Manufacturers of digital watches used a skimming approach in the 1970s. Once other manufacturers were tempted into the market and the watches were produced at a lower unit cost, other marketing strategies and pricing approaches are implemented. New products were developed and the market for watches gained a reputation for innovation.

Psychological Pricing

This approach is used when the marketer wants the consumer to respond on an emotional, rather than rational basis. It's strange how consumers use price as an indicator of all sorts of factors, especially when they are in unfamiliar markets. Consumers might practice a decision avoidance approach when buying products in an unfamiliar setting, an example being when buying ice cream. What would you like, an ice cream at Rs.10, Rs.25, Rs.50? The choice is yours. Maybe you're entering an entirely new market. Let's say that you're buying a lawnmower for the first time and know nothing about garden equipment. Would you automatically by the cheapest? Would you buy the most expensive? Or, would you go for a lawnmower somewhere in the middle? Price therefore may be an indication of quality or benefits in unfamiliar markets.

Product Line Pricing

Where there is a range of products or services the pricing reflects the benefits of parts of the range. If you buy chocolate bars or potato chips (crisps) you expect to pay X for a single packet, although if you buy a family pack which is 5 times bigger, you expect to pay less than 5X the price. The cost of making and distributing large family packs of chocolate/chips could be far more expensive. It might benefit the manufacturer to sell them singly in terms of profit margin, although they price over the whole line. Profit is made on the range rather than single items.

Optional Product Pricing

Companies will attempt to increase the amount customers spend once they start to buy. Optional 'extras' increase the overall price of the product or service. For example airlines will charge for optional extras such as guaranteeing a window seat or reserving a row of seats next to each other. Again budget airlines are prime users of this approach when they charge you extra for additional luggage or extra legroom.

Captive Product Pricing

Where products have complements, companies will charge a premium price since the consumer has no choice. For example a razor manufacturer will charge a low price for the first plastic razor and recoup its margin (and more) from the sale of the blades that fit the razor. Another example is where printer manufacturers will sell you an inkjet printer at a low price. In this instance the inkjet company knows that once you run out of the consumable ink you need to buy more, and this tends to be relatively expensive. Again the cartridges are not interchangeable and you have no choice.

Product Bundle Pricing

Here sellers combine several products in the same package. This also serves to move old stock. Blu-ray and videogames are often sold using the bundle approach once they reach the end of their product life cycle. You might also see product bundle pricing with the sale of items at auction, where an attractive item may be included in a lot with a box of less interesting things so that you must bid for the entire lot. It's a good way of moving slow selling products, and in a way is another form of promotional pricing.

Promotional Pricing

Pricing to promote a product is a very common application. There are many examples of promotional pricing including approaches such as BOGOF (Buy One Get One Free), money off vouchers and discounts. Promotional pricing is often the subject of controversy. Many countries have laws which govern the amount of time that a product should be sold at its original higher price before it can be discounted. Sales are extravaganzas of promotional pricing!

Geographical Pricing

Geographical pricing sees variations in price in different parts of the world. For example rarity value, or where shipping costs increase price. In some countries there is more tax on certain types of product which makes them more or less expensive, or legislation which limits how many products might be imported again raising price. Some countries tax inelastic goods such as alcohol or petrol in order to increase revenue, and it is noticeable when you do travel overseas that sometimes goods are much cheaper, or expensive of course.

Value Pricing

This approach is used where external factors such as recession or increased competition force companies to provide value products and services to retain sales e.g. value meals at McDonalds and other fast-food restaurants. Value price means that you get great value for money i.e. the price that you pay makes you feel that you are getting a lot of product. In many ways it is similar to economy pricing. One must not make the mistake to think that there is added value in terms of the product or service. Reducing price does not generally increase value.

See also eMarketing Price and international Marketing price.

Our financial objectives in terms of price will be secured on how much money we intend to make from a product, how much we can sell, and what market share will get in relation to competitors. Objectives such as these and how a business generates profit in comparison to the cost of production, need to be taken into account when selecting the right pricing strategy for your mix. The marketer needs to be aware of its competitive position. The marketing mix should take into account what customers expect in terms of price.

Premium Pricing

Use a high price where there is a unique brand. This approach is used where a substantial competitive advantage exists and the marketer is safe in the knowledge that they can charge a relatively higher price. Such high prices are charged for luxuries such as Hotel rooms, first class air travel, etc.

Sales Promotion

Sales promotion is a set of marketing technologies aimed to stimulate the demand in particular products and increase brand awareness. Limited in time, it creates a feeling of time-sensitiveness, generates new leads, and keeps existing customers engaged.

Benefits of Sales Promotion

- It helps to generate new leads. Sales promotion can boost your product image since it encourages sharing information about it within social groups related to your business. If you sell training football shoes, people keen on playing football will share the message.

- Allows re-engaging with your existing audience. Once a person subscribed to a brand's email newsletters, they will receive regular sales promotions. It is a way to keep the audience engaged and maintain a close connection with the company, which is crucial for building loyalty.
- Skyrockets revenue. Sales promotions help companies to increase the number of sold goods, even though they need to lower the price to achieve that goal. Of course, merely reducing the price is not enough, people should need your product, while the discount is only another reason to make a purchase.
- Increases brand awareness. Sales promotion is a way to make a name for your brand because people are more likely to talk about a company that proposes benefits and saves their money. That's what sales promotion does.

Sales Promotion Objectives

- Launch a new product. If you're going to expand and turn your small coffee shop into a bakery, you need to reach new market segments. You can attract new customers by offering a free cookie with each cup of coffee or suggest visitors set their own price once in a while.
- Attract new clients. This objective should be your long-term goal since it allows your business to grow. Your potential clients are likely your competitors' customers, so analyzing their product and benefits, you can offer something more valuable.
- Stay competitive. Researching and analyzing your competitors will not only help you attract new clients but constantly improve your product and customer service.
- Make existing customers buy more. It's always easier to make an existing customer buy more than attract new clients. Provide each client with a personalized approach — it will help you build customer loyalty. As a result, clients will promote your brand organically.
- Sell during the off-season. Goods like swimwear, boats, tents, air conditioners, refrigerators are definitely more popular in summer but you should consider special strategies to sell them throughout the year. Offer time-limited discounts, "1+1=3" campaigns, and other marketing tricks.
- Run clearance campaigns. They're especially popular before summer and winter. As dealers need to make room for a new collection, they

often run total clearance campaigns when users can buy goods from old collections at extremely reduced prices.

Types of Sales Promotion

- **Price deal.** It is a temporary cost reduction, for instance, 20% off for a coffee for a week.
- **Loyalty reward program**. This means that customers collect points or credits when they buy coffee. If they get 10 points, for example, they will have one coffee for free.
- **Bonus-pack deal**. It means that a customer can get more products paying the original price. For instance, they pay a dollar for one cup of coffee and get free candy, which gives some positive emotions and makes them come back in the future.
- **Giveaways**. These tactics aim to increase brand awareness. It means giving some items for free in exchange for personal information to use in further marketing. For example, offer a free cup of coffee in exchange for a phone number, which you can use for many purposes: promoting new sales, sharing updates and news with short text messages, etc.
- **Coupons.** You can sell coffee for the original price and give a coupon, which will make the next purchase 5% cheaper.
- **Mobile couponing**. It stands for coupons received on mobile phones via SMS. To get a discount, a customer needs to show the coupon on their smartphone.
- **Sampling.** Choosing this promotion type, companies give a sample of the product; for instance, the first cup of coffee to promote a new taste.

Sales Promotion Techniques

1. **Discounts:** This technique is as old as the hills. Small companies and big corporations use this method to sell more. One of the reasons it›s so popular, even today, is that discounts are great for both consumers and retailers. Sellers can clear room in their warehouse for new arrivals and customers can buy more at reduced prices. Keep in mind that a normal discount should be between 5-20% since clients won›t even notice less than 5% discount, but more than 20% off will make them feel suspicious about your brand.
2. **Time-limited offers:** This technique works even better than a big discount. With this trick, marketers manage to create a sense of urgency

and fear of missing out on their products. You can give clients 24 hours to grab this special offer. To make this technique perform better, you need to advertise your promotion on each channel you use. This will bring more sales and increase your site traffic.

3. **Seasonal promotions:** People often buy ski suits in summer and air conditioners in winter to save money. Selling products during off-seasons can be a real challenge, so we strongly recommend you to run seasonal promotions. Sell items from old collections at reduced prices and dont forget to advertise your campaign via email and social media.
4. **"1+1=3":** «Buy one and get one for free» and «Buy 2 items and get the third one for free» are very familiar marketing tricks. Such campaigns help you sell products at a low price or save money shopping together with a friend. Retailers can significantly boost sales with this technique reinforcing clearance sales.
5. **Holiday promotions:** Christmas, New Years Eve, Halloween, International Womens Day, and Valentines Day are great chances to skyrocket sales. People are extremely generous when buying presents for their friends and family. Launch your holiday campaigns in advance, and invest in advertising via email, PPC, social media, and other channels. This will help you increase brand awareness and site traffic.
6. **Gifts:** Who doesnt like freebies? If you are a startup or about to launch a new product, go for this technique. It will help you reach big audiences fast, build brand recognition, and collect user-generated content which is especially valuable for every type of business. Let users try your service for free for 7 days, launch a campaign that will let each client who spends $100+ receive a gift, or give away free samples with each order.
7. **Contests:** Competitions are a great opportunity to boost user engagement and increase brand awareness and sales. You can let your audience to create a slogan for your brand, a new advertising message, design, or share creative ideas on how to use your product in an unusual way. Make sure that the prize correlates with the effort spent on participating in your contest.
8. **Reward points:** You definitely should reward clients who buy from you regularly - people love brands that appreciate their choice. So, with this technique, you can start building customer loyalty. Give points to each client who makes a second purchase or spends a certain amount of money. Then, let them exchange those points for a product they like.

9. **Special prices:** Marketers usually run a 1-day campaign when users can buy everything at a fixed price. These prices usually look tempting for users and they can't overcome the feeling of missing out. The goal may be an annual clearance of goods. You can set a fixed price for each product category of your store. For example, sweaters for $5.99, jeans for $9.99, coats for $15.99. This technique works.

10. **First-purchase coupons:** It always takes time for people to give money to a new store especially when buying expensive products. To make them think over the purchase faster, offer a special incentive. You can send a welcome email to a new visitor with a coupon to get a 10 or 15% discount off their first purchase. For better performance, limit this appealing offer to a couple of days.

11. **Free shipping:** Very often users leave your site without buying just because of expensive delivery options. To win back these potential clients, you can run a time-limited campaign that allows them to receive their orders for free if they spend a certain amount of money. If you sell medium-priced goods, do not make this fixed sum too high. Otherwise, people won't fall for this trick.

Sales Promotion Examples

- Email marketing
- Facebook marketing
- SMS marketing

Risk Management

- "Risk is an event or injury that can cause damage to an institution`s income and/or reputation".
- "It is like energy that cannot be crated nor destroyed but only can be passed on or managed".
- "There is direct relationship between risk and reward and the quest for profit maximization has given rise to accelerated risk taking for enhanced rewards".
- "Whatever be the type of risk, impact is primarily financial. Ultimately risk manifest in the form of loss of income and reputation".

Risk is part of any business`s lexicon and understanding and subsequently managing it is the most important concern.

- The risk is inherent in the business.
- Given the importance of risk management, it is no wonder that it is today receiving scrutiny from the world`s top most organizations, banks, financial institutions, regulators , governments and so on.
- Organizations and institutions put tangible assets (such as funds, technology, processes and people) and intangible assets (such as reputation, brand and information) at risk to achieve their objective.
- Whether the organizations are for profit or not for profit the task of management is to manage these risks in the uncertain environment.

Organizational management has thus become synonymous with risk management

Sources of risk

- Interest rate risk Interest rate risk is the risk of an adverse effect of interest rate movements on a firm`s profit or balance sheet. Interest rates affect a firm in two ways by affecting the profits and by affecting the value of its assets or liabilities.
- Exchange risk Exchange risk is a possibility of adverse effect on the value of firm`s assets, liabilities or income, as a result of exchange rate movements.
- Default risk It is the risk of non-recovery of sums due to from outsiders, which may arise either due to their inability to pay or un-willingness to do so.
- Liquidity risk Liquidity risk refers to the risk of possible bankruptcy arising due to the inability of firm to meet its financial obligations.
- Business risk It is the risk faced by business from its external and internal environment. Internal factors like labour strike, death of key personnel, machinery break-down etc. External factors like government policy, changes in customer preference etc
- Financial risk It refers to bankruptcy arising from possibility of firm not being able to repay its debts on time. Higher the debt-equity ratio of firm, higher the financial risk faced by it. Liquidity risk and wrong capital structure are the prime reasons for financial risk .
- Market risk It is the risk of value of a firm`s investments going down as a result of market movements. It also referred as price risk.

- Marketability risk This is the risk of the assets of a firm not being readily marketable.

The changing form of risk

- We all know is risk is associated with every business activity. In a repressed financial system risk is not apparent.
- The earlier ethos inspect/detect/react have been substituted with new concepts like anticipate/prevent/monitor/mitigate.

Risk management process

Determining objectives

- It is a first step, may be profits, or to develop competitive advantage.
- It is to be decided by management.

Identifying risks

- Each corporate needs to identify the possible sources of risk and the kinds of risk faced by it.

Risk evaluation

- Once the risk is identified, they need to be evaluated for ascertaining their significance.
- The significance depend upon the size of loss that it result in, and the probability of the occurrence of such loss.

Development of policy

- Based on tolerance level of the firm, the risk management policy needs to developed.
- The time frame of policy should be comparatively long, so that the policy is relatively stable.

Development of strategy

- The tenure of a strategy is shorter than policy it needs to factor in various parameters that keep changing.
- A strategy is essentially an action plan, which specifies the tools, techniques and instruments that can be used to manage these risks.

Implementation

- This is the operational part of risk management
- It is finding the best deal in case of risk transfer, providing for contingencies in case risk retention, designing and implementing risk control programs, etc.

Review

- The function of risk management needs to be reviewed periodically. • Monitor effectiveness of the decision taken previously.

Risk management techniques

Two kinds of techniques used for management of various categories of risk

1. Internal techniques are those that are a part of the day-to-day operations of the firm.
2. External risk are those that require the company enter into some kind of financial contract with a market entity
    - Management of business risk Some of business risks are not manageable, i.e. they have to be borne Operational risks can be managed by building flexibility into operations
    - Asset-liability management Marshall & Bansal describes ALM as " an effort to minimize exposure to price risk by holding the appropriate combination of assets and liabilities so as to meet the firm`s objective and simultaneously minimizing the firm`s risk" To manage interest rate risk and exchange risk

Guidelines for risk management

- Common goal of risk management and financial management
- To create shareholder wealth
- To generate Net present value
- Proper mix of risk management techniques
- No risk management is fool proof or complete in itself
- Employs most optimum mix of risk control, risk prevention, risk transfer and risk retention
- Proactive risk management
    - Number of uncertainties involved in financial markets

    - Continuous changes in interest rate, exchange rates, commodity prices, economic variables and external environment is a reality
    - Risk management cannot be done after the happening of an event, it has to be done in its anticipation.
- Flexibility
    - Risk management strategies should not be too rigid
    - They should be flexible enough to allow risk manager to make most appropriate decision in according to the circumstances
- Bringing risk to the optimal level
    - The maintenance of risk at the level of optimal (The risk bearing capacity of the firm)
    - Firm should not be exposed to risks which may results in its liquidation
- Risk substitution
    - In general, risk management techniques do not eliminate the risk completely but substitute it by another kind of risk

Part F
Accountancy

32

Book Keeping

What is book keeping?

Book keeping is defined as;

1. The art of recording business transactions (pecuniary transactions) in a regulator and systematic manner.
2. Book keeping is the science and art of correctly recording in books of accounts all those business transactions that result in the transfer of money or money's worth.
3. Book keeping is an art of recording day to day business transactions in a set of books in a most systematic manner.
4. It is the process of analysing, classifying and recording transaction in accordance with pre-conceived plan.

Objectives of book keeping

How much have we earned this year?

How much during the past year?

Is our business improving?

Also, how much cash do we have?

How much our customers owe us?

Are they paying us regularly?

How much do we owe to our suppliers and other creditors?

How much we have invested in our business?

How much of it is retained so that we can expand the business?

Objectives of book keeping and its advantages

1. To have permanent record of mercantile transactions – replacing the memory.
2. To keep the records of income and expenditure of the business in such a way, net profit or net loss for any related period is readily ascertained.
3. To keep records of (a) assets, (b) liabilities in such a way that the financial position of the business undertaking is readily obtained. This helps in the sale or purchase of the business. It helps in insolvency position.
4. To keep track of all changes in the value of assets and liabilities.
5. To enable the business man to review and revise his policies in the light of past experiences brought to light by the analytical and interpretive records and reports.
6. To show the composition of capital, its size, its increase or decrease and whether the maximum utilization is made.
7. To know whether the line of business is profitable? If not reasons for the same.
8. To keep control on expenses with a view to minimize the same.
9. To know the names of customers and other debtors who owe money to the business.
10. To know the names of creditors and suppliers to whom the business owes money.
11. To have important information for legal purposes like claims against the firm can be established in the court of law (income tax calculation),

Who are the persons interested in financial information?

1. Owners of the business: May be the individual owner, partners of the business or even share holders. They all have their interest in the capital of the business and its profits or losses.
2. Creditors: Persons, companies, etc., who have supplied material to the business.
3. The management i.e., the official machinery that is running the business wants to know the positions of the business so that they can the business more efficiently.
4. Prospective investors like those persons who intend to invest in the

business but not yet decided. They will decide after going through the business records. They may be individual partners or share holders.

5. Buyers of the firm or a per cent of share in the retiring partners and heirs of the deceased partners also want to know the accounting information.
6. Government wants the accounting information to levy tax on the firm.
7. Students and researchers are immensely helped in gaining and interpreting accounting knowledge.

What is accounting?

Accounting is the science of recording and classifying business transactions and events primarily of a financial character and then of making significant summaries, analysis and interpretations of those transactions and events and communicating the results to decision making persons.

Types of accounting work

Accountant or account keeper has to perform following types of accounting work.

1. Constructive work: Formulation of principles of details of procedures of accounting. This is called 'Accountancy'.
2. Recording work: Actual recording of day to day transactions of business according to the laid down principles and procedures. This is called 'Book Keeping'.
3. Interpretive work: This is preparing of analytical statement of a business regarding various aspects of the dealings. This is helpful to the management, buyers, investors, etc. This branch is called 'Reporting'.
4. Critical work: This is concerned with verification of different records of book keeping of the business to check the correctness of the records. This is called 'Auditing'.

Division of the field of accounting or specialised fields of accounting

1. Financial accounting: Book keeping, accounting and auditing.
2. Administrative or management accounting: Interpretive work and reporting to the management.
3. Cost accounting and budget accounting: Cost of operation and to plan the whole work for better targeting.

4. Tax accounting: Details with the intricacies of computation of tax of a business on the basis of cost of purchases and sales.
5. Special investigations: Establishing the price of a business or valuation of goodwill of a firm, profitability or otherwise of a product, feasibility of bonus plans, etc.

Different books used in accountancy

Book of Accounts

A	B
Books of original entry or prime entry	Books of final entry or Principal book
a. Statistical records	or Ledger accounts
b. Journal or General journal	or 'T' accounts
c. Special journals or subsidiary journals	or Personal Real or Nominal accounts

1. Cash book
2. Purchases book (purchase daybook)
3. Sales book (sales daybook)
4. Purchases returns book
5. Sales returns book
6. Bills payable book (Bills of exchange book)
7. Bills receivable book (Bills of exchange book)
8. Journal proper
9. Petty cash book

A. What is a journal?

Journal is the primary or original book of entry is which all transactions are recorded in the form of 'entries'. These entries are entered in the order of their happening of occurrence in a chronological order. From these journals, entries are transferred to ledger.

B. What is a ledger?

It is a book of final entry wherein the transactions that are finally entered in Memorandum book or journals are finally entered in ledger. It is also called the 'Principal Book of Accounts'. Transactions relating to different persons are recorded separately in the name of each person in a ledger.

C. What is a cash book?

This is an account book where only cash transactions i.e., both receipts and payments of cash are recorded.

D. Purchase book or Purchase Daybook or Daybook of Purchase, Bought Daybook, Invoice book, Credit Purchase book, Purchase Journal, Purchases register

This book records only credit purchase of goods in which trends deals.

E. Sales book of Daybook of Sales or Sales daybook

In this book only credit sales of goods dealt by the traders are entered.

F. Purchase returns book

It contains the records of returns of goods purchased by the trader for which no cash is received. This happens when the goods are purchased but, the purchased goods are;

a) Defective,

b) Damaged during transit,

c) Qualities delivered or received may not agree with invoice,

d) The price charged may be too high,

e) Goods may have been received quite later (say-off season),

f) Substandard,

g) Terms and conditions may not be suitable.

G. Sales returns book

It records the goods returned by customers out of the sales already made and for which no cash is paid.

H. Bills payable book

In this book bills passed or pronotes passed or accepted are recorded.

I. Bills receivable book

In this book bills already drawn or acceptance received are entered.

J. Journal proper

Is the journal in which (this is like miscellaneous journals) those entries are entered, which cannot be entered in any of the above listed subsidiary journals or books.

Glossary of commercial terms

1. Business

It is an establishment for the conduct of trade or commerce. It denotes activities of person or group of persons, undertaken to exchange goods and/or services with a view to earn income and profit.

Eg: i. A manufacturing business,

ii. Banking business,

iii. Insurance business, etc.

Business is a semi-agent or a medium which accepts money from the proprietor or investor, pays him if profit is earned and demands from him, if loss is incurred.

2. Proprietor

He is the owner of the business. He invests capital in the business with the invention of earning profit. He undertakes all risks involved in the business. He enjoys all the incomes and profits and bears all expenses and losses if any. He has the claims against net assets of the business i.e., total assets minus liabilities to outsiders.

3. Assets

These are the material and non-material things or possessions or properties of the business including the amounts due to it from others.

Eg: Land, buildings, furniture, equipment, plant, machinery, fixtures, cash, bank balance, debtor's bills receivable, stock of goods, investments, etc., are all assets.

3A. Tangible assets

These are assets having physical existence like – cash, furniture, land, building, etc.

3B. Intangible assets

These are assets with no physical existence. But, their possession gives rise to some benefits to owners. Eg: Goodwill, patents, trademarks, etc.

4. Liabilities

These denote the amounts, which a business owes to others (other than the proprietor/s) on different accounts such as;

a. Loan from bank, b. Loan from other persons, c. Creditors for goods supplied, d. Creditors for services rendered to the business, etc.

Liabilities are also called Creditors equity i.e., Creditors claims on assets.

5. Capital

It is the amount invested by the proprietor/s in the business. For the business capital is a liability towards the owner. It is also called net worth or net assets, i.e., Assets – Liabilities = Capital. Capital is also called owner's equity or owner's claim against assets.

Assets = Capital + liabilities

$$A = C + L$$

or Capital = Assets – Liabilities

$$C = A - L$$

Residual value of assets is called capital

Reserves and undistributed profits increase the capital

Losses (which are not transferred to capital) also increase capital.

6. Equity

Any rights or claims to assets or any interest in property or in a business is known as equity. Therefore, it denotes liabilities. An equity holder may be a creditor, a partner, a shareholder or a proprietor. Therefore, all liabilities of a business are the creditors equity and the capital is owner's equity.

Therefore, Assets = Capital + Liabilities

= Owners equity + Creditors equity

7. Accounting equation

It is a mathematical form of saying that in any business the total assets always equal to owners equity + creditors equity.

Assets = Owners equity + creditors equity

8. Balance sheet

It is a statement of financial position of a business at any given time. It discloses the assets, liabilities and owners equity or capital of a business at a given time. The equation i.e., accounting equation is sometimes referred to as Balance Sheet equation. This balance sheet equation is always maintained in the accounts book keeping. That is a position of equality (in values) between assets on one hand and capital and liability on the other hand.

9. Debtor

One who owes debt or money is a debtor, i.e., one who owes money to a business is a debtor.

10. Creditor

One to whom a debt is owed or creditor is a person to whom some money is to be paid for the loan taken, service obtained or goods bought.

11. Drawings

It is the value of the cash or goods withdrawn by the owner or proprietor for his personal or domestic purposes or use. It is opposite of capital.

12. Revenue and income

Sales of products, merchandise (goods for sales and services) earnings by way of interest, rents, wages, salaries, commission, etc., are revenues. 'Revenue' is the gross money receipts which increases owners equity (capital) on one hand and also the assets (cash or account receivables) on the other hand.

'Income' is the money or money's equivalent earned or accrued during an accounting period increasing the total of previously existing net assets (net worths) and arising from the sales and rentals of any types of goods or services.

Eg: When goods of Rs.10,000/- are sold to Rs.15,000/-, the sum of Rs.15,000/- is the revenue, whereas Rs.5,000/- is earned over and above the original asset value of Rs.10,000/- is the income. Similarly the receipts and amounts receivable for services rendered like rent, wages, salary, interest, commission, dividend, etc. are income.

13. Expense

It is the money spent in conducting business activities. It is the expenditure in return for which some benefit i.e., service is received. Eg. expenditure on clerk's salary for clerical services, money spent to pay the wages to labourers for the labour received to the business.

14. Loss

It is depletion or decrease in the value of any asset without resulting in any revenue or benefit.

15. Service

It is the work performed by the business to get revenue or the work obtained from others by spending for the same. Thus, rendering the service results in income and receiving service results in expense.

16. Goods

These are articles bought for resale to earn profit.

17. Transaction

It is the exchange of cash, goods or services in a business.

a) Cash transaction: is one where cash receipt or payment is involved in any exchange.

b) Credit transaction: It is the transaction wherein cash is neither received nor paid at the time of transaction, but involves exchange on credit or debit.

c) Non cash transaction: is one where the question of receipt of cash or payment of cash does not arise at all. Eg: Depreciation, return of goods, etc.

18. Books of accounts and entry

The various books wherein transactions of varied nature of a business are entered are the books of account.

19. Entry

Entry is the record of a transaction of a business in a journal.

20. Gross profit

Difference between selling price and the cost price of the goods is the gross earning or gross profit of the businessman.

21. Gross loss

Difference between cost price and selling price of goods.

22. Net profit (net income)

Surplus remains after charging against gross profit all expenses including depreciation and other provisions properly attributable to the normal activities of the particular group.

23. Account

Summary of similar elements in the transactions relating to a person, thing or service. Eg: Cash account, goods account, persons account, income and expenses account, etc., short form A/c or a/c.

24. Debit and credit

These are symbols used while recording transactions. Debit (Dr) refers to the receiving account and credit (Cr) to giving account. If any benefit is received or a person is a receiver of benefit the receiving or receivers account is said to be debited. If benefit is given or a person is a giver of benefit, the giving account or givers account is said to be credited.

25. Voucher

It is a written document in support of a business in respect of a transaction, represented on a carbon or counter copy of a cheque or a receipted bill or an acknowledgement receipt received.

26. Receipt

It is a written acknowledgement of a receipt of cash/money/ goods, etc. It is an accounting document recording physical receipt of something acquired/got.

27. Folio

If means the page (number) of a journal or a ledger (J.F. and L.F.).

Accountancy

Accountancy, systems of accounting, systems of book-keeping and methods of double entry

Book-keeping and accountancy or Accounting although appear to be same, in reality, they are two different terms.

Book keeping refers to merely recording of business transactions in a set of books in a most systematic manner.

Accounting or accountancy on the other hand refers to not only book keeping, but also extends its scope to summerising, analysing, classifying, interpreting and finally reporting the results to the concerned for decision making.

Systems of accounting

Accounting system is a basis for designing polices for accounting business transactions. There are three systems.

a) Cash system or cash receipt and cash payment system.

b) Mercantile system or accrual system.

c) Mixed or hybrid system.

a. **Cash system:** Here only actual cash receipts and actual payments are recorded. Credit systems are not recorded as long as they are not converted to cash. This system is used by non-trading concerns like school, college, clubs, associations, service persons like doctors, lawyers, etc. Under this system, a statement of receipts and payments containing only cash transactions are entered. This is not a complete system as it ignores accruals.

b. **Mercantile system or accruals system:** Under this system all items of income and expenditure i.e., receipts and payments of both cash and noncash items of a particular period are recorded. The income earned but not received and expenses incurred, but not paid i.e., all accrued items are considered here.

c. **Mixed or hybrid system**: This is partly a mercantile and partly a cash system. Here income or receipt items are recorded in cash system, but cash expenses and noncash expenses are recorded in mercantile system.

Systems of book keeping

Business transactions can be recorded in any system which provides to the businessman, the necessary financial position of his business and the result of his transactions. The following systems of book keeping are followed.

1. Single entry system: It is a method which recognises cash and personal items of the transaction and ignores the impersonal items. In that it is incomplete, inaccurate and unscientific.

2. Double entry system: (i) It is most scientific, (ii) It recognises both the aspects of each transaction and records each aspect, (iii) It is complete, accurate and scientific.

Illustration of double entry: Eg. Suppose Mr.Ravikumar owns a retail egg shop and sells goods worth Rs.500 to Mr.Monish and Mr.Monish pays cash of Rs.500/-.

In any transaction there are always two parties. Each party has two aspects of transaction and both of these aspects have to be recorded in the double entry system.

Eg: Goods → Sells goods → worth Rs.500

Ravikumar (Businessman) → Monish

-(Goods) +(Ravikumar)

Cash ← Pays ← 500

+500 Cash of Rs.500

i.e., Ravikumar
- Goods of 500/-
+ Cash of Rs.500/-

Monish
+ Goods of Rs.500/-
- Cash of Rs.500/-

i.e., each party has two aspects.

3.Indian system: This is almost same as double entry system.

Methods of double entry

Double entry system can be recorded either by (i) Balance sheet or accounting equation method or American method or by (ii) Basic book keeping method or British method.

i. Balance sheet or accounting equation method

Illustrative problem No.1

Transaction-1: Suppose Mr.Jayadeva starts a retail egg shop investing Rs.30,000/- in cash on 1st May 2004. What does it mean to the business?

Assets = { Capital + Liabilities } Liabilities in broad sense

= 30,000 + Nil

{owners claim + creditors claim}

When the above equation is written in the form of conventional balance sheet.

Mr. Jayadeva's balance sheet as on May 1st 2004

Liabilities	Rs.	Assets	Rs.
(Jayadeva's claim) Capital	30,000/-	Cash	30,000/-
	30,000/-		30,000/-

Illustrations – 2

On May 2, Mr.Jayadeva buys a building for the shop from Mr.Ravikumar for Rs.40,000/- on credit, what does that mean?

Assets = Capital + Liabilities

Owner's claim + Creditor's claim

Cash + Building = Jayadeva's claim + Ravikumar's claim

30,000 + 40,000 = 30,000 + 40,000

When the above equation is expressed in conventional balance sheet, it will be –

Balance sheet of Jayadeva as on May 2, 2004

Liabilities	Rs.	Assets	Rs.
Jayadeva's claim (Capital) Ravikumar's claim (Creditors)	30,000/- 40,000/-	Cash Building	30,000/- 40,000/-
	70,000/-		70,000/-

Illustration – 3

On May 3rd Mr. Jayadeva buy's furniture worth Rs.1,000/- for cash.

A = C + L
Cash 30,000 – 1000
Building 40,000 = 30,000 + 40,000
Furniture 1,000

Here increase in the value of one asset (0→1,000) has decreased the value of another asset (30,000→29,000) when the above equation is written in the conventional balance sheet way →

Balance sheet as on May 3rd, 2004

Liabilities	Rs.	Assets	Rs.
(Capital) Owner's claim Creditors claim	30,000/- 40,000/-	Cash Building Furniture	29,000/- 40,000/- 1,000/-
	70,000/-		70,000/-

Transaction May 4th

Mr. Jayadeva withdrew Rs.600/- for his personal use.

A = C + L
Cash 29,000 – 600
Building 40,000
Furniture 1,000
= 28,400 + 1,000 + 40,000
} = owner's claim + Creditors claim
= 29,400 + 40,000
69,400 = 69,400

When the above equation is written in a conventional balance sheet way →

Balance sheet as on May 4rd, 2004

Liabilities	Rs.	Assets	Rs.
(Capital) Owner's claim Creditors claim	(29,000+1,000) - 600 = 29,400/- 40,000/-	Cash Building Furniture	28,400/- 40,000/- 1,000/-
	69,400/-		69,400/-

In the above example, it is clear that the two aspects of every transaction are straight away recorded through the 'Accounting equation', which has two sides.

Assets = Liabilities

Assets = Owner's claim + Creditors claim

= Capital + Liabilities

LHS	RHS
Records any increase or decrease in the value of assets	Recording increase or decrease in the value of liabilities and claim

1. Increase in the value of one asset may increase the value of total liability.
2. Increase in the value of one asset may decrease the value of another asset.
3. Decrease in the value of one asset may decrease the value of total liability.
4. Decrease in the value of one asset may increase the value of total liability.

Just like the accounting equation has two sides namely LHS & RHS, each transaction also two aspects.

Like the equation each item whether an asset or a liability, each has two sides namely a left hand side or debit (Dr) and the right hand side or credit side (Cr).

In the case of assets – the left side indicates the acquisition of asset i.e., increase in the value of assets and the right side denotes the disposal and therefore a decrease in the value of assets.

Assets	
Dr.	Cr.
Left side (+) Acquisition of assets and increase in their value	Right side (-) Disposal or reduction in assets and decrease in the value of assets

In the case of liabilities (Creditors equity)

Liabilities (Creditors equity)	
Dr.	Cr.
Settlement of claims or Decrease in the liabilities or decrease in the value of liabilities	Creation of new claims or Increase in the liabilities or increase in the value of liabilities.

i.e., in the case of liabilities, the left side denotes settlement of claims i.e. decrease in the value of liabilities. Right hand indicates creation of new claims or increase in the liabilities or increase in the value of liabilities.

In case of the capital: Any profit earned by the business or fresh capital brought will increase the amount of capital and loss of withdraw's will decrease it. Therefore, profit is recorded on right hand side of capital and loss on the left hand side.

Capital = Owner's equity	
Dr.	Cr.
Left side (-)	Right side (+)
Business loss and withdrawals for personal use and reduction in capital	Profits and introduction of funds and increase in capital

Accounting equation is written as Revised Accounting Equation

Assets = Liabilities and Capital

Dr Assets Cr　　　　Dr Liability Cr　　　　Dr Capital Cr

Assets		=	Capital	+	Liability	
Dr	Cr		Dr	Cr	Dr	Cr
Left (+) Acquisition leads to increase in the value of assets	Right (-) Disposal leads to decrease in the value		Left (-) Drawings and losses (decrease)	Right (+) Investment and profit (increase)	Left (-) Settlement of liabilities (decrease the liability)	Right (+) Creation of new liabilities (increase the liabilities)

Rules of double entry according to accounting equation method

For asset a/c → a. Debit acquisition of and increase in asset

b. Credit disposal of and decrease in asset

For capital a/c → a. Debit withdrawl from and decrease in capital

b. Credit addition to and increase in capital

For liabilities a/c → a. Debit any reduction in the liability

b. Credit any increase in the liability or creation of liability

Expenses and income a/c → a. Debit the expenses or losses

b. Credit the income or profits

Assets		=	**Capital**		+	**Liabilities**	
Dr (+)	Cr (-)	=	Dr (-)	Cr (+)		Dr (-)	Cr (+)
Acquisition of assets and increase in assets	Disposal or decrease in assets or in their value	=	Loss, withdrawals and decrease in capital	Profits and increase in the capital		Settlement of claims and decrease in value	Creation of new claims and increase in value

Changes in the value of capital

In the course of recording transactions pertaining to income expenditure, profit, loss, drawers, etc., finally the capital also gets changed along with the other assets and liabilities.

1. Income earned and received, increase the value of cash asset if received in cash or creates a new asset as 'Income receivable' if not received in cash, at the same time the capital gets increased as such income means profit to proprietors.
2. Expenses incurred cause reduction in the value of cash asset if paid in cash and create a new liability as outstanding expenses, if not paid in cash. At the same time they reduce the capital as such expenses ultimately mean loss to proprietor.
3. Drawings in cash by the proprietor mean reduction in cash asset as well as in capital.

Practical method of accounting income and expenses

Expenses and losses cause decrease in capital and income and profits cause increase in capital. However, as there are many types of expenses and income which repeat several times during the accounting period, it is not advisable to record each and every item through capital. Instead they are summarised first in a statement called 'Profit and loss account' and only the net result i.e. either net profit or net loss is ultimately recorded through capital.

Points of Distinction	Book Keeping	Accounting
Meaning	An art of recording financial transactions in a systematic way	A science of making plans & polices for recording financial dealings and also for their classification, analysis, interpretation, finalisation and reporting their results for decision making.
Scope	Narrow scope, only of recording the transactions	Broader scope of recording as well as presentation of results
Nature of work	Primary work of maintaining basic records, simple work of recording	Finalisation of basic records to obtain results thereof – complex work of finalising
Staff involved	Junior staff of clerks and book keepers without special skills	Special staff with professional skill and knowledge
Importance	Helps in making permanent record	Helps in decision making
Users	Internal users, namely owners and managers	Internal and external users

Classification of Accounts

Personal accounts
(relating to person)

Impersonal accounts
(relating to property, things and services)

Relating to accounts of *natural* persons like Ram, Shyam or X, Y, Z etc., or *artificial* persons like firms, clubs, school, Govt. a/c or accounts of *representative* persons of these institutions	**Real accounts** or accounts of assets like real and tangible things of impersonal nature like furniture, machinery etc., or invisible and intangible assets like copy right, patents, trade marks, etc.	**Nominal or fictitious accounts** relating to services rendered or received and to those items which do not exist in reality. All expenses losses, incomes and gains are entered here.

Recording of an accounting element

The double entry system requires the recording of both the aspects of each transaction. Each aspect of a transaction being an accounting element for recording each aspect in the account books, an account is opened in the name of each accounting element or the aspect. For recording each type of the goods, each expense and income, a separate account has to be opened in account books.

Illustration

Give classification of the following accounts

a)	Ram a/c → P	i)	Rent a/c → N
b)	Syndicate bank a/c → P	j)	Motor van a/c → R
c)	Govt. of India a/c → P	k)	Travelling expenses → N
d)	Outstanding salary a/c → P	l)	Goods a/c → R
e)	Machinery a/c → R	m)	Loan a/c → P
f)	Copy right a/c → R	n)	Metro stores a/c → P
g)	Salary paid a/c → N	o)	Capital a/c → P
h)	Dividend a/c → N		

P = Personal a/c; R = Real a/c; N = Nominal a/c

Philosophy of 'debit' and 'credit' (British system)

1. The worlds 'debit' and 'credit' have no specific meaning. They are used only as accounting symbols.
2. In accounting terminology the left side of an account is called 'debit' side and the right side called 'credit' side.
3. Every transaction has two aspects.
4. Inflow of benefit is recording on the left hand side or 'Dr' side and out flow of benefit is recorded on the right hand side or 'Cr' side.

Inflow of benefit is also termed as 'charge to or receiving value' by an account. Outflow means discharge or 'giving' of money value. Therefore, receiving account is debited. Outflow means giving or sacrificing and hence giving a/c is credited.

Principles of double entry

i. Personal accounts: When the person receives something write it on the debit side and when he gives write it on the credit side.
ii. Real account: Debit what comes in and credit what goes out.
iii. Nominal or fictions account: Debit expenses and losses credit income and gains or profits.

Personal a/c
- Debit (receiver)
- Credit (giver)

Real a/c
- Debit Assets acquired or received
- Credit Property or assets reduced or parted

Cash a/c
- Debit (receipts)
- Credit (payments)

Nominal or fictions a/c
- Debit Expenses & loses
- Credit Profit & gains

Accounting cycle or accounting process

1. Writing transactions in the memorandum or waste book.
2. Journalising or entering the transactions in the journal.
3. Ledger posting and balancing.
4. Preparation of a trial balance.
5. Drafting final accounts and balance sheets closing i.e., trading a/c and profit and loss a/c.

Accounting cycle or accounting process

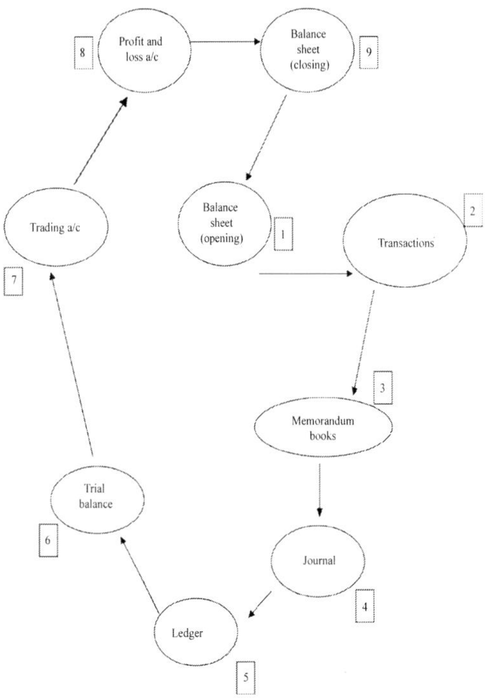

Journalising

Journal

'Journ' is Latin word means 'a day'. Journal means a day book. The day to day business transactions are first recorded in this book in chronological order and in two fold aspects namely 'Dr' and 'Cr' aspects.

Journalising is the process of making journal entries into the journal in a systematic manner.

Memorandum or Waste Book

All the business transactions are first recorded through a diary or a waste book or rough book known as 'Memorandum Book', before they are entered into a journal.

Subsequently as and when time permits, they are recorded in the journal after analysing each aspect of the transaction using the principles of double entry.

Form of Journal

Date	Particulars	L.F. (Ledger folio)	Dr	Cr
Year, month and day	By name of a/c debited To name of a/c credited	LF No.	Amount	Amount

Illustration of waste book and Journal entries of Sri Manoj.

Waste book or rough book entries of Sri Manoj.

Date	Particulars	Amount
2004 April, 1	Started business with cash	20,000
2	Bought goods for cash	8,000
5	Sold goods to Hemanth (on credit)	4,000
6	Sold goods for cash	6,000
9	Received cash from Hemanth	3,000
13	Purchased furniture from Tarique (on credit)	5,000
18	Paid office rent	200
20	Purchased goods from Raja (on credit)	7,000
30	Cash paid to Raja	1,000
30	Received commission	600

Journal of Sri Sri Manoj

Date	Particulars	L.F.	Dr	Cr
2004 April 1	By cash a/c Dr To Sri Manoj.'s capital a/c (cash invested to start business)	45 3	20,000 -	- 20,000
2	By goods a/c Dr To cash a/c (cash purchased vide cash memo No.)	22 45	8,000 -	- 8,000
5	By Hemanth's a/c Dr To goods a/c (Credit sales, per outward invoice No.)	5 22	4,000 -	- 4,000
6	By cash a/c Dr To Goods a/c (cash sales per cash Memo No.)	45 22	6,000 -	- 6,000
9	By cash a/c Dr To Hemanth's a/c (cash received on a/c per receipt No.)	45 5	3,000 -	- 3,000
13	By Furniture a/c Dr To Tarique a/c (bought furniture on credit per bill No.)	18 30	5,000 -	- 5,000
18	By rent a/c Dr To cash a/c (Paid office rent for the month of .... Bill no.)	42 45	200 -	- 200
20	By goods a/c Dr To Raja a/c (credit purchases as per invoice No.)	22 15	7,000 -	- 7,000
30	By Raja's a/c Dr To cash a/c	15 45	1,000 -	- 1,000
30	By cash a/c Dr To commission a/c Total	45 37	600 54,800	- 600 4,800

Steps in journalising

1. Decide the nature of transaction from business point of view and study its effect on the business. Eg: Cash or credit transactions.
2. Find out the two aspects or two sides of transaction i.e., which two accounts are involved. Give each a name.
3. Know the type of each a/c – Real, Personal or Nominal.

4. See what comes in or what goes out, or who is the receiver or who is the giver or whether there is expense or loss and income or gain.

Ledger posting and balancing

Ledger: It is a book of final entry because the transactions that are first entered in memorandum books and journals are finally written in the ledger. It is a book wherein transactions of similar nature pertaining to a particular person, article or a service are grouped in an account through a process called posting, i.e, transferring entries from journal to the ledger. It is also known as 'Principal book of accounts' because it is from this book that the final financial information relating to profit and loss and balance sheet is derived by the businessman.

Process of posting journal entry to ledger

The student/accountant should read the journal entry twice or thrice as it is, and then copy it down in the ledger as he utters or reads. Thus, if he reads "By cash account debit" he should debit to cash account and so on. For example, if we say Sri Manoj. started his business with Rs.20,000 on 1st April 2004, this transaction will appear in journal as waste book of Sri Manoj.

Date	Particulars	Amount
1.4.04	Started business with cash	20,000

Ledger of Sri Manoj

Cash A/c

Dr Cr

Date	Particulars	JF	Amount	Date	Particulars	JF	Amount
1.4.04	To Manoj's capital a/c		20,000				

Sri Anand's

Capital A/c

Dr Cr

Date	Particulars	JF	Amount	Date	Particulars	JF	Amount
				1.4.04	By cash a/c		20,000

In the ledger we have debited 'Cash a/c' as we read it with Rs.20,000 with the particulars 'To capital a/c' (the credit part of journal entry) on the debit side of cash a/c. Similarly we credit Rs.20,000 to 'Capital a/c' as we read it so, with the particulars. By cash a/c (the debit part of the journal entry) on the credit side of capital account).

Accounting elements

1. Cash A/c	Cash a/c
2. Manoj.'s capital A/c	Personal a/c
3. Goods a/c	Real a/c
4. Hemanth's a/c	Personal a/c
5. Furniture a/c	Real a/c
6. Tarique's a/c	Personal a/c
7. Rent a/c	Nominal a/c
8. Raja's a/c	Personal a/c
9. Commission a/c	Nominal a/c

Ledger entries of Sri Manoj

Dr Cr

Date	Particulars	JF	Amount		Date	Particulars	JF	Amount
1.4.04	To Manoj's capital a/c		20,000					
					2.4.04	By goods a/c		8,000
6.4.04	To goods a/c		6,000					
9.4.04	To Hemanth's a/c		3,000					
					18.4.04	By rent a/c		200
					30.4.04	By Raja's a/c		1,000
30.4.04	To commission a/c		600					

Sri Manoj's Capital a/c

Dr Cr

Date	Particulars	JF	Amount		Date	Particulars	JF	Amount
					1.4.04	By cash a/c		20,000

Goods a/c

Dr Cr

Date	Particulars	JF	Amount		Date	Particulars	JF	Amount
2.4.04	To cash a/c		8,000					
					5.4.04	By Hemanth's a/c		8,000
					6.4.04	By cash a/c		6,000
20.4.04	By Raja's a/c		7,000					

Hemanth's a/c

Dr Cr

Date	Particulars	JF	Amount		Date	Particulars	JF	Amount
5.4.04	To goods a/c		4,000					
					9.4.04	By cash a/c		3,000

Furniture a/c

Dr Cr

Date	Particulars	JF	Amount		Date	Particulars	JF	Amount
13.4.04	To Tarique a/c		5,000					

Tarique a/c

Dr Cr

Date	Particulars	JF	Amount		Date	Particulars	JF	Amount
					13.4.04	By furniture a/c		5,000

Rent a/c

Dr Cr

Date	Particulars	JF	Amount		Date	Particulars	JF	Amount
18.4.04	To cash a/c		200					

Raja's a/c

Dr Cr

Date	Particulars	JF	Amount		Date	Particulars	JF	Amount
					20.4.04	By goods a/c		7,000
30.4.04	To cash a/c		1,000					

Commission a/c

Dr Cr

Date	Particulars	JF	Amount		Date	Particulars	JF	Amount
					30.4.04	By cash a/c		600

Balancing and checking of Accounts by trial balancing

After ledger posting, the next stage is (a) Balancing the account, and (b) checking the arithmetical accuracy of the work through trial balance.

Balance is the difference between the total debits and the total credits of an account or the total of an account containing only debits or credits.

Balancing means insertion of writing of the difference between the debit amount and credit amount on the side where the total is less than the other, so that the grand total of the two sides become equal.

Personal accounts are generally balanced regularly to know the amounts due to or due from the persons. Sometimes personal accounts are balanced after every transaction as in bank ledgers.

Real accounts are generally balanced at the end of financial period.

Cash accounts are invariably balanced every day to know the cash on hand at the end of every day.

Nominal accounts are not balanced as they are to be closed by transferring them to final accounts. However, for trial balancing even these nominal accounts are also balanced. When the totals of credits and debits are same, it means the account is squared or closed.

When there is only one entry on either debit or credit side of an account, that amount itself is the balance of that account. Similarly when an account has only one sided entries, the total of the entries on that side itself is the balance of that account.

Steps in balancing

1. Take the totals of both the sides on a rough sheet.
2. Find the difference between bigger total and smaller total. This difference is called balance.
3. Record the above balance as the last item on the side having smaller total. The date should be the last date of the period.
4. If the balance is written on debit side, write 'To balance c/d' (carried down) and if the balance is to be placed on the credit side write 'By balance c/d' in the particular column.

Dr. The account Cr			Dr. The account Cr	
To total of Dr side 6000 -------- Grand 6000 Total	By total of Cr. Side 4500 By Balance (debit) c/d 1500 -------- Grand 6000 Total		To total of Dr side 3000 To balance (Cr.)c/d 5000 ------- Grand 8000 Total	By total of Cr. Side 8000 -------- Grand 8000 Total
To balance debit b/d 1500				By balance Cr b/d 5000

Example of debit balance Example of credit balance1

5. Write the total of each side in the a/c. These totals are written at the same level.
6. Lastly the amount of closing balance as recorded in the account should be brought down as the opening balance at the beginning on next day at the appropriate side.

Meaning of ledger balances in different types of accounts

a) Personal Accounts: (I) debit balance indicates that the person is debtor, (ii) Credit balance indicates money is payable to person.

b) Real account: (I) Debit balance indicates the excess of what comes in than what goes out, (ii) Credit balance represents profit on sale of assets which should be transferred to profit and loss account.

c) Cash account: Always shows debit balance or a nil balance as one cannot spend more than the receipts.

d) Nominal account: (I) Debit balance indicates expense or loss (ii) Credit balance indicates income or gain from that account

c/d – carried down; c/f - carried forward

b/d – brought down; b/f - brought forward

c/o – carried over; b/o – brought over

Cash A/c

Dr			Cr
To Total of Dr side	29,600	By total of Cr side By balance (debit) c/d	9,200 20,400
Grand total	29,600	Grand total	20,400
To balance (Dr) b/d	20,400		

Debit balance

Manoj s capital a/c (P)

Dr			Cr
To Total of Dr side To balance Cr c/d	0 20,000	By total of Cr side	20,000
Grand total	20,000	Grand total	20,000
		By balance c/d	20,000

Credit balance

Goods a/c ®

Dr			Cr
To Total of Dr side	15,000	By total of Cr side By balance (debit) c/d	10,000 5,000
Grand total	15,000	Grand total	15,000
To balance (Dr) b/d	5,000		

Debit balance

Hemanth's a/c

Dr			Cr
To Total of Dr side	4,000	By total of Cr side By balance (debit) c/d	3,000 1,000
Grand total	4,000	Grand total	4,000
To balance (Dr) b/d	1,000		

Debit balance

Furniture a/c (R)

Dr			Cr
To Total of Dr side	5,000	By total of Cr side By balance (debit) c/d	0 5,000
Grand total	5,000	Grand total	5,000
To balance (Dr) b/d	5,000		

Debit balance

Tarique a/c (R)

Dr			Cr
To Total of Dr side	0	By total of Cr side	5,000
To balance (Cr) c/d	5,000	Grand total	5,000
Grand total	5,000		

Credit balance

Rent a/c (R)

Dr			Cr
To Total of Dr side	200	By total of Cr side By balance (debit) c/d	0 200
Grand total	200	Grand total	200
To balance (Dr) b/d	200		

Debit balance

Raja's a/c

Dr			Cr
To total of Dr side To balance (credit) c/d	1,000 6,000	By total of Cr side	7,000
Grand total	7,000		
		By balance (Cr) b/d	6,000

Credit balance

Commission a/c

Dr Cr

Date	Particulars	JF	Amount		Date	Particulars	JF	Amount
30.4.04	To total of Dr. To balance C/d Grand total		0 600 600		30.4.04	By cash a/c		600 600

Credit balance

Trial balance of Mr.Manoj

Sl. No.	Name of account	LF	Dr.	Cr.

1	Cash a/c		20,000	-
2	Manoj's capital a/c		-	20,000
3	Goods a/c		5,000	-
4	Hemanth's a/c		1,000	-
5	Furntiure a/c		5,000	-
6	Tarique's a/c		-	5,000
7	Rent a/c		200	-
8	Raja's a/c		-	6,000
9	Commission a/c		-	600
	Grand total		31,600	31,600

Final accounts

After the business transactions are entered in journals, ledgers and after the completion of trial balance, the trader prepares the final accounts to know the net profits or loss of the business. This is done by (a) Trading account, (b) Profit and loss a/c and (c) By balance sheet.

All nominal accounts and goods accounts (i.e., goods bought for resale or consumable goods in the office) are closed at the end of an accounting period by making what are called closing entries, whereas all personal and real accounts pertaining to property, assets, debtors and creditors are just shown in the form of a statement called – Balance sheet.

A. Trading account (real account)

It is a good account prepared mainly to know the profitability of the goods bought and sold by the businessman. It is an account that shows the result of trading that is buying and selling known as gross profit. The difference between selling price and cost price of the goods is the gross earning.

1. Gross profit = Net sales – Net purchases
2. Gross profit = Net sales – Net purchases + purchases expenses
3. Gross profit = Sales – returns {opening stock + (purchases – returns) – closing stock + purchase expenses}
4. Gross profit = {(sales –returns inwards) + (closing stock)} – {Opening stock + (purchases – returns outwards) + purchase expenses}

The 'gross earning' or 'gross profit' dictates the terms of business i.e., whether the trader should continue to trade in the same line of goods or to change over to different type of goods. Such 'gross earning' is called 'gross profit'. However, when the cost of buying is more than the selling price the results is 'gross loss'.

The cost price or buying price includes/

a. Purchase price

b. Bringing expenses (carriage, cartage, freight, duty, etc.)

c. Conversion expenses, if raw materials are converted into salable products.

Preparation of trading account

Trading account is a ledger account. As the trading account contains the results of operations over a period, the reading should be Trading a/c for the period ……….

The format of trading a/c is as follows;

Name of the business or proprietor)

Trading a/c for the period ended ……..

Dr				Cr
Particulars	Amount		Particulars	Amount

What to debit in a trading a/c?

1. Opening stock.
2. Purchases done during the period – returns outwards.
3. Purchase expenses.
4. Manufacturing expenses.

What to credit in a trading a/c?

1. Sales during the period – returns inwards.
2. Issue of goods as samples.
3. Goods damaged or lost or destroyed or consumed personally.
4. Closing stock.

Example

In January Mr. Ravikumar bought 120 kg of certain goods at Rs.5.50 per kg and sold the same during the half year ending on 30th June at average price of Rs.7.50 per kg. Find the gross profit taking Rs.7 as purchase expenses.

Mr. Ravikumar

Trading Account for the half year ending 30th June

Dr				Cr
Particulars	Amount		Particulars	Amount
To purchases To purchase expenses To profit and loss a/c (gross profit transfer)	660 7 233		By sales	900
	900			900

From the following figurers find out the gross profit of Monish Kumar and Brothers.

	31.12.2004	31.12.2004
Purchases	26,000	34,000
Sales	20,000	38,000
Stock (closing)	12,000	16,000
Purchase expenses	500	700

Mr. Monish Kumar and Bros.

Trading Account for the year ending 31.12.2004

Dr				Cr
Particulars	Amount		Particulars	Amount
To purchases To purchase expenses To profit and loss a/c	26,000 500 5,500		By sales By closing stock (31.12.2004)	20,000 12,000
	32,000			32,000

Mr. Monish Kumar and Bros.

Trading Account for the year ending 31.12.2004

Dr				Cr
Particulars	Amount		Particulars	Amount
To opening stock To purchases To purchase expenses To profit and loss a/c (gross profit transfer)	12,000 34,000 700 7,300		By sales By closing stock (31.12.04)	38,000 16,000
	54,000			54,000

B. Profit and loss account

Profit and loss a/c is one which shows either the net profit or net loss or the ultimate profit or ultimate loss. The primary aim of profit and loss account is to ascertain the net profit or net loss of a particular accounting period.

To find out net profit, a trader has to deduct many expenses other than for goods purchase and manufacture, from gross profits. These other expenses include;

a. Administrative expenses – salaries, bonus, bank charges, stamps.

b. Selling expenses – Salesman's commission, etc.

c. Distribution expenses – Delivery van, etc.

d. Depreciation costs

Therefore the net profit is the surplus remaining after deducting from the gross profit all expenses, including depreciation and other provisions, properly attributable to the normal activities of a business. When the total of all these expenses exceeds the gross profit the difference between the two is 'net loss'

Format of profit and loss a/c

(Name of the proprietor)

Profit and loss account for the year ending ……

Dr				Cr
Particulars	Amount		Particulars	Amount

What to record on the Dr side of profit and loss a/c

1. Administrative expenses: (a) office salaries and wages (b) insurance, rent, printing stationary, heating and lighting, repairs and renewals, telephone charges, a/c fees, legal fees, audit fees, bank charges, bank commission, interest paid and interest on capital, etc.

2. Selling expenses: Salesman's salaries, travelling expenses, advertising, discount allowed, bad debts, rates and taxes, selling commission, brokerages, free samples, trading expenses, etc.

3. Distribution expenses: Carriage outward, warehouse expenses, warehouse insurances, delivery van expenses, packing expenses, etc.

4. Depreciation and other provisions: (a) Depreciation of different assets, (b) provision or reserve for doubtful debts, (c) discount on debtors, (d) provision or reserve for any other expenses.

On the credit side

1. Miscellaneous incomes: (a) Discount received, (b) commission received, (c) rent received, (d) interest received, (e) bonus received, (f) profit on sale of assets, and (g) bad debts recovered etc.
2. Provision or reserve for discount on creditors.

Example: Mr. Ram found his gross profit on 31st March 2004 to be Rs.5,600. His other expenses were as under:

Salaries - 1,200

Lighting - 120

Rent and taxes - 625

Bank charges - 26

Postage's - 15

Find out the profit for the year ending 31 March 2004.

M/s. Ram

Profit and loss account for the year ending 31.3.2004

Dr				Cr
Particulars	Amount		Particulars	Amount
To Salaries To Rent and taxes To Lighting To Bank charges To Postage To Capital a/c (net profit transferred)	1200 625 120 26 15 3614		By trading a/c (gross profit transferred)	5600
	5600			5600

Balance sheet

Balance sheet is a simple statement about a business enterprise, prepared at regular intervals showing what a business owns and what it owes. In other words, it is a sheet of all those ledger 'balances' pertaining to the 'properties' and 'assets' owned and liabilities owed by the business on a particular day.

It contains all the unclosed balances of 'real' and 'personal' accounts. The important aspect of balance sheet is that it always balances i.e, the total value of assets is always equal to the total value of the claims or liabilities. This is because the liability to the owner 'capital' is always made up of difference between assets and liabilities to outsiders. Or in other words;

Assets = Liabilities + capital

Or Assets - Liabilities = capital

Drafting a balance sheet

1. Trading and profit and loss accounts are prepared with the help of closing entries and all the 'goods' accounts and the nominal accounts in the ledger are closed.
2. The accounts that remain still 'open' in the ledger are real accounts and personal accounts.
3. The book keeper should pick up such accounts showing Dr or Cr balances and put them on a sheet of paper.
4. After the closure of all nominal accounts when balance of all the real and personal accounts are written on a sheet of paper in a standard form, it is termed as 'balance sheet', which means a sheet containing balances of real and personal accounts.

Here a point to be noted that the balance of personal and real accounts are not transferred by passing closing entries but merely extracted in the form of a statement.

Form of balance sheet

It has two sides, the left side and the right side. But, these two sides are not comparable with Dr and Cr of a ledger account because the balance sheet is not an account. No words such as Dr or Cr and To or By should be used in the balance sheet. The left hand side is liabilities side and contains credit balance of all personal accounts remaining in the ledger and on the right hand side (which is assets side) are listed the debit balance of real and personal accounts standing in the ledger.

(Name of the business or proprietor) as on _____________ (date, month and year)

Capital and liabilities	Amount	Property and assets	Amount
Personal accounts showing credit balance		Real and personal accounts showing debit side	
Total		Total	

Specimen Balance sheet (General trading company)

Balance sheet as on ---------------

Capital and liabilities	Amount	Property and assets	Amount
Liability to the owner		Fixed assets	
(Proprietors investment)		Land & building (premises)	
Capital account		Plant and Machinery	
Current account		Tools	
		Investments	
Fixed liabilities		Furniture and fixtures	
(Long term loans)		Vehicles, goodwill	
Bank loans		Patents and pattern	
Loan on mortgage		Trade marks	
Loan from parties		Long term loan (advance)	
Current liabilities		Current assets	
(Short term loans and other		Closing stock of finished goods	
liabilities)		Raw materials	
Sundry creditors		Work in progress	
Bills payable		Stationary	
Bank over drafts		Goods sent for consignment, etc.	
Outstanding or accrued		Sundry debtors	
expenses		Bill receivable	
Income received in advances		Prepaid expenses	
Etc.		Accrued income or	
		Income due but not yet received	
		Cash at bank	
		Cash on hand	
		Fictitious assets	
		Preliminary expenses	
		Advertising expenses	
		Underwritten commission	
		Other expenses not written ….	
a. Current liability		a. Current liability	
b. Fixed liability		b. Fixed liability	
c. Liabilities to owner		c. Liabilities to owner	

Balance sheet as on ___________

Capital and liabilities	Amount	Property and assets	Amount
a. Current liability		a. Current liability	
b. Fixed liability		b. Fixed liability	
c. Liabilities to owner		c. Liabilities to owner	

1. Liability to the owner: His investment in the form of capital.
2. Fixed liability: Liabilities payable by the business not in the near future but are long term nature.
3. Current liability: (a) Trade creditors for purchase of goods, (b) Loan creditors for short term loan, (c) Outstanding creditors for salaries wages etc.
4. Fixed assets: Assets of permanent nature having long period of life and cannot be converted in cash in a short period.
5. Current assets or floating assets: Can be converted into cash in the ordinary course of business and are held for a short period.
6. Fictitious assets or intangible assets: Debit balance of certain amounts which are not yet written off.

Eg: For the year ended 30th Sept 2004, M/s. Pande and Sons have earned a net profit of Rs.13,469. Other balances in their ledger are as under.

Cash in hand	3,600	Plant & Machinery	8,500
Cash at bank	9,327	Sundry debtors	5,678
Bills payable	2,800	Sundry Creditors	4,736
Capital	15,000		

You are requested to draw their balance sheet as on 30th Sept.

Solutions

M/s. Pande and Sons

Balance sheet as on 30th Sept. 2004

Capital and liabilities		Amount	Property and assets	Amount
Capital	15,000	26,069	Plant & Machinery	8,500
Less drawing	2,400		Sundry debtors	5,678
	----------		Stock	6,500
	12,600	4,736	Cash at bank	9,327
Add net profit		2,800	Cash on hand	3,600
for the year	13,468			
	----------	33,605	Total	33,605
Sundry creditors				
Bills payable				
	Total			

Note:(1) Drawings is the personal account of the owners for having withdrawn money from the business for personal use

1994 Sept. 30	Capital Account Dr To drawing account (transfer of balance on drawing a/c to capital account	2400 - -2400

(2) The balance on the profit and loss account is also transferred to the capital account to the credit side – if there is net profit, to the debit side – if there is net loss. In this case also a closing entry is necessary

1994 Sept. 30	Profit and loss Account Dr To capital account (net profit transferred to capital account)	2400 - -2400

If there is net loss, however, the entry is reversed as under

1994 Sept. 30	Capital account Dr To Profit and loss Account (net loss transferred to capital account)	xxxx xxxx

Cash book

Cash book is also known as '*Cash account book*'. It is a practical necessity. Sale of goods for cash, cash purchases, payment to creditors and for different expenses and receipt from debtors, etc., are few examples involving cash. Therefore, to record all cash transactions separately from noncash transactions, special book is maintained called 'Cash book'. This book helps the trader to know regularly the cash and bank balance on hand.

Dual purpose: Cash book basically a subsidiary journal, but it serves both as a subsidiary journal i.e., at the book of primary entry and also as a ledger i.e., as a book of final entry, i.e, it has dual role as a journal and ledger. It is a principal book wherein the cash truncations are entered as original entries. From these entries a separate ledger can be made, but such a necessity does not arise as the cash entries are not entered in any other subsidiary journal. Hence, the cash book itself serves as a ledger for cash account. Thus, it fulfils the dual role.

Rulings of cash book: Like an account it has left hand side and right hand side. On the left hand side called debit side or 'Dr', all amounts received are entered. Left hand side is also known as the receipt side. Right hand side or 'Cr' is also known as credit side and Payments made' are entered here. The Dr and Cr side always face each other.

Type of cash book

1. Simple or single column cash book: i.e., only one amount column on each side either cash at office or cash at bank.

Simple Cash Book: Simple cash book is like an ordinary cash account.
Its proforma is given below.

Dr. Cr.

Date	Particu-lars	L.F.	Amount	Date	Particu-lars	L.F.	Amount

1. Double column cash book: i.e, having two amount columns on each side as under (I) cash and discount column, (ii) cash and bank column, (iii) bank and discount column.

Two columnar cash book

a. *Cash book with Cash and Discount Columns only:*In this case, a separate bank account will be maintained in the general ledger. However all transactions involving cash and / or bank must be passed through the cash book.

Model : Cash book with Cash and Discount Columns only

Dr Cr.

Date		Re-ceipts	V.No.	L.F.	Dis-count Rs.	Amount Rs.	Date	Pay-ments	V.No.	L.F.	Dis-count Rs.	Amount Rs.

The entries for cash receipts and payments are made in the usual manner. However, wherever discounts are involved, they are entered in the discount column in the same line. The other point is to be noted that the transactions involving cheque payments are first treated as withdrawals of necessary cash from bank and subsequent payment in the form of cash. It is also noted that at the end of each period, the cash book is balanced with the words 'Bybalance c/d'. However, the discount columns are merely totalled but not balanced.

Procedure for posting from the cash book

- For every item appearing in the debit side, other than the opening balance, a credit is given in the corresponding account. If there is discount, it will also be credited to that account.
- Likewise, items appearing on the credit side of cash book will have their debits in the corresponding accounts together with discount if any.

- As for the discount columns, they are totalled at the end of each period, and the debit and credit totals carried respectively to the debit and credit sides of the discount account and posted as ' To Sundries' respectively.

b. Cash book with Bank and Discount Columns only: This type of cash book is maintained where all cash received is banked at once and all payments other than petty items (which met out of petty cash) are made by cheques. As for postings from the above cash book, the procedure is similar to that in case of other cash book. The Discount Columns are not balanced; instead their totals, as in the previous case, are taken to the two sides of the Discount Account.

Model: Cash book with Bank and Discount Columns only

Dr. Cr.

Date	Receipts	V.No.	L.F.	Discount Rs.	Bank Rs.	Date	Payments	V.No.	L.F.	Discount Rs.	Bank Rs.

Three column cash book: i.e, with three amounts columns on each side. (a) for cash at office, (b) for cash at bank and (c) for discount.

Three columnar cash book

*Cash book with Cash, Bank and Discount Columns only:*This is most common and the best from all points of view. Here, the entries are made in the respective columns according as whether they increase / decrease the cash or bank balance. At the end of the period, the cash bank balances are balanced, while the discount totals are dealt with as in the case of other types of Cash Book.

Model : Cash book with Cash, Bank and Discount Columns only

Dr. **Cr.**

Date	Receipts	V.No.	L.F.		Discount Rs.	Cash Rs.	Bank Rs.	Date	Payments	V. No.	L.F.	Discount Rs.	Cash Rs.	Bank Rs.

Multicolumn cash book: Receipts and payments recorded either department wise or article wise. i.e., printing dept. cutting dept. dyeing dept, etc. and radios, TVs, fans, services, etc., or bank-wise such as Canara Bank, Vijaya Bank, SBI, etc.

Petty cash book: For recording cash payments for petty expenses.

Note: (a) cash book being a journal book, each entry must be supported by a suitable narration or at least by cash memo or voucher No. etc., where entry is self explanatory.

(b) since the cash book is cash account book, it should be balanced regularly. Many traders balance daily, some weekly and others monthly.

(c) It must be remembered that we can never pay more cash than what we have received. Therefore, the debit total (receipts) is always more than or at least equal to but never less than the credit (payments) total and the cash book always shows a debit balance or nil balance but never credit balance.

Subsidiary journals

For business having a large number of transactions, it is practically impossible to write all the transactions in one journal. Further, the transactions are usually of similar nature and take place repeatedly. Therefore, transactions can be classified into cash and non-cash transactions.

Cash transactions are entered in one category, credit purchases in another category and credit sales in yet another category.

In practice, the main journal is subdivided in such a way that a separate book is used for each category or group of transactions, which are repetitive and sufficiently large in number. Thus, when the main journal is subdivided into special or subjournals they are called subsidiary journals.

Subsidiary books

1. Cash book
2. Day book of purchases or purchase day book
3. Sales book
4. Purchases return book
5. Sales return book
6. Bills receivable book
7. Bills payable book (item 6 and 7 are called bills of exchange)
8. Journal proper

Uses of subsidiary book

1. Cash book records only cash transactions.
2. Purchases book records only credit purchase of goods in which the trader deals.
3. Sales book records only credit sales in which the trader deals.

4. Purchase return book records return of goods purchased by the trader for which no cash is received.
5. Sales payable book where in bills accepted or passed are entered.
6. Bills payable book where in bills accepted or passed are entered.
7. Bills receivable book, wherein bills drawn or acceptances received are entered.
8. Journal proper is the journal in which are entered those entries, which cannot be entered in any of the above listed subsidiary books.

Proforma of Purchase Day Book

Bought Day Book, Invoice Book, Credit Purchases Book, Purchases Journal or Purchase Register

Date	Name of the supplier	LF	Inward invoice or details	Amount
Year, month, day Date of purchase			Bills No. or Invoice No. or details of purchase	Net amount of the bill
Closing date	By purchases a/c Dr		Grand total Rs.	

Posting the entries of purchases Day Book to ledgers

1. Debit purchases a/c with the periodical total as To Sundry a/c's (various a/c's) as per purchases day book (PDB), Date of posting will be the date on which the total is made.
2. Credit suppliers a/c with the individual's amount against his name as 'by purchases a/c' with the date of purchase and not the date on which the total is made.

Proforma of Sales Day Book (SDB), Day Book of Sales,

Sales Day Book, Sales Journal, Sales Registers

Date	Name of the customer	LF	Outward invoice No.	Amount
Year, month, day Date of sale	Name of the customers to whom goods are sold		Invoice No. or details of Invoice	Net amount of the invoice
Closing date	To sales a/c Cr		Grand total Rs.	

Posting the entries to ledger

1. Debit to customer's a/c with the individual amount against his name 'To sales accounts' with the date of sale.
2. Credit to 'sales a/c' with the periodical total as By Sundry a/c's as per sales day book with the date on which a/c is closed.

Proforma of purchases returns or returns outward book

Date	Name of the suppliers	LF	Inward invoice or details	Amount
Year, month, day YMD	Names of persons or suppliers to whom goods are returned		Details calculations or no. of debit note sent to supplier	Net amount
Closing date	To returns outwards a/c Cr		Grand total Rs.	

Posting the returns outward book

1. Debit to suppliers a/c to whom debit note is sent for goods returned as 'To returns outwards a/c' with individual amount.
2. Credit to 'returns outward a/c' with the periodical total as 'By sundry a/c' as per Returns Outwards Book (RPB)

Proforma of Sales Returns Book or Returns Inward Book

Date	Name of the supplies	LF	Credit note	Amount
Date of receipt or returns	Names of customer, who have returned the goods		Credit note no. or details	Net amount of the bill
Closing date	By return inwards a/c Dr		Grand total Rs.	Amount

Posting to ledger

1. Debit returns inward a/c with the periodical total as 'To Sundry a/c' as per returns inward book putting the date of the totaling date.
2. Credit to individual a/c or customer's a/c with the individual amount as 'By returns inwards a/c mentioning the date of return.

Some Important Types of Bank Accounts

1. Receiving of deposits
   a) Current accounts and current deposits
   b) Savings bank accounts

   c) Fixed deposit accounts
   d) Recurring deposit accounts
   e) Multiple optional deposit accounts.

2. Lending of funds
   a) Loans
   b) Over drafts
   c) Cash credits
   d) Discounting of bills

Receiving of deposits

Current accounts: These accounts are generally opened by business and industrial concerns, public authorities, etc., which have frequent and numerous transactions. They can be opened with a minimum deposit of Rs.500/- to Rs.3000/- depending on the bank rules. These accounts are opened by customers neither for the purpose of earning interest nor for the purpose of saving, but for the convenience of making payments by cheques proper and satisfactory introduction is necessary for opening current accounts. Current accounts are active or running accounts, which are continuously in operation. In current accounts customers can deposit any amount of money and any number of times and also withdraw any number of times as long as there is enough money in their credit.

Current deposits or demand deposits or demand liabilities are the deposits made by the current account holders and these deposits can be withdrawn by the depositor any time without any fixed time frame. For this reason current deposits cannot be invested by the banks elsewhere to learn profits. Also current deposit do not attract any interest generally.

Savings bank accounts: Generally saving bank accounts are opened by middle and low income groups who wish to save a part of their current incomes for their future needs and earn fair interest on them. Proper introduction of the customer is required for opening these accounts. The deposits can be made by the use of a pay-in-slip and withdrawals can be made by issuing a cheque if the SB a/c is with cheque facility or by issuing a withdrawal slip when the SB a/c is without cheque facility. A minimum of Rs.500/- for SB a/c without cheque and minimum of Rs.1000/- deposit is required to open SB a/c with cheque facilities. As the deposits are invested by the banks, they will be in a position to pay interest to the customers. Usually SB accounts are given 4.5 to 5 % annual interest. The interest is calculated on the basis of the amount outstanding in the account between 10th and last working day of the month. There are certain restrictions on the operation of SB a/c.

1. There can be more than 50 withdrawals in a period of six months.
2. Generally not more than Rs.10,000/- is allowed to be withdrawn on any day. However banks are usually liberal on these restrictions.
3. Further, when the withdrawal has to be done involving more than Rs.10,000/- a prior notice may have to be given to the bank.

Fixed deposit accounts or time deposit or term deposit account: They are opened by investors who do not want to invest their money in risky industrial or other business securities, but wish to deposit their money in banks and earn good and steady income. No introduction is normally necessary to open fixed deposit accounts as they are not operated by cheques. In these accounts fixed amounts are deposited by customers for fixed periods at fixed rates of interest. The minimum amount that should be deposited in a fixed deposit account is more than Rs.50/-. There is no maximum limit. The period of deposits ordinarily varies from 45 days to five years. The fixed deposits can be withdrawn only after the expiry of fixed periods. That is why it is called time deposit or term deposit. The rate of interest normally varies between 9 to 13% depending on the duration of deposit.

Lending of funds

Loans: Banks will advance loans to borrowers normally on certain securities and usually for productive purposes by opening a separate account called 'loan account' for an agreed period. A loan is generally granted for a period of 1 to 3 years. However, there are specialised banks like housing banks, industrial banks, etc., which advance loans on long term up to 10 to 15 years. The rate of interest charged on these loans by the banks may vary between 18 to 22%. It may be as less as 14% and as high as 36% in some banks. For example, Citi Bank which is a credit bank charges as high as 2.95% per month or approximately 36% annually.

Overdrafts

An Overdraft is a financial arrangement under which a Current a/c holder is permitted by the bank to overdraw i.e., draw more than the amount standing to his credit up to an agreed limit. After the expiring of agreed period the customer is expected to settle the overdraft in his account. In the case of an overdraft interest is charged only on the amount actually utilized by the borrower.

Cash credits

A cash credit is a financial arrangement under which a borrower is allowed an advance under a separate account called the Cash Credit a/c up to a specified limit called cash credit limit. As it is a separate account by itself, it does not require a current account. A cash credit is usually granted against the security of agricultural or industrial products like rice, wheat, pulses, sugar, cotton textiles, etc. Sometimes it is given against a guarantee i.e., a bond of credit signed by one or more sureties. It is very rarely given against the personal security of the borrower.

Discounting of bills of exchange

Discounting is an arrangement under which a bank takes a bill of exchange maturing within a short period of 60 to 90 days from an approved customer and pays him or credits his current account or even a SB a/c immediately the present value of the bills ie., the face value of the bill minus the discount charges. Then on the due date of the bill, the bank receives the face value of the bill from the acceptor of the bill. In case the bill is dishonoured by the acceptor the bank recovers the amount from the customer who has discounted the bill. The interest charged for this kind of financial accommodation is called the discount and is charged on the face value of the bill for the unexpired period of the bill i.e., from the date on which the bill is discounted to the date on which the bill matures.

Partial budgeting

Partial budgeting is a statement of anticipated changes in costs, returns and profitability for a minor modification. It consists of four important elements viz., added costs, added returns, reduced returns and reduced costs. Partial budgeting technique is generally used to evaluate the profitability of input substitution, enterprise substitution and scale of operation.

1. Added costs : Additional costs are incurred, if the proposed modification is the introduction of a new enterprise or increase in size of the existing enterprise.
2. Added returns : Additional returns could be received when the proposed modification is the addition of a new enterprise or increase in size of the existing enterprise or adoption of technology that results in higher productivity.
3. Reduced returns : Decrease in the returns is observed when the proposed modification involves the elimination of an existing enterprise or reduction in size of the enterprise.

4. Reduced costs : Decrease in the costs is found when the proposed modification involves the elimination of existing enterprise or reduction in the size of the enterprise or adoption of technology that uses fewer amounts of resources.

Example

Estimate the net gain for introduction of machine milking over manual milking

S.No.	Particulars	Existing practice Manual milking (in Rs.)	New practice Machine milking (in Rs.)
1	Depreciation on equipment	2000	2500
2	Interest on investment	10000	15000
3	Repair and maintenance	5000	10000
4	Electricity expenses	1200	2400
5	Labour expenses	20000	5000
6	Returns through milk	200000	220000 (Premium price for clean milk)

Partial budgeting

A	Added cost	in Rs.	C	Added returns	in Rs.
1	Depreciation on equipment	500	1	Returns through milk	20000
2	Interest on investment	5000			
3	Repair and maintenance	5000			
4	Electricity expenses	1200			
B	Reduced returns		D	Reduced costs	
	Nil		1	Labour expenses	15000
A+B	Total of Added costs and Reduced returns	11700	C+D	Total Returns and Reduced costs	35000
	Net change (C+D) – (A+B) = Rs. 23300/-				

Economics of A 10 Cross-Bred Cow Unit

Non-recurring expenditure

1. Land available
2. Purchase of 10 crossbred cows
3. Housing

   Total livestock units = 10 cows = 10 units

   female calves x 0.5 unit = 2.5 units

   Total = 12.5 units

   Space required = @ 48 sq.ft./cow unit = 48 x 12.5 = 600 sq.ft.

4. Equipments:

   a. Sanitary milking pail   b. Milk can

   c. Chaff cutter   d. Cow chains, ropes

   e. Buckets

Recurring expenditure

1. Non-variable recurring expenditure:

   a. Interest on capital

   b. Depreciation on cow's values @ 12% per lactation per year

   c. Depreciation on buildings values @ 5% per year

   d. Depreciation on equipments @ 10% per year

2. Variable recurring expenditure:

   a. Fodder for 12.5 L.U. (Dry fodder @ 7 kg/LU/day ~ 32 tons

   (if green fodder 10% of the body weight)

   b. Concentrate feed requirements:

i. 10 cows in milk x 5 kg x 305 days	= 15,250 kg
ii. 10 dry cows x 2 kg x 60 days	= 1,200 kg
iii. 5 female calves x 2 kg x 275 (365-90) days	= 2,750 kg
Total	= 19,200 kg

c. Feeding milk for 5 female calves 5 x 90 days x 3 lit x cost of one litre of milk

d. Labour: One milker cum attendant @ Rs........ per month

e. Health coverage for 12.5 LU

f. Insurance @ 4.5% of the value of cows

g. Miscellaneous expenditure

Total recurring expenditure = (i) + (ii)

Receipts

1. Sale of milk
2. Sale of 5 heifers = 0.5 LU value x 5
3. Sale of cow dung = 12.5 LU x 15 kg x 365 = 68,437.5 kg (roughly 70 tonnes).
4. Sale of male calves at birth

Net profit = Total Receipts – Total recurring expenditure

Note: i. Profit increases, if self labour is possible

ii. Profit varies, if the milk value fluctuates

Economics of 1000 broilers

Non-recurring expenditure

1. Building: 1 sq.ft./bird @ Rs. .... Per sq.ft.
2. Equipments: Brooders, chick guard, waterers, feeders, etc. @

   Rs.....per bird

Recurring expenditure

1. Cost of 1000 broiler chicks @ Rs..........per chick
2. Cost of feed for 42 days i.e, 6 weeks at 3.1 kg/bird:

   3.1 x 1000 = 3.1 tonnes @ Rs......per kg
3. Brooding charges, medications, vaccinations, paddy husk and other miscellaneous expenses @ Rs......per bird
4. Labour charges @ Rs...../per month for 2 months

5. Interest on capital @ Rs...../year for 2 months
6. Depreciation on buidling @ 5%/annum for 2 months =

$$\frac{\text{Cost of building x 0.5}}{12} \times 2$$

7. Depreciation on equipments @ 10%/annum for 2 months.

$$\frac{\text{Cost of equipments x 0.1}}{12} \times 2$$

Income

1. Sale of 970 birds = 1.5 kg/bird @ Rs.... per kg
2. Sale of gunny bags @ Rs....per bag for 45 bags
3. Sale of manure = 2 tons of litter @ Rs..... per ton

Net profit = Total Receipts – Total recurring expenditure

Note: i. If self labour – profit increases

ii. Mortality rate 5%

Economics of 1000 Layers in Cage System

Non-recurring expenditure

1. One brooder cum grower house

   25 x 20 = 500 sq.ft. @ Rs. .... Per sq.ft.
2. Equipments during growing period @ Rs.....per bird
3. Cage layer house = 50 x 20 = 1000 sq.ft. @ Rs.....per sq.ft.
4. Cages for 1000 birds @ Rs.....per bird

Recurring expenditure

I. Growth period (0-20 weeks)

   a. Day old chicks @ Rs.....per bird for 1000 chicks

   b. Feed @ Rs.....kg. per bird i.e., 8 tonnes @ Rs.....per ton

   c. Brooding charges, medications, vaccinations, etc. @ Rs.....per bird

d. Labour charges @ Rs...../per month for 5 months

e. Depreciation on building (brooder house) @ 5%/annum for 5 months =

f. Depreciation equipments @ 10% per annum for 5 months

II. Laying period (20-72 weeks)

a. Feed for 980 birds @ 40 kg/bird, i.e., 39.200 kg = 39.2 tones @ Rs..../ton

b. Medicines @ Rs.....per bird, etc.

c. Labour charges @ Rs.....per month for one year

d. Depreciation on building (cage, layer house) @ 5%/annum

e. Depreciation on cages @ 16%/annum

III. Interest on capital cost @....% annum for 17 months

Income

1. Sale of eggs: 300 eggs / bird /year
2. Sale of spent hens @ Rs..../bird
3. Sale of manure @ Rs..../ton
4. Sale of gunny bags @ Rs....per bag for 600 bags

Net profit = Total Receipts – Total recurring expenditure

Note: If self labour – profit increases

Economics of 1000 Layers Under Deep Litter System

Non-recurring expenditure (Capital expenditure)

a. Land – available

b. Building:

1. One brooder cum grower house

   25 x 20 = 500 sq.ft. @ Rs. .... Per sq.ft.

2. Cage layer house = 2 sq.ft./bird for 1000 birds

   2000 sq.ft. @ Rs.....per sq.ft.

3. Equipments @ Rs.....per bird

Recurring expenditure (working capital)

I. Growth period (0-20 weeks)

a. Cost of Day old chicks @ Rs…..per bird for 1000 chicks

b. Chick mash, grower mash etc. @ 6.5 kg per bird

i.e., 45 g/bird/day for 140 days @Rs…..per ton

c. Brooding charges, medications, @ Rs…..per bird

d. Labour charges @ Rs…../per month for 5 months

II. Laying period (20-72 weeks)

a. Feed for 980 birds @ 40 kg/bird,

i.e., 110 g/bird/day = 39.2 tones @Rs…./ton

b. Medicines @ Rs…..per bird

c. Labour charges @ Rs…..per month for one year

III. Interest on capital @ …% /annum

Income

1. Sale of eggs: 300 eggs / bird /year = 300 x 980 x egg value
2. Sale of spent hens @ Rs…./bird for 980 birds
3. Sale of manure 30 tones @ Rs…./ton
4. Sale of gunny bags @ Rs….per bag for 600 bags

Net profit = Total Receipts – Total recurring expenditure

Note:Profit increases in case of self labour

Economics of Sheep Farming [100 Ewes and 5 Rams]

Non-recurring expenditure

1. Housing : 12 sq.ft./animal
2. Cost of ewes: @ Rs./ewe
3. Cost of rams @ Rs./ram
4. Equipments, etc.

Recurring expenditure

1. Feed cost @ Rs...../animal /day
2. Labour charges @ Rs...../months (one labourer)
3. Medicines and miscellaneous expenditure @ Rs....animal
4. Depreciation on building @ 5%/annum
5. Interest on capital @..% / annum
6. Insurance premium @ 5% of animal cost

Income

1. Sale of sheep at the age of 6 months @ Rs..../animal for 120 sheep
2. Sale of manure

Net profit = Total Income – Total recurring expenditure

Note:

1. Lambing rate : 3 lambing in 2 years
2. Fertility rate : 90%
3. Mortality rate : 5-10%

Economics of Goat Farming

[100 DOES AND 5 BUCKS]

Non-recurring expenditure

1. Housing : 12 sq.ft./animal
2. Cost of does: @ Rs./does
3. Cost of bucks @ Rs./bucks
4. Equipments, etc.

Recurring expenditure

1. Feed cost @ Rs...../animal /day
2. Labour charges @ Rs...../months (one labourer)
3. Medicines and miscellaneous expenditure @ Rs....animal
4. Depreciation on building @ 5%/annum

5. Interest on capital @..% / annum
6. Insurance premium @ 5% of animal cost

Income

1. Sale of goats at the age of 6 months @ Rs…./animal for 200 goats
2. Sale of manure

Net profit = Total Income – Total recurring expenditure

Note:

1. Kidding rate : 3 kidding in 2 years
2. Fertility rate : 90 %
3. Twinning rate : 40%
4. Mortality rate:5-10%

Economics of piggery farming [Unit of 10 Sows and one boar]

Non-recurring expenditure

1. Housing : 800 sq.ft. @ Rs…../sq.ft.

   [Farrowing pens = 3, 6'x10'x3 = 180 sq.ft.

   Mating pens = 1, 18'x10'x1 = 180 sq.ft.

   Dry stock pens = 5, 8'x10'x5 = 400 sq.ft.

   Store room = 1, 8'x10'x1 = 40 sq.ft.

   Total = 800 sq.ft.

2. Borewell
3. Wallowing tank
4. Weighing balance and other equipments
5. Purchase of parent stock (10+1) @ Rs…../pig

Recurring expenditure

1. Feed cost
2. Labour charges (one labourer)
3. Medicines and miscellaneous expenditure

4. Depreciation on building @ 5%/annum
5. Interest on capital @..% / annum
6. Insurance premium @ 5% of animal value for adult animal

Income

1. Sale of pigs = 130 piglet/year
2. Sale of manure
3. Sale of gunny bags

Net profit = Total Receipts – Total recurring expenditure

Note:

1. Litter size = 8/farrowing
2. Fertility rate : 90%
3. Mortality rate : 10%
4. Number of farrowing = 2/sow/year

Economics of Broiler Rabbits

Non-recurring expenditure

1. Construction of shed: 30'x40' @ Rs..../sq.ft.
2. Cages 150 nos. @ Rs.../cage
3. Equipment, feeders, waters.
4. Purchase of parent stock: @ Rs..../rabbit

Recurring expenditure

1. Feeding
    i. @ Rs./day/adult rabbit for 1 year
    ii. @ Rs./day/ young rabbit for 45 days
2. Labour charges @ Rs...../months (one labourer)
3. Medicines, electricity charges, etc.
4. Depreciation on sheds @ 5%/annum

5. Depreciation on equipments and cages @ 10%/annum
6. Insurance premium (adult rabbits) @ 5% of animal value
7. bank interest on capital @ …..%/annum

Income

1. Sale of young rabbits (2284) @ Rs…./rabbit
2. Sales of adult (20) @ Rs…/rabbit
3. Sale of manure
4. Sale of gunny bags

Net profit = Total Income – Total recurring expenditure

Note:

1. No. of kindling /year
2. Fertility rate : 90%
3. Mortality rate : 20%
4. Litter size : 8

Project on Dairy Farming with 10 Crossbred Cows

Techno-Economic Assumptions

	Techno-Economic Assumptions						
1	Type of animal	Crossbred (HF cross & Jersey cross)					
2	Number of animals	12	6 in I hallf& 6 in II half of first year				
3	Cost of animals (Rs./animal)	40000					
4	Floor space requirement (Sq. ft/cow)	60					
5	Cost of construction of animal shed (Rs./Sq.ft)	600					
6	Floor space requirment of store room (Sq.ft)	300					
7	Cost of construction of store room(Rs./Sq.ft)	450					
8	Cost of equipment (Rs./animal)	300					
9	Cost of milking machine	60000					
10	Insurance premium/animal (%) 6						
11	Rate of Interest (%)	12					
12	Depreciation on building (%)	10					
13	Depreciation on feeding equipment (%)	20					

14	Depreciation on milking machine (%)	15					
15	Margin money requirement(%)	20					
16	Repayment period in years	6					
17	Veterinary aid/animal/year (Rs.)	300					
18	Unit labour cost per month (Rs.)	10000					
19	Electricity charges (Rs./year)	12000					
20	FEEDING						
21	a.Concentrate feed requirement (Kg/day)						
	Total lactating days	305					
	-For lactating animals	5					
	Total dry period in days	60					
	-For dry animals	1.5					
	Cost of concentrate	25					
	b.Dry fodder requirement (Kg/ animal/day)	5					
	Cost of dry fodder (Rs./Kg)	4					
	c. Fodder area requirement	3					
	Fodder cultivation cost in first year (Rs. /Acr)	25000					
	In subsequent years (Rs. /Acr)	7000					
22	Returns						
	Milk yield (lit/day/animal)	10					
	Sale price of milk(Rs./litre)	35					
	Number of heilfer calves	6					
	Sale price of heifer calves (Rs./ animal)	5000					
	Number of bull calves	6					
	Sale price of bull calves(Rs./ animal)	2000					
	Sale of manure and gunny bags (Rs./animal)	250					

	Details of Bankable Investment	
S.No.	Particulars	Value in Rs.
A	Fixed Investment	
1	Cost of Animals	480000
2	Cost of Building	567000
3	Cost of Equipment	3600
4	Cost of Milking Machine	60000
	Total Fixed Investment	1110600

B	Working Capital (For 3 Months)	
1	Insurance Charges for Animals	28800
2	Labour Charges	30000
3	Cost of Concentrate Feed	45000
4	Cost of Green Fodder	18750
5	Cost of Dry Fodder	21600
6	Veterinary Aid	900
7	Electricity Charges	3000
8	Miscellaneous Charges	600
	Total Working Capital	148650
	Total Cost of the Project	1259250
	Cost of the Project	
	Loan from Bank	1007000
	Margin amount from entrepreneur	252000
	Total Cost of the Project	1259000

		Production Detail				
			I. Lactation period				
Particulars	I year	II year	III year	IV year	V year	VI year	VII year
First batch	1620	1830	1830	1830	1830	1650	1650
Second batch	1080	1650	1650	1650	1650	1650	1650
Total	2700	3480	3480	3480	3480	3300	3300
			II. Dry Period				
Particulars	I year	II year	III year	IV year	V year	VI year	VII year
First batch	570	360	360	360	360	540	540
Second batch	0	540	540	540	540	540	540
Total	570	900	900	900	900	1080	1080

Income-Expenditure Statement

Particulars	I year	II year	III year	IV year	V year	VI year	VII year
Income							
From Sale of milk	945000	1218000	1218000	1218000	1218000	1155000	1155000
From sale of manure & gunny bags	3000	3000	3000	3000	3000	3000	3000
From sale of heifer calves	30000	30000	30000	30000	30000	30000	30000
From sale of bull calves	12000	12000	12000	12000	12000	12000	12000
Total Income	990000	1263000	1263000	1263000	1263000	1200000	1200000

Expenditure							
On concentrate feed	358875	468750	468750	468750	468750	468750	453000
On green fodder	75000	21000	21000	21000	21000	21000	21000
On dry fodder	65400	87600	87600	87600	87600	87600	87600
On veterinary aid	3600	3600	3600	3600	3600	3600	3600
On labour	120000	120000	120000	120000	120000	120000	120000
On insurance	28800	28800	28800	28800	28800	28800	28800
On electricity	12000	12000	12000	12000	12000	12000	12000
On depreciation							
-Building	56700	51030	45927	41334	37201	33481	30133
-Equipment	12720	10176	8141	6513	5210	4168	3334
On interest	120840	100700	80560	60420	40280	20140	0
Total Expenditure	853935	903656	876378	850017	824441	799539	759467

Profit and Loss Statement

Particulars	I year	II year	III year	IV year	V year	VI year	VII year
Expenditure							
Total Expenditure	853935	903656	876378	850017	824441	799539	759467
Net Expenditure (TE- Dep &Int)	663675	741750	741750	741750	741750	741750	726000
Income							
Total Income (TI)	990000	1263000	1263000	1263000	1263000	1200000	1200000
Net Profit(TI-NE)	326325	521250	521250	521250	521250	458250	474000

Repayment Schedule

	Repayment Schedule			
	Loan Amount	1007000		
	Rate of Interest per annum	12.00	1.00	per month
	Term of loan in Years	6	72	months
	Payment due per year	244928.30		
	Payment due per month	19687.00		
Month	Payment Due	Principal	Interest	Balance
				1007000
1	19687	9617	10070	997383
2	19687	9713	9974	987670
3	19687	9810	9877	977860
4	19687	9908	9779	967951
5	19687	10007	9680	957944
6	19687	10108	9579	947836
7	19687	10209	9478	937627
8	19687	10311	9376	927317
9	19687	10414	9273	916903
10	19687	10518	9169	906385

11	19687	10623	9064	895762
12	19687	10729	8958	885032
13	19687	10837	8850	874196
14	19687	10945	8742	863251
15	19687	11054	8633	852196
16	19687	11165	8522	841031
17	19687	11277	8410	829754
18	19687	11389	8298	818365
19	19687	11503	8184	806862
20	19687	11618	8069	795243
21	19687	11735	7952	783509
22	19687	11852	7835	771657
23	19687	11970	7717	759686
24	19687	12090	7597	747596
25	19687	12211	7476	735385
26	19687	12333	7354	723052
27	19687	12456	7231	710596
28	19687	12581	7106	698014
29	19687	12707	6980	685308
30	19687	12834	6853	672474
31	19687	12962	6725	659511
32	19687	13092	6595	646420
33	19687	13223	6464	633197
34	19687	13355	6332	619842
35	19687	13489	6198	606353
36	19687	13623	6064	592730
37	19687	13760	5927	578970
38	19687	13897	5790	565073
39	19687	14036	5651	551036
40	19687	14177	5510	536860
41	19687	14318	5369	522541
42	19687	14462	5225	508080
43	19687	14606	5081	493474
44	19687	14752	4935	478721
45	19687	14900	4787	463822
46	19687	15049	4638	448773
47	19687	15199	4488	433573
48	19687	15351	4336	418222
49	19687	15505	4182	402717
50	19687	15660	4027	387058
51	19687	15816	3871	371241
52	19687	15975	3712	355267
53	19687	16134	3553	339132

54	19687	16296	3391	322837
55	19687	16459	3228	306378
56	19687	16623	3064	289755
57	19687	16789	2898	272965
58	19687	16957	2730	256008
59	19687	17127	2560	238881
60	19687	17298	2389	221583
61	19687	17471	2216	204112
62	19687	17646	2041	186466
63	19687	17822	1865	168643
64	19687	18001	1686	150643
65	19687	18181	1506	132462
66	19687	18362	1325	114100
67	19687	18546	1141	95554
68	19687	18731	956	76822
69	19687	18919	768	57904
70	19687	19108	579	38796
71	19687	19299	388	19497
72	19692	19497	195	0

	Cash Flow Statement						
Particulars	I year	II year	III year	IV year	V year	VI year	VII year
Income							
From Sale of milk	787500	1015000	1015000	1015000	1015000	962500	962500
From sale of manure & gunny bags	2500	2500	2500	2500	2500	2500	2500
From sale of heifer calves	15000	15000	15000	15000	15000	15000	15000
From sale of bull calves	5000	5000	5000	5000	5000	5000	5000
Total Cash Inflow	810000	1037500	1037500	1037500	1037500	985000	985000
Outflow							
On concentrate feed	299062.5	390625	390625	390625	390625	390625	377500
On green fodder	50000	14000	14000	14000	14000	14000	14000
On dry fodder	27250	36500	36500	36500	36500	36500	36500
On veterinary aid	3000	3000	3000	3000	3000	3000	3000
On labour	120000	120000	120000	120000	120000	120000	120000
On insurance	42000	42000	42000	42000	42000	42000	42000
On electricity	10000	10000	10000	10000	10000	10000	10000
Total Outflow	551313	616125	616125	616125	616125	616125	603000
Net Cash Inflow	258688	421375	421375	421375	421375	368875	382000
	IRR	50%					

	Financial Analysis of The Project						
Particulars	I year	II year	III year	IV year	V year	VI year	VII year
Capital Investment	1259000						
Working Capital	663675	741750	741750	741750	741750	741750	726000
Total Cost	1922675	741750	741750	741750	741750	741750	726000
Total Benefit	990000	1263000	1263000	1263000	1263000	1200000	1200000
Depreciation-Buildi	56700	51030	45927	41334	37201	33481	30133
Depreciation-Equip	12720	10176	8140.8	6513	5210	4168	3334
Interest	120840	100700	80560	60420	40280	20140	0
Total (A)(NOI)	1180260	1424906	1397628	1371267	1345691	1257789	1233467
Interest	120840	100700	80560	60420	40280	20140	0
Loan Intalment	167833	167833	167833	167833	167833	167833	0
Total (B)	288673	268533	248393	228253	208113	187973	0
DSCR(A/B)	4	5	6	6	6	7	
Net Cash Flow	-932675	521250	521250	521250	521250	458250	474000
DCF at 20%	0.833	0.694	0.579	0.482	0.402	0.335	0.279
Disc. Benefit	825000	877083	730903	609086	507571	401878	334898
Disc.cost	1602229	515104	429253	357711	298093	248411	202613
NPV at 20% DCF	-777229	361979	301649	251374	209479	153467	132285
DCF at 25%	0.800	0.640	0.512	0.410	0.328	0.262	0.210
Disc. Benefit	792000	808320	646656	517325	413860	314573	251658
Disc.cost	1538140	474720	379776	303821	243057	194445	152253
NVP at 25% DCV	-746140	333600	266880	213504	170803	120127	99405
				Ave. DSCR		6	
NPV at 20%	633004			B:C ratio at 20%		1.173	
NPV at 25%	458180			B:C ratio at 25%		1.139	

References

A Text Book of Commerce – By B.S.Raman (1988) (United Publishers, Mangalore)

Agricultural Economics by S. Subba Reddy, P. Raghu Ram, T.V. Neelakanta Sastry and I. Bhavani Devi; ISBN 81-204-1596-5

Agricultural Marketing in India by S.S. Acharya and N. L. Agarwal; ISBN No.: 81-204-1636-8

Anjani kumar, 2009 India's livestock sector trade: Opportunities and challenges

Anjani Kumar. 2010. Exports of Livestock Products from India: Performance, Competitiveness and Determinants. Agricultural Economics Research Review, Vol. 23 January-June 2010 (57-67).

APEDA (2014) http://apeda.gov.in/apedawebsite/Announcements/plants-2- approved-meat-processing-plants.pdf.

APEDA. www.apeda.gov.in

Basic Principles of Economics and Marketing – By M. Thirunavukkarasu & R. Prabhakaran, Dept. of A.H.Economics, Madras Veterinary College, Chennai.

Bharti S K, Pathak V, Anitha and Singh V P. 2015. An overview of Indian Meat Marketing: Challenges and Scope. Indian Journal of Agriculture Business, 1(1), 2015.

Business Management – By B.S.Raman (1993) (United Publishers, Mangalore)

CME Group, Self-Study Guide to Hedging with Livestock Futures and Options, 2020.

Currency & Banking – By A.V.Ranganadhachary & R.R.Paul (1990) (Kalyani Publishers, New Delhi)

Deepak Shah. 2012. Trade Performance of India in Livestock Products: Prospects and Issues under WTO Regime. Munich Personal RePEc Archive (MPRA) Paper No. 39275, Jun 2012.

Deepak Shah. 2012. Trade Performance of India in Livestock Products under WTO Regime. Munich Personal RePEc Archive (MPRA) Paper No. 56636, Jun 2014.

Department of Agriculture, Cooperation & Farmers Welfare.

Department of Animal Husbandry, Dairying & Fisheries, Ministry of Agriculture & Farmers Welfare, Government of India.

DHAD, (2012) 19th Livestock census–All India report, Ministry of Agriculture Department of Animal Husbandry, Dairying and fisheries. Krishi Bhawan, New Delhi.

e- Krishi Shiksha - http://ecoursesonline.iasri.res.in/course/view.php?id=379

Economicsdiscussion.net.

Elements of Economics) - B.S.Raman (1989) (United Publishers, Mangalore

Essentials of Marketing Management – By S.A.Sherlekar, P.N.Reddy and H.R.Appannaiah (1990) (Himalaya Publishing House, Bombay, Delhi, Nagpur)

FAO Food outlook, (2014) www.fao.org/docrep/019/i3751e/i3751e.pdf.

Global Agricultural Information Network, 2019. Assessments Of Commodity And Trade Issues made by USDA staff and not necessarily statements of official U.S. Government Policy, Livestock and Products Annual, India.

https://sendpulse.com/support/glossary/sales-promotion

https://www. businessmanagementideas. com/management/approaches-to-management/approaches-to-management-classical-modern-scientific-and-system-approach/19527

https://www.agrifarming.in/dairy-farm-project-report-for-bank-loan-project-proposal#Appraisal_of_dairy_farm_project